Community and Public Health Education Methods

A Practical Guide

FOURTH EDITION

Robert J. Bensley, PhD, MCHES
Western Michigan University
Kalamazoo, MI

Jodi Brookins-Fisher, PhD, MCHES
Central Michigan University
Mount Pleasant, MI

JONES & BARTLETT
LEARNING

World Headquarters
Jones & Bartlett Learning
5 Wall Street
Burlington, MA 01803
978-443-5000
info@jblearning.com
www.jblearning.com

Jones & Bartlett Learning books and products are available through most bookstores and online booksellers. To contact Jones & Bartlett Learning directly, call 800-832-0034, fax 978-443-8000, or visit our website, www.jblearning.com.

Production Credits

VP, Product Management: David D. Cella
Director of Product Management: Cathy L. Esperti
Product Assistant: Rachael Souza
Director of Vendor Management: Amy Rose
Vendor Manager: Nora Menzi
Director of Marketing: Andrea DeFronzo
VP, Manufacturing and Inventory Control: Therese Connell
Composition and Project Management: SourceHOV LLC
Cover Design: Scott Moden
Rights & Media Specialist: Robert Boder
Media Development Editor: Troy Liston
Cover Image: © mammuth/E+/Getty
Printing and Binding: Edwards Brothers Malloy
Cover Printing: Edwards Brothers Malloy

Library of Congress Cataloging-in-Publication Data
Names: Bensley, Robert J., editor. | Brookins-Fisher, Jodi, editor.
Title: Community and public health education methods : a practical guide / [edited by] Robert J. Bensley and Jodi Brookins-Fisher.
Other titles: Community health education methods.
Description: Fourth edition. | Burlington, MA : Jones & Bartlett Learning, LLC,
[2019] | Revised edition of: Community health education methods : a practical guide. 3rd. ed. c2009. | Includes
bibliographical references and index.
Identifiers: LCCN 2017036582 | ISBN 9781284142174 (pbk. : alk. paper)
Subjects: LCSH: Health education--Handbooks, manuals, etc. | Community health services--Handbooks, manuals, etc.
Classification: LCC RA440 .C66 2019 | DDC 362.1--dc23 LC record available at https://lccn.loc.gov/2017036582

6048

Printed in the United States of America
21 20 19 18 17   10 9 8 7 6 5 4 3 2 1

This book is dedicated to the memory of
Loren B. Bensley, Jr.—husband, father, friend, and
consummate health educator who touched many,
many lives during his life. He meant the world to us
and not a day passes where either of us do not use
some of the wisdom or guidance he taught us.
He was our mentor, as he guided our professional
development and infused within us the belief that
it truly is possible to be all you can be and do all you
can to make the world a better place. He embodied
this philosophy and we are forever grateful for having
been touched by the true character of a man who
epitomized what a health educator truly should be.

Brief Contents

SECTION 3   **Applying Community and Public Health Education Methods and Strategies at the Community and Policy Level**   **189**

Contents

Chapter 4 Exploring Social Marketing Concepts 53

Mike Newton-Ward, MSW, MPH
Karen Denard Goldman, PhD, MCHES

Chapter 5   Building a Health Communication Framework ..69

Gary L. Kreps, PhD
Rosemary Thackeray, PhD, MPH
Michael D. Barnes, PhD, MCHES

SECTION 2   Acquiring the Tools for Applying Community and Public Health Education Methods and Strategies   93

Chapter 6   Developing Effective Presentation and Training Skills 95

Heather M. Wagenschutz, MBA, MA
Keely S. Rees, PhD, MCHES

Chapter 9   Working with Media Outlets 169

David Fouse, BA

SECTION 3   Applying Community and Public Health Education Methods and Strategies at the Community and Policy Level   189

Chapter 10   Facilitating Groups 191

Kathleen M. Roe, DrPH, MPH
Kevin Roe, MPH
Frank V. Strona, MPH

Chapter 11 Building and Sustaining Coalitions 217

Frances D. Butterfoss, PhD, MSEd

Chapter 12 Advocating for Health Policy 243

Cicily Hampton, PhD, MPA
Sue Lachenmayr, MPH, CHES

Chapter 13 Using Media Advocacy to Influence Policy 267

Lori Dorfman, DrPH, MPH
Michael Bakal, MPH, MEd

Preface

Robert J. Bensley, PhD, MCHES
Western Michigan University
Jodi Brookins-Fisher, PhD, MCHES
Central Michigan University

Welcome to the fourth edition of *Community and Public Health Education Methods: A Practical Guide*. This text is designed to assist you in effectively communicating messages and affecting norms and behaviors of individuals and communities. It is a book about the methods we use as health education specialists—the ways in which we tell a story, impact the social and political environment that influences population health, and empower others to seek healthy lifestyles. It explains the basic tools we need in order to communicate messages to those we are trying to serve and it provides an understanding of the skills needed for making a difference.

This text is unique because many of the chapters are written by and for health education specialists who have years of experience developing and applying skills to impact health. Much of the material within this text comes straight from the trenches, where real health education occurs. It is a guide designed to assist the health education specialist who exists on a shoestring budget and is attempting to implement the strategies theorists and researchers have found to be effective. It is for the overburdened practitioner who is working with multiple populations, across multiple settings, experiencing multiple problems. It is a guide to assist those on the front lines of health education in completing their mission.

▶ What is New to this Edition

This edition has been expanded in several ways, all of which are designed to provide both students and practitioners with an expanded understanding of the application of skills related to the practice of health education.

- Includes a new chapter focusing on using social media tools, such as Facebook, twitter, Instagram, Pinterest, Snapchat, texting, blogging, smartphone apps, and internet channels (e.g., YouTube)
- Incorporates the new CHES competencies throughout the book, so that users understand what to expect in terms of CHES with each chapter
- Each chapter includes key terms, additional resources, interesting "Did You Know?" facts, and a series of "Community Connections" vignettes designed to provide readers with an easy-to-understand, practical application on the concepts presented

As should be expected, all chapters have been revised to reflect both current and timely practices. In addition, each chapter continues to be user friendly by conforming to a common chapter format.

Organization of the Text

The text is divided into three sections, each containing chapters that center on a common theme.

Section 1 focuses on building the foundation for selecting and applying community and public health education methods, including chapters focusing on theories and models, becoming a professional, promoting multicultural diversity, social marketing concepts, and health communication strategies.

Each chapter in Sections 2 and 3 follow a similar format that includes an introduction to the topic, steps for implementing the skill, tips, and techniques for successful implementation, strategies for overcoming challenges, and expected outcomes.

Section 2 comprises chapters that focus on acquiring tools necessary for applying community and public health education methods strategies. These skills include developing presentation and training skills, developing and selecting resources, using social media, and working with media outlets.

Section 3 comprises chapters that pertain to building the framework where methods and strategies can be applied in impacting population health. These chapters focus on facilitating groups, building and sustaining coalitions, and using skills for influencing the health policy. It is our intent that this fourth edition will continue to assist students and practitioners in the acquisition and delivery of health education skills.

Acknowledgments

This updated edition has been a long time coming and there are many individuals to thank for the past and present editions. The original text came to fruition in the late 1990s with the help of various health educators from our beloved State of Michigan and we want to thank them for their passion for keeping the people of our state on a path toward health. To work with you all is a great reward for us!

We also want to thank the present authors of this text. Your contributions have made this the "go to" methods text in our profession, and we thank you for providing your expertise and wisdom to the content. We appreciate your dedication, timeliness, and willingness to go with the flow as we edited the chapters to find a unified voice throughout the text.

We also acknowledge the dedication and patience of our publisher and editors who worked on segments of the book while we refined other sections. Your contributions to the text will only make it look more polished and professional.

To past authors of chapters who are no longer part of the project, we thank you for the building blocks of which this text has grown to meet the needs of an ever-changing profession. We especially want to acknowledge two authors who have passed since the last edition: Karen Denard Goldman and Loren B. Bensley, Jr. One was boisterous and the other was refined, but they were both giants in our personal development and in the field of health education. We happily acknowledge them here and as authors of their respective chapters.

Finally, we thank our families, who have grown and multiplied since the last edition. Family is central to all we do and who we are, and all of you make life good.

Contributing Author Biographies

M. Elaine Auld, MPH, MCHES

Elaine Auld is chief executive officer of the Society for Public Health Education (SOPHE), where she oversees the organization's portfolio in professional preparation, professional development, publications, and advocacy. She has devoted her career to elevating the profession of health education by contributing to research, publications, and resources; serving as a principal investigator to numerous public and private grants and contracts to advance health education and health promotion; acting as a national and international spokesperson and advocate for the field, including testifying before Congress; and serving in volunteer and elected leadership roles for alumni and professional organizations. Elaine helped to inaugurate the Health Education Advocacy Summit in 1997, which has trained thousands of health professionals during the last two decades. In addition to policy advocacy, her passions include advancing health equity and contributing to national and international workforce development and competencies. Elaine is a charter CHES (#0056) and has been honored with awards from SOPHE, American Public Health Association (APHA), Eta Sigma Gamma, the Health Education Directory (HEDIR), and the National REACH Coalition. As the 2010 recipient of the Distinguished Alumni Award from the University of Michigan School of Public Health, she proudly admits to bleeding maize and blue.

Michael L. Bakal, MPH, MEd

Michael Bakal is a strategic communications specialist at Berkeley Media Studies Group (BMSG), a project of the Public Health Institute, where he provides training and consultation in media advocacy. His workshops help build the strategic communications capacity of nonprofit groups, public health professionals, youth, and university students. A certified bilingual science teacher, Michael has worked as a classroom teacher and a facilitator of informal education programs in Berkeley, Los Angeles, and Guatemala. As Fulbright scholar to Guatemala, Michael worked as a science teacher and researcher studying youth empowerment. He is cofounder of Voces y Manos, a nonprofit organization that facilitates youth-led advocacy and sustainable development projects.

Michael D. Barnes, PhD, MCHES

Dr. Barnes is a professor of public health and associate dean in the College of Life Sciences at Brigham Young University. Dr. Barnes' research and teaching interests include health communication interventions and policy advocacy, for which he has garnered many publications and received notable grants. Barnes and his colleagues cofounded the Computational Health Science (CHS) at BYU, a collaborative research group between public health and computer science. CHS examines the role various social media and technology play in both health surveillance and communication. Dr. Barnes has received numerous honors and awards, including BYU's *Wesley P. Lloyd Award* for distinction in graduate education, the Society for Public Health Education *National Public Health Fellow* and *Health Education Advocate Achievement* awards, and New Mexico State University's *Donald C. Roush Excellence in Teaching Award*. He actively contributes to the public health profession through dedicated service on international, national, and local boards. His passion for the profession is constantly sparked by training and mentoring students, interacting with colleagues throughout the world, and is rivaled only by spending time with family, being active outdoors in Utah's mountains, and growing and harvesting fruit from his backyard trees and vines.

Loren B. Bensley, Jr., EdD, CHES

Dr. Bensley was a professor emeritus at Central Michigan University, where he served 33 years in the professional preparation of health educators. His interest in learning theory and its relationship to methodology had its origin during his first years in teaching in secondary schools. As a university professor, his research and teaching reflected this continued interest in helping students understand theory and applying it to the selections of school and community health education methods. During his career, Dr. Bensley was highly active in professional associations at the state, national, and international levels, including president of the American School Health Association, a member of the original role delineation and health education unified code of ethics project, and numerous committee chair and member roles in almost every prominent health education association. In addition, Dr. Bensley was a longtime supporter and advocate for Eta Sigma Gamma, the national health education honorary, which now bears his name on the student *Gamman of the Year* award. Dr. Bensley, who spent a lifetime committed to the advancement of the health education profession and is the patriarch of three generations of health educators, passed away on November 21, 2016.

Robert J. Bensley, PhD, MCHES

Dr. Bensley is a professor of public health and the director of the eHealth Innovations Group at Western Michigan University. Over the past 25 years, his research interests have focused on using technology modalities as a means for influencing health behavior change. He is the founder of *wichealth.org*, which has impacted parent-child feeding behavior change in over four million WIC clients across 35 states, and the author of the patent-pending *Behavioral Intelligence Framework*. In addition, Dr. Bensley has served as principal investigator on over 200 externally funded grants and contracts, totaling over USD 12 million, supporting the development and implementation of technology-based health behavior change programming. Dr. Bensley was a Fulbright Senior Scholar in 2003 focusing on health promotion activities at the Nelson Mandela Metropolitan University in South Africa. Prior to his career in health education, he was employed by IBM, where he served as a systems engineer providing technical assistance and education to educational institutions, hospitals, and local government agencies. He resonates with the concept of being a "third culture kid," having spent significant time living in various countries around the world.

Jodi Brookins-Fisher, PhD, MCHES

Dr. Brookins-Fisher is a professor in the Division of Community Health within the School of Health Sciences at Central Michigan University. She is foremost considered a human rights advocate who believes everyone should experience life as they want to live it. She developed a diversity course for health professionals and enjoys the opportunity to contribute to the understanding of how culture influences health. Dr. Brookins-Fisher has been involved in health education at the local, state, and national levels, most recently serving a six-year term as Eta Sigma Gamma's vice president, president, and past president. She currently serves as the Advocacy Committee cochair for the Society for Public Health Education. Previously, she was on the board of Great Lakes Chapter SOPHE and the Michigan Organization for Adolescent Sexual

Health. She is owner of JBF Health Consulting, LLC, of which she serves as an evaluation consultant to many state projects. Dr. Brookins-Fisher is a passionate Michigander, who believes the beauty of her state rivals anywhere in this awesome country.

Frances D. Butterfoss, PhD, MSEd

Dr. Butterfoss is a health educator committed to building, sustaining, and evaluating partnerships to promote health and social justice. In her past lives, she was a visiting nurse, high school biology teacher, and an army wife. Currently, she is president of *Coalitions Work*, a consulting group that helps coalitions and partnerships reach their full potential, and an adjunct professor at Eastern Virginia Medical School. Dr. Butterfoss founded and directed several coalitions and received research support from many agencies and foundations. She has published widely and her books, *Coalitions and Partnerships in Community Health* and *Ignite! Getting Your Community Coalitions Fired Up for Change*, are great resources for academics and practitioners alike. Dr. Butterfoss is a past president and Distinguished Fellow of the Society for Public Health Education. She is a nationally recognized expert on coalition building and organizational development, with more than 25 years of experience training and consulting with organizations, coalitions, and communities across America. You can usually find Fran in an airport on the way to a coalition engagement, hiking in Shenandoah National Park, or cruising on *Moonshadow* in the Chesapeake Bay.

Lori Dorfman, DrPH, MPH

Dr. Dorfman cofounded Berkeley Media Studies Group (BMSG), a project of the Public Health Institute, in 1993. She directs BMSG's research on how public health issues appear in the media, which BMSG applies to its media advocacy training with community groups and to its professional education for journalists. Her research and media advocacy across a range of public health issues—from alcohol and tobacco to nutrition and food marketing to violence prevention, trauma, and sexual assault—focuses on how we can widen the frame from portraits of individuals to the landscapes that surround them. Dr. Dorfman is also Associate Adjunct Professor at the School of Public Health at the University of California, Berkeley, where she teaches a course on mass communication and public health. She consults on strategic communications with foundations, public health groups, and government agencies and writes frequently on media advocacy. Her passion for media advocacy has not waned over the years, though social media frenzies can make her a little dizzy. She rests her mind by painting in her basement.

David Fouse, BA

David Fouse is director of communications at the American Public Health Association, where he oversees media relations, *The Nation's Health* newspaper, online strategy, social media, branding, and more. He has over 25 years of experience in communications and marketing with national nonprofit organizations. He works with journalists and others to raise awareness of public health issues, communicate the value of public health work, and share the latest research and news from APHA, the *American Journal of Public Health*, National Public Health Week, and others. He is a graduate of the National Public Health Leadership Institute and is certified in Crisis and Emergency Risk Communications from the Centers for Disease Control and Prevention.

Karen Denard Goldman, PhD, MCHES

Dr. Goldman was a health educator for over 20 years, whose career included experience as a frontline public health educator, manager, executive, teacher, author, principal investigator, researcher, speaker, and profession leader. Until her death in 2014, she worked in local health agencies, voluntary nonprofit organizations, schools, hospitals, private industry, and colleges and universities.

As director of KDG Health Education Consulting, Dr. Goldman provided health education and social marketing technical assistance, training, and keynote presentations for over 15 years. She served as an associate editor of *Health Promotion Practice*, which published columns known as *Health Education Tools of the Trade*. She was SOPHE president, coordinator of the New York State Coalition for Health Education, and coordinator of the Professional Development Board of the National Commission for Health Education Credentialing (NCHEC). Dr. Goldman conducted the first federally funded, nationally broadcast conference on social marketing in New York City, and conducted social marketing orientation and training for community and public health personnel across the country. Her whit, courage, leadership, passion, and voice touched many lives. In 2016, SOPHE renamed the SOPHE Mentor Award, which honors an individual who has made a significant contribution to the preparation and/or performance of health educators, in Dr. Goldman's honor.

Cicily Hampton, PhD, MPA

Dr. Hampton is the senior director of Health Science & Policy at SOPHE, where she leads the association's legislative and regulatory advocacy activities that address public health, health disparities, school health, and health education, in addition to planning and conducting advocacy trainings. Prior to her current position with SOPHE, Dr. Hampton worked as a policy analyst evaluating health outcomes for North Carolina's Medicaid program and at a healthcare advocacy firm lobbying on behalf of healthcare reform. Dr. Hampton has experience in federal and state advocacy, as well as the development and execution of state and national lobbying strategies around delivery system and payment reform, quality metrics, and health disparities. Dr. Hampton is also an assistant research professor at the University of North Carolina at Charlotte, where she continues her health disparities research.

Gary L. Kreps, PhD

Dr. Kreps is a University Distinguished Professor and director of the Center for Health and Risk Communication at George Mason University. He studies the use of strategic evidence-based communication to promote public health, with a focus on the dissemination of relevant health information via a broad range of health communication channels and technologies to reduce health inequities for vulnerable populations. Dr. Kreps' well-funded research program is reported in more than 400 publications. He was the founding chief of the Health Communication and Informatics Research Branch at the National Cancer Institute, where he introduced major cancer communication research initiatives such as the Health Information National Trends Survey (HINTS) research program and the Centers of Excellence in Cancer Communication Research (CECCR) initiative. He serves on the Food and Drug Administration's Risk Communication Advisory Committee and is a special advisor to the Veterans Health Administration. Over the past decade, he introduced a number of international health communication projects to promote global health, including the HINTS-China research program, the HINTS-Germany research program, and the Global Advocacy Leadership Academy (GALA). In the past, Dr. Kreps served as dean of the School of Communication at Hofstra University, executive director of the Greenspun School of Communication at UNLV, and as a professor at Northern Illinois, Rutgers, Indiana, and Purdue Universities. He has received many honors for his work, including the 2015 *Research Laureate Award* from the American Academy for Health Behavior.

Sue Lachenmayr, MPH, CHES

Sue Lachenmayr is a past president of SOPHE and served as chair of the national SOPHE's Advocacy Committee and as Advocacy Committee chair and president of the New Jersey SOPHE. She is a health education consultant in the areas of advocacy training and program implementation at the local, state, and national levels. Sue is coauthor of *Amplifying Our Voices: Training for Public Health Advocacy* and winner of SOPHE's 2001 *Program Excellence Award*. She recently spent four years in Washington D.C. as senior director of the National Council on Aging's Chronic Disease Self-Management Technical Assistance Center. Now in her fourth retirement, she is a consultant for the MAC, Inc. Living Well Center of Excellence, where she advocates for older adult wellness and trains individuals and professionals in evidence-based behavior change programs. Sue is committed to empowering older adults through self-management skills to take charge of their health, which is especially important to her, as she is one herself.

Mike Newton-Ward, MSW, MPH

Mike Newton-Ward has worked with social marketing since 1997. He has consulted with state, federal, and international governmental and nonprofit organizations on the incorporation of a social marketing approach into their work, and has presented numerous trainings and conference offerings on social marketing. He has reviewed and contributed to social marketing textbooks and journals for major publishing houses and is on the editorial board of *Social Marketing Quarterly*. He is a founding member of both the International Social Marketing Association and the Social Marketing Association of North America. Mike currently teaches the social marketing course at the University of North Carolina-Chapel Hill Gillings School of Global Public Health; is a part time contractor at RTI International, as the lead social marketer in the Center for Communication Science; and consults independently. Additionally, Mike has provided social marketing consulting with CDC, and worked with state and local public health departments on the use of Web 2.0 and e-Health technologies. The 5th World Social Marketing Conference recently presented Mr. Newton-Ward with an award for *Outstanding Contributions to Social Marketing*, during the first occurrence of the award being given. Mike is a self-professed snob about three things: well-brewed coffee, high quality dark chocolate, and well-done social marketing.

Mike Perko, PhD, MCHES

Dr. Perko is a professor in the University of North Carolina, Greensboro (UNCG) Department of Public Health Education, with prior appointment as chair of the Department of Health Science at the University of Alabama. Dr. Perko also currently serves as the chief Wellness Advisor to the National Rural Electric Cooperative Association, where he has trained over 2,000 Benefits Administrators responsible for managing the health of 35,000 association members throughout the country. In 2015, Dr. Perko was named one of the top 100 Worksite Health Promotion Specialists by a national panel of experts, and has been invited as keynote speaker on health and wellness at many national forums, including the Institute for Organizational Management, the U.S. National Chamber of Commerce Executive Training Seminar's, and the National Safety Leadership Summit. In 2008, he was the inaugural speaker for a health promotion initiative for U.S. Army forces stationed at the 173rd Airborne division in Vicenza, Italy. Dr. Perko received the 2017 and 2011 UNCG *Excellence in Teaching Award* and the same award at UNC Wilmington in 2002. His fifth children's book, *How to EAT, LEAP, and SLEEP like a SUPERHERO!* was published in April 2015 by the Wellness Council of America. Dr. Perko enjoys spending every minute of his free time with his family and coaching his kid's sports. When not doing that, he is playing ice hockey.

Kathy Delavan Plomer, MPH

Kathy Delavan Plomer has been in the field of health education for the last 25 years. Her experience includes work at two local health departments, four nonprofit health agencies, including a cancer research center and extensive community volunteer work. She has a diverse professional background, including experience in materials design, e-learning, in-person training design and delivery, school health policy development, program implementation, and professional development. Kathy currently is the head of Odyssey Consulting and works with ETR as a professional development consultant. She also works at the Tri County Health Department,

Colorado, in the area of fall prevention for older adults. As a community volunteer and elected official, she serves as president of the Board of Education for the Adams 12 Five Star Schools and on the Board of Directors for the Colorado Association of School Boards, where she advocates for schools to serve not only the academic needs of students, but also their physical, emotional, and mental health needs as well.

Keely S. Rees, PhD, MCHES

Dr. Rees is director of the Public Health-Community Health Education program and professor in the Department of Health Education and Health Promotion at the University of Wisconsin-La Crosse. Over the past 20 years, Dr. Rees' has focused her career on prenatal care, exercise prescription and behaviors during and after pregnancy, social support for preconception and prenatal nutrition, tobacco use during pregnancy, and sexuality education and advocacy for young children, teens, and parents, and schools as community outreach for nutrition and exercise. She has been working in collaboration with Pine Ridge Indian Reservation and Global Partners of Gundersen Health System to provide education and advocacy with Native American youth and leaders. In addition to her teaching career at UW-LaCrosse, Dr. Rees has worked internationally in Ireland and Spain with other universities, researchers, and organizations identifying ways to better prepare health educators for the field. Dr. Rees has been a faculty cosponsor for the Beta Phi Eta Sigma Gamma Chapter since 2003 and served on the Board of Trustees for SOPHE.

Kathleen M. Roe, DrPH, MPH

Dr. Roe is professor of Public Health and Community Health Education at San José State University in Northern California. As founder and director of the Community Health Studies Group and Salud Familiar en McKinley, Dr. Roe has been involved in community health promotion efforts for over 35 years, including HIV prevention planning, school-based community health promotion, neighborhood capacity building for health, and

community support for relative caregivers. She is also cofounder of the Intercambio, a longstanding university partnership with the artisans in a pueblo in Oaxaca, Mexico. Dr. Roe is a past president of SOPHE and a former member of the Governing Council of APHA. She is grateful for her career in health education and always inspired by Dorothy Nyswander's description of health educators: "We are dreamers, and our dreams have to do with the basic purposes of an open society."

Kevin Roe, MPH

Kevin Roe currently teaches at San Jose State University (SJSU) in the Health Science and Recreation Department after spending more than 25 years in public health and health education practice. His areas of professional expertise include community organizing, LGBT health, HIV/AIDS prevention and treatment, community planning, and evaluation. Kevin's areas of emphasis at SJSU include program planning and evaluation, community organizing, and he is on the team developing the new BS degrees in public health. Kevin lives with his husband and their two rescue cats.

Liliana Rojas-Guyler, PhD, CHES

Dr. Rojas-Guyler has combined academic, community, and corporate industry work experience. She is committed to health education initiatives that enrich the lives, health, and well-being of women, particularly those women who may be in vulnerable or disadvantaged positions. Dr. Rojas-Guyler is currently an associate professor of Health Promotion and Education at the University of Cincinnati. Dr. Rojas-Guyler has published and presented widely on minority health issues, particularly those relating to Latina health. Her research agenda includes determinants of health among vulnerable populations, health behaviors, the influence of culture, and professional preparation needs of future health educators to address cultural appropriateness in health program planning. Liliana is a native of Colombia, has lived in the United States for nearly 30 years, and in Ohio since 2002, where she resides with her family—her husband and two sons.

Michael Stellefson, PhD

Dr. Stellefson is an associate professor in the Department of Health Education and Promotion at East Carolina University (ECU). His research focuses on developing and evaluating patient-centered technology to improve patient self-management in chronic disease, specifically Chronic Obstructive Pulmonary Disease (COPD. Dr. Stellefson has published over 60 peer-reviewed articles, and he has served as principal investigator on a R36 Health Services Dissertation Award, KL2 Mentored Career Development Award, and several pilot awards from the University of Florida (UF) Clinical and Translational Science Institute. His research has focused on examining how technology can enable healthcare stakeholders to collaborate and share information on patient behavioral tasks critical for improving disease management and health outcomes. He is the author of *COPDFlix*, a low computer literate social media website for patients, informal caregivers, and clinicians to collaborate and share patient education videos on self-management, for which he received the 2016 Society for Public Health Education *Technology Award*. Prior to joining the ECU faculty, Dr. Stellefson served as an assistant professor and associate chair in the Department of Health Education and Behavior at UF.

Frank V. Strona, MPH

Frank Strona has been working in gay men's health, community organizing, and substance use concerns for almost 20 years and has established himself as a nationally recognized frontline specialist in HIV/STD harm reduction techniques, sexual health, Internet interventions, and prevention education. He has served as the 2006 and 2007 community cochair for the California HIV/AIDS Prevention Planning Group, in addition to being a member of the San Francisco HIV Prevention Planning Council from 2004 to 2014. During 2015–2016, Frank expanded his reach to include emergency operations and assisted as a health communications lead for Ebola-affected countries. Most recently, he served as the senior communication analyst on the *President Commission for Bioethical Issues* (PCBI) under President Obama. In addition to his communications efforts, he was charged with cocreating curriculum and serving as a training lead for a new public health capacity training on democratic deliberation decision making methodology for high impact health departments. As owner and lead strategic coach for MentorSF. com, Frank is providing training nationwide on adapting curricula for online learning, blogging, and social media, and helps answer the question of "How do I tell my story?" with his Storytelling Technology Bootcamps.

Rosemary Thackeray, PhD, MPH

Dr. Rosemary Thackeray is a professor in the Department of Health Science at Brigham Young University (BYU), where she teaches undergraduate and graduate courses in program evaluation and research methods. Her research has focused on social marketing, social media, and prevention of cytomegalovirus. Prior to joining the BYU faculty, Dr. Thackeray was employed for nine years at the Utah Department of Health, Bureau of Health Education. Her experience included program development and management, research and evaluation, worksite wellness, violence prevention, coordinated school health, and physical activity. Dr. Thackeray also worked part time as a health educator with Salt Lake Community Health Centers and FHP Health Care, and facilitated weight management classes for the American Heart Association. While on a sabbatical, Dr. Thackeray worked for the Centers for Disease Control and Prevention National Center for Health Marketing in Atlanta. In her spare time, Dr. Thackeray enjoys traveling, spending time with family, reading, collecting antique glassware, and eating ice cream.

Heather M. Wagenschutz, MBA, MA

Heather Wagenschutz currently serves as a course codirector for Leadership and the Paths of Excellence at the University of Michigan Medical School. Her career started in 1994 as a public health educator with a tri-county health department, and later worked in sales and marketing for two pharmaceutical companies before transitioning to university positions. Heather's teaching experience has been with Kellogg Community College, Davenport University, and leadership skill building sessions for medical students. Heather loves to golf (although golf does not always love her back), dancing until her knees "can't take it anymore," learning new things, and laughing with friends and family.

Kathleen J. Young, PhD, MPH

Dr. Young is a professor in the Public Health and Masters of Public Health Program in the Department of Health Sciences at California State University, Northridge (CSUN), where she serves as a health policy and cultural assessment specialist, coordinates university-community partnership service learning programs with public health organizations and agencies, and previously served as the coordinator of the COUGH-Northridge tobacco control policy assessment organization. Dr. Young's research interests include women's health issues, specifically in primary prevention strategies in healthcare services, cultural competence for the healthcare practitioner, and health policy assessment. Dr. Young served on the Board of Directors and as cochair of the Health Policy Advocacy Committee for the American Association for Health Education, and was the recipient of the American Public Health Association Alcohol, Tobacco & Other Drugs Section *College-Based Leadership*, the CSUN *Distinguished Faculty Visionary Community Service-Learning*, and the National Institutes for Health & CSUN *Research Infrastructure in Minority Institution Scholars Program* awards. In addition, she served as a Fulbright Scholar at Zhejiang University in the School of Medicine in Hangzhou, China, in 2015.

Building the Foundation for Selecting and Applying Community and Public Health Education Methods and Strategies

CHAPTER 1

Foundations for Selecting Community and Public Health Education Strategies

Loren B. Bensley, Jr., EdD, CHES
Robert J. Bensley, PhD, MCHES
Jodi Brookins-Fisher, PhD, MCHES

▶ Author Comments

This chapter introduces the reader to foundations underlining why we select the methods and strategies we do for implementing health education programs. The role of health education specialists is to understand the underlying causes, or determinants, of negative health behaviors and outcomes and how to select methods and strategies that are most likely to motivate and educate individuals, families, organizations, and communities. Through training, health education specialists are equipped with skills and empowered to change environments and behaviors to improve the quality and quantity of people's lives. The existence of this power to make a difference creates the burden of responsibility to practice theoretically sound health education. How can health education specialists, then, implement health education with some assurance that specific health problems are being addressed in the best possible way? It is by focusing on the real determinants impacting health and following appropriate theory when selecting and applying methods that will yield positive results.

⌕ CHES COMPETENCIES

1.4.1   Identify and analyze factors that influence health behaviors.
2.4.1   Use theories and/or models to guide the delivery plan.
3.3.2   Apply theories and/or models of implementation.*
7.1.1   Create messages using communication theories and/or models.

*Advanced level competency

Reprinted by permission of the National Commission for Health Education Credentialing, Inc. (NCHEC) and Society for Public Health Education (SOPHE).

▶ Introduction

Health education specialists cannot assume nor take for granted that everyone is motivated and learns the same. There is no generic way to educate about health. If there were, there would be no use for this book. One of the most difficult tasks for behavioral scientists and health education specialists is changing and sustaining individual or group behavior. At the same time, it is important to understand how behavior fits into a broader social ecology world, where focus is not only on individual behavior change, but also interpersonal, organizational, community, and policy. This model affirms the importance of using multipronged approaches when attempting to change and sustain behaviors, and it is through this broader intervention perspective that the greatest likelihood for influential change on the individual can occur.

Selection of health education methods needs to consider the focus of influence or what level the intervention is geared toward. Central to the application of the social ecological model is that health status and behaviors are shaped by various levels of influence following a macro- to micro-level approach, where broader spheres of influence have the capability to reaching and supporting greater change in health status or behavior.[1] This model can be visualized as a series of concentric circles, with the innermost circle focusing on intrapersonal factors associated with the individual. At this level, efforts are made to influence the individual in adopting specific positive health behaviors. These behaviors can then be supported or encouraged

through interpersonal relationships via family, social groups, or other social networks. Organizational structures such as health and medical plans, population health-serving organizations, and the like provide mechanisms for ensuring individual ability to engage in and sustain behaviors. Community-level influence coming from employers, media, community-based organizations, businesses, and other community structures assists in providing a broader level of support for engaging in and maintaining positive behavior changes. At the broadest end, policy initiatives such as laws, policies and regulations, health prevention strategies and goals, and state or national guidelines drive the focus on ensuring whatever positive behaviors are being sought can thrive. Each level has influence on the circles contained within it, so that the widest net is cast at the furthermost circle (i.e., policy level), which has great influence on community and organization, which has influence on interpersonal and so forth (**FIGURE 1.1**).

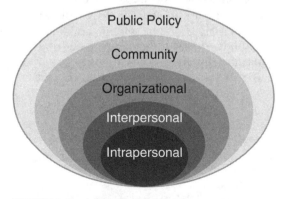

FIGURE 1.1 Social Ecologial Model.

When considering how best to impact individual change, it is important to consider which strategies and methods will have the greatest likelihood of ensuring that change can be sustained. Along with the need for individual change, a good health education specialist will also try to affect change in the social determinants of health within the individual's broader environment. As previously stated, this might include instituting methods for change in a policy or community. Method selection is, therefore, defined broadly and different methods work in different situations for different groups. A "one method fits all" does not exist, and there is rarely a singular method for behavioral or environmental change to occur.

Planning models are helpful to health education specialists because they map out not only which methods are appropriate considering the individual, program, and environment but also ensure method selection occurs only after program goals and objectives have been developed. It is always exciting to get to the method selection; however, it is of utmost importance methods are selected based on the program's desired outcomes. Otherwise, it is difficult to determine if and when change occurs. As always, previous scientifically based research should be consulted to help determine which methods have been tested and show the best possibility of success.

This book is a collection of different methods that can be used at various levels to impact the

COMMUNITY CONNECTIONS 1.1

Kara has 10 years of experience working in public health, 6 of which were as a registered dietitian working in the Women, Infants, and Children (WIC) program and the last 4 as supervisor of the maternal and infant section of the Northwest County Health Department. She received a master's degree in health education and is very active in the state's chapter of the Society for Public Health Education (SOPHE) serving as its president. As a supervisor, she is highly organized and considered a "pro" by her peers.

Keisha is a graduate of a respected undergraduate community health education program and recently received CHES status. She has been employed by the health department for one and a half years and is considering starting on her master's degree in health education at a nearby university. Her colleagues know her as a creative person with a solid understanding of professional issues. Like many health education specialists, she tries to balance her commitments and responsibilities to her family, employment, and potential graduate studies.

Hector is a recent graduate with a bachelor's degree in health education from one of the state's universities known for its excellent professional preparation program. As an undergraduate, he was active in Eta Sigma Gamma, the National Health Education Honorary, serving as chapter president. Hector was hired six months ago as a health education specialist, where he shares time between the maternal and infant, chronic disease and health promotion and community assessment sections of the department.

If you ask Keisha, with her one and a half years' experience, she will tell you that at times she becomes frustrated and disappointed with the lack of success in motivating individuals to make changes in their health behaviors. She often feels disillusioned with her chosen profession. As an undergraduate, she believed she could make a difference in people's lives by helping them live healthy lifestyles. At times, there seems to be progress toward this belief, which gives her hope.

Kara can identify with Keisha's disillusionment because she went through a similar experience as a dietitian. It was after attending a state SOPHE conference and starting her master's degree that she realized there was more to improving population health than just one-on-one transference of content, knowledge, and behavior change skills. As a dietitian, Kara had integrated her personal strengths such as her organizational and communication skills into her practice at the expense of applying theory to the selection of methods. She could see where Keisha, like herself, would use motivational and behavioral change methods without a sound theoretical foundation. Kara knows that Keisha needs help and encouragement, as well as applying theory within a social ecology framework.

Hector, on the other hand, is doing all he can to make health education work. Like many young professionals, he and Keisha are hardworking, enthusiastic, and idealistic in their pursuits. Though, being spread across sections, they had much to learn.

greatest likelihood of success with positive health. Each chapter is designed to present different models and methods that can be used within interventions designed to influence change. The remainder of this chapter focuses on an introduction to change theory—the backbone necessary for implementing any of the methods appearing in this book.

▶ Health Education Theories

Methods selected by health education specialists should be grounded in behavior change theory. The health education profession has subscribed to a number of theories, which take into consideration variables that influence individual behavior and population health. These theories serve as a foundation and structure from which community health education methods can be applied. Selecting methods without considering theory is like building a house without a foundation. The potential for the house to collapse will always be a threat. Likewise, methods chosen without a theoretical base will be vulnerable to failure. Can health education specialists afford to take these risks? Of course not! Health education specialists are concerned about individual lifestyles that cause real or potential health problems. As a result, programs with the greatest potential for success must be designed and implemented. The understanding and application of theory to practice is an insurance policy that this will occur.

It is important to understand the meaning of theory. A **theory** is a general explanation of why people act or do not act to maintain and/or promote the health of themselves, their families, organizations, and communities.[2] There are numerous theories commonly used by health education specialists. It is not the intent of this chapter to explain all the theories in health education, but to discuss a limited number—those commonly used. Unfortunately, theories do not work in some situations, which is why researchers and theorists are constantly trying to improve and develop new theories and models. In time, new theories will evolve that will continue to help better understand the most effective approaches for affecting change in individuals and communities.

Within the context of behavior change, theories can generally be classified in two groups, depending on their focus. Intrapersonal theories focus on individuals as the units of change, whereas interpersonal and community theories focus on social systems, organizations, and cultures. Intrapersonal theories are based on the premises that behavior is determined by (1) what we know, which in turn results in how we act; and (2) perceptions, attitudes, beliefs, levels of motivation, self-efficacy, skills, resiliency, and environmental variables. Interpersonal and community models are designed to support healthy lifestyles by reducing or eliminating hazards in social and physical environments. These models center on community-level change, including community organization, theories of organizational change, and diffusion of innovation, and are important in planning comprehensive community-based programs.

Although there are numerous theories and models that have been used to promote individual and population health changes, the following three intrapersonal and two interpersonal-focused theories and models are commonly used by health education specialists. The following section contains a simple description of each theory and its practical application, as displayed in the ongoing vignette found in the Community Connections sections of this chapter. The intent is not to provide a detailed and complex discussion of each theory, as there are numerous existing resources that serve this purpose. Rather, the intent is for the reader to recognize that many different theories and models exist, each of which should be identified and applied based on the overall need and goal associated with the health-related issue.

Intrapersonal Theories
The Health Belief Model

The Health Belief Model (HBM), as its title suggests, has to do with beliefs surrounding health and was one of the first designed to encourage people to take action toward positive health.[3] The model emphasizes the role of perceptions of vulnerability to an illness or condition and the potential effectiveness in treatment or action. It means health education specialists should take into consideration an individual's perception that he or she is vulnerable to a negative health condition and the actions on the part of individuals that could prevent the threat and eliminate possible illness or negative condition.

COMMUNITY CONNECTIONS 1.2

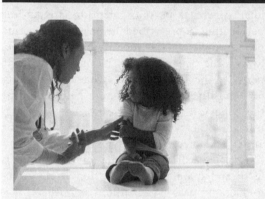

© LWA/Dann Tardif/Blend Images/Getty.

One of the health education programs Keisha was concerned about was motivating low-income mothers to immunize their infants. The method she used was direct communication through a brochure she developed and distributed to mothers who had just delivered or that were clients participating in WIC. Keisha decided on applying the Health Belief Model (HBM), because she knew it addresses a belief in perceived severity of illness and that, if informed of this severity, people would respond to prevention messages. The perception that their babies were at risk would surely motivate mothers to have their children immunized.

When the results of Keisha's efforts were 40% less than the program's goal, she turned to Kara and asked for help. In analyzing the plan, Kara assured Keisha the choice of method was appropriate, the group identified was at high risk, and that Keisha's goals and objectives along with her evaluation methods were reasonable. The problem was in implementing the theoretical model. Kara could clearly see that the HBM, as used, was incomplete. In her explanations to Keisha, she pointed out that she only used one of the four principles of the model, which was to inform mothers of the potential severity associated with their infants not being immunized. After realizing the mistake of not implementing all the components of the model, Keisha asked Kara how the model should have been applied to this situation.

Kara explained the program overemphasized the perceived severity associated with not protecting infants. What was missing was the perception of why and how children were susceptible. Another mistake was the failure to anticipate barriers that would discourage mothers from having their infants immunized. These might include cost, perceived threat to the infant's health if immunized, religious beliefs, or accessibility to services. The third, and probably most serious mistake, was neglecting the questions of what, where, when, and how services could be obtained. Keisha did not anticipate barriers and failed to plan services around the difficulties these barriers created. For example, she failed to make clear what the cost would be, who would qualify for free services, when infants should be immunized, the low risk of possible reactions, and where mothers could take their children to be immunized.

Kara suggested Keisha conduct a random sample of the priority population to determine if they had their children immunized and, if not, why. The results confirmed Kara's assumptions. Keisha found that 65% of mothers did not have their babies immunized because of a perceived threat to the child's health, inconvenience, lack of time, and not knowing where they could receive services. Keisha realized that if the HBM had been fully applied to the methods she chose, more information would have been conveyed that may have addressed these perceptions.

The HBM is based on the belief that health-related behavior is determined by whether individuals (1) perceive themselves to be susceptible to a health problem, (2) see the health problem as serious, (3) are convinced they will benefit from treatment or prevention activities, and (4) recognize the need to take action and any barriers that would interfere with this action. Four questions dictate whether or not a person is convinced actions that can be taken are likely to prevent negative health conditions:

- Am I susceptible?
- Is it serious?
- Do the benefits in taking action overcome the emotional, financial, social, or other costs?
- Are services or help available?

The perceived need to take action is influenced by variables that affect a person's perceptions and, as a result, indirectly influence health behavior. These modifying factors include level of educational attainment, cultural differences, demographic characteristics, personal experiences, economic status, and other social determinants, all of which can influence the perception of susceptibility, severity, benefits, and barriers.

Theory of Planned Behavior

The Theory of Planned Behavior is based on the assumption that behavior, or the intention to behave in a certain way, is determined by the person's attitude toward the behavior, subjective norms, and perceived behavioral control. In other words, if a person perceives a given outcome will be a positive experience, and that others positively view it, and that it is not difficult to perform, the person is more likely to exhibit that behavior.[4]

The health education specialist needs to identify what a person's intention is regarding performing a prescribed behavior. This could be accomplished by identifying (1) attitudes toward the behavior—why he or she wishes to perform the behavior and what expectations, both positive and negative, are held regarding the behavior, (2) subjective norms—what significant others will think about the behavior, and (3) perceived behavioral control—how difficult it will be for the individual to perform and maintain the behavior. If an inventory of the person's intentions is positive, it is more likely he or she will perform the intended

---

COMMUNITY CONNECTIONS 1.3

Keisha had received a request from a local church to talk to a group of teenage girls about postponing sexual intercourse. Knowing peers often influence teens, she looked for an approach that would use positive influence as a motivator. Keisha knew the Theory of Planned Behavior focused on identifying behavioral intent and so decided that could be the foundation for her presentation.

Keisha asked the girls questions in order to clarify the level of intent the girls had to perform the desired behavior. Specifically, Keisha asked about attitudes regarding this behavior, who they admired and respected, and what they would expect those they admired to do in the same situation. What she discovered, much to her delight, was the girls' intentions to postpone sexual intercourse were generally positive. The questions Keisha asked really worked in helping the girls define the importance of the desired behavior and in identifying who might have difficulty in performing the behavior. She felt that if these girls identified significant others and thought about what they would do under similar circumstances, it would help them think twice and reconsider their actions. Keisha was pleased, as the use of the theory seemed to work. As she mentioned to Kara, "I think I really made a difference." Kara was also pleased with Keisha's success, but reminded her that the Theory of Planned Behavior is a predictor of behavior. There are a lot of variables such as self-efficacy, self-esteem, and communication skills that will determine if the girls' intentions will result in the desired behavior. As a result, methods can be designed for these individuals based on theories related to the variables.

behavior. Key to this theory is the concept of reasoned action. A person needs to reason or think logically about an intended behavior. This is a cognitive process—discovering or finding reasons or intentions to behave in a certain way.

Transtheoretical Model (Stages of Change)

The Transtheoretical Model is based on the assumption that behavior change is a process and individuals are at varying levels of motivation or readiness to change. People at different stages in the process of change can benefit from different interventions. In other words, the methods used for a desired outcome are not generic because individuals are not always at the same stage or level of readiness to change. The model also assumes people may **relapse** or return to a previous stage, which can often happen. The model identifies five stages or levels of readiness that could be applied to any type of behavior change.[5]

- **Precontemplation**. Those in this stage either have no interest or capability to initiate change. This could be due to lack of knowledge, previous failures at change, or other barriers that make it difficult to consider behavior change (e.g., lack of any understanding of the impact of calories associated with pizza and fast foods).
- **Contemplation**. These individuals are considering changing behavior someday, but just not yet ready due to one or more barriers that prevent initiating the behavior. These barriers can include time, social support, money, fear, and many other difficult-to-overcome issues (e.g., desire to change eating habits but do not have support from family).
- **Preparation**. This stage includes individuals who are preparing for and experimenting with behavior change but lacking self-efficacy to actively engage in the process (e.g., setting a New Year's resolution or "next Monday" to begin eating healthier).
- **Action**. Individuals who are actively engaging in the behavior change process, but hav-

ing done so for less than a given period time needed to turn the action into a habit fit this stage of readiness change (e.g., following a 21-day healthy eating program).
- **Maintenance**. Those who have made change and are sustaining the behavior change over time are considered to be in maintenance (e.g., having followed healthy eating guidelines for the past year).

⑦ DID YOU KNOW?

According to its creators, James Prochaska and Carlo DiClemente, the Transtheoretical Model can also be used for addiction treatment and recovery.

Data from Fitzgerald, K. (2016, Nov. 1). 6 ways to understand the changes in addiction and treatment recovery. *The Recovery Village*. Retrieved from http://www.therecoveryvillage.com/recovery-blog/six-stages-change-recovery/

The model should be easy to remember because the key word *stage* is what the model encompasses; individuals move through many stages in their attempt to change behaviors. Because the theory is based on stages, it is necessary to determine the stage in which an individual or group resides. This is important, as the intervention provided must match the stage of readiness to change. Asking a few simple questions, as demonstrated in Community Connections 1.4, can be one means of determining the appropriate stage.

Ten processes of change, categorized as either cognitive and affective experiential processes or behavioral processes, are the mechanisms in which people engage in change.[5] Some processes such as those focusing on getting the facts and noticing effects on others are more akin to earlier stages of change, whereas those that focus on support systems, reinforcement, and managing the environment are more helpful with more active stages of readiness to change. Central to stages of change movement is the concept of decisional balance, focusing on the pros and cons associated with the change. As the pros start to outweigh the cons, the behavior is more likely to advance along the stage of change continuum.

COMMUNITY CONNECTIONS 1.4

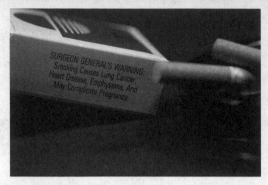

Courtesy of Debora Cartagena/CDC.

Hector was given the responsibility of designing a smoking cessation program for employees of a small automotive parts manufacturing company. In taking on this task, he was concerned some individuals would sign up for the program with different levels of readiness to change. For example, he assumed some had stopped smoking, but within a short period of time started again. Some would have a support system of family and friends who would encourage their efforts. Others would be lifetime smokers who would find giving up smoking very difficult. Levels of readiness would range from a sincere desire to quit to a "been there, done that" attitude. Hector needed to know the stage of change for each participant, but how? That was the question.

Hector remembered that when he worked on a county tobacco policy coalition, the director of the community cancer agency had mentioned his experiences with smoking cessation programs. Hector had been impressed with the materials from the cancer agency, and now he thought they might provide some helpful information. All it took was one phone call. The director shared stage-based questions that could be used to determine the stages of readiness to change associated with smoking behavior. What a find! Hector's networking pays off and his job was going to be much easier.

Hector developed a questionnaire based on examples provided by the director of the cancer agency, to determine the stages of participants' readiness. Questions focused on the following five stages of change:

- Interest in trying to quit
- Thinking about quitting soon
- Ready to plan a cessation attempt
- In the process of cessation
- Trying to stay smoke free

Hector was able to arrange the participants into five groups according to their stage of readiness to engage in smoking cessation. As a result, different strategies and methods such as personal testimonies, analysis of smoking behaviors and failed attempts, text messaging, determination and individualization of cessation approaches, use of online support systems, and use of medical personnel were designed to help the participants implement changes over time.

Hector felt good about applying the Transtherotecial Model in planning the smoking cessation program. He told Keisha, "I feel like I have individualized the approach in helping people give up a very unhealthy behavior."

Interpersonal and Community Theories

Social Cognitive Theory

Central to social learning theory is the belief that human behavior is explained in terms of a three-way, dynamic, and reciprocal phenomenon, in which personal factors, environmental influences, and behavior continually interact and influence each other. As such, a basic premise of Social Cognitive Theory (SCT) is that people not only learn through their own experiences, but also by observing the actions of others and the results of those actions.[6] This theory is one of the most widely used among health education specialists to both describe human behavior and develop interventions for positively impacting change. Although at first SCT seems easily understandable, the theory is actually rather complex. The scenario in Community Connections 1.5 can be used to apply six concepts essential to understanding SCT:

- **Reciprocal determinism** means behavior changes are determined from interactions between a person and his or her environment. The environment can influence or discourage a person in a healthy way or can be detrimental, depending on whether the environment is supportive or corrosive. Conversely, people can influence the environment so that it is more conducive to a healthy lifestyle. For example, some of the individuals in Hector's program may experience environmental factors that are supportive of healthy eating and exercise, while others may not. If negative forces exist, it may be necessary to change the environment to provide opportunities for choosing healthy foods and for engaging in exercising. Hector applied this concept by having each participant identify positive and negative forces in their work and living environments that helped or hindered their desire to lose weight.

- **Behavioral capability** is a person's capability to change a behavior by having the knowledge and skills necessary to enact a desired behavior. Applied to Hector's program, it means that education is necessary to learn about healthy foods and its preparation as well as about types of exercises designed for flexibility, body tone, strength, cardiovascular fitness, and endurance. Skills also need to be developed such as analyzing labels, counting calories, preparing food, taking one's target heart rate, lifting weights safely, and planning exercises for body tone and flexibility.

- **Expectations** include what a person expects as a result of modifying behavior. This is usually referred to as the positive value of the desired behavior. For Hector's program, this would include expectations of improved physical appearance, becoming more physically fit, having more energy, and being more disciplined. These expected outcomes must counter the pleasures that come from poor choices such as eating foods that taste good but are unhealthy, or avoiding the pain of exercise by not exercising. This is especially true early in a program before a person experiences results or the value of his or her predetermined expectations. Personal goals that are accomplished become rewards and are considered pleasurable. In attempting to help participants identify their expectations, Hector, in the beginning, asked them to list their expectations as a result of losing weight and becoming more fit. These could then be developed into their personal goals.

- **Reinforcement** is the response to a person's behavior that will increase the continuance of the behavior. Positive reinforcement would be experienced in how individuals feel about the way they look and feel. The reinforcement of their expectations motivates them to continue with the program. External reinforcement methods used by Hector were praise, before-and-after photos, and rewards.

- **Self-efficacy** can be defined as believing that one has the ability to take action and persist.

COMMUNITY CONNECTIONS 1.5

Frustrated with the failure of individuals who signed up for their healthy eating and exercise program to change, Hector considered talking with a health psychologist who specialized in behavior change. Hector had previously met Dr. Hill, a nationally respected health education consultant, who specializes in counseling clients with undesirable health behaviors. Hector decided to call him and see if he could help him out. After a brief video conference with Dr. Hill, Hector was enlightened regarding the potential of applying Social Cognitive Theory to his attempt to help participants with healthy eating and exercise behaviors. Dr. Hill had warned him though, "Changing behavior is not easy because everyone comes from different environments and experiences. If, however, you apply program objectives and methods to theory, you will have a better chance of success."

Accomplishing obtainable goals establishes a person's degree of efficacy. People who fail to accomplish predetermined goals become part of the history of failed attempts, causing self-defeating behavior. Hector attempted to build efficacy by identifying and sharing personal strengths of the participants. Strengths such as perseverance, positive attitude, and a willingness to learn can go a long way in building self-efficacy.

- **Observational learning** includes the ability to learn by observing others. In so doing, a person can see success as well as failure, and the positive or negative effects of these results. In Hector's program, those who had been successful in both losing weight and maintaining weight loss provided personal testimonies, which Hector chose to use as positive examples for his participants. Leaders need to serve as role models so they do not cause participants to think, "I can't hear what you say because of what I see."

Diffusion of Innovation

Diffusion of Innovation (DOI) is a community-level change versus intrapersonal or interpersonal change, theory that provides a process for disseminating and implementing innovations. The word *diffusion* means to integrate, distribute, or spread widely. *Innovation* is something that is new or different. Applied to health education, DOI means integrating innovative ideas, products, or best practice programs into health education initiatives.

As new programs and materials are developed, innovative ideas and methods become available that improve the delivery of health education. Health education specialists need to keep abreast of new developments and apply them when appropriate. The question is how to select the best innovations and diffuse or integrate them into program implementation. Diffusion of Innovation incorporates established criteria for selecting innovations, which include the following:

- **Relative advantage** is the degree to which an innovation is seen as better than the idea, practice, program, or product it replaces.

- **Compatibility** refers to how consistent the innovation is with the values, habits, experiences, and needs of potential adopters.
- **Complexity** refers to how difficult the innovation is to understand or use.
- **Treatability** is the extent to which the innovation can be experimented with before a commitment to adopt it is required.
- **Observability** is the extent to which the innovation provides tangible or visible results.

---

⑦ DID YOU KNOW?

The tobacco industry has used Diffusion of Innovation Theory to promote flavored cigarettes to youth, as they attempt to stay ahead of public health practitioners by finding new tobacco users.

Data from Greenberg, M. R. (2006). The diffusion of public health innovations. *American Journal of Public Health, 96*(2), 209–210. http://doi.org/10.2105/AJPH.2005.078360

DOI also explains people's readiness to accept an innovation once they buy into it. Individuals accepting an innovation are known as *adopters* and can be characterized as follows[7]:

- **Innovators** are the first to adopt.
- **Early adopters** are interested, but do not want to be the first to adopt.
- **Early majority adopters** accept innovations once others they respect have done so.
- **Late majority adopters** include individuals who are skeptical and late to adopt.
- **Late adopters (laggards)** are the last to get involved, if they get involved at all.

Understanding the readiness of adopters is the key to selecting the best method for motivating individuals to subscribe to a new idea, product, or program. The early adopters and early and late majority, who combined are the largest group, will need to be convinced that the idea, product, or program would be to their advantage. It is up to the health education specialist to determine what methods and strategies can be used to communicate the innovation to the priority population, considering use of opinion leaders, media and social media channels, health communication campaigns, and other techniques described in this book.

COMMUNITY CONNECTIONS 1.6

One of Hector's initiatives for the year was to work with local public schools on a violence prevention program. This was the result of a needs assessment compiled by a county commission on violence that indicated a 35% increase in school violence over the past five years. The most common acts identified by the assessment were bullying, fighting, and threatening violence with intent to do harm.

Hector was committed to the task and looked forward to the challenge. The problem was where to start. Should he develop a violence prevention curriculum with teacher training or should he work with schools in developing school policy? To what extent should law enforcement agencies and the county prosecutor be involved? After using a program planning model and establishing goals and objectives, Hector thought a curriculum with teacher training was the best approach. When he approached Kara with his idea, she suggested he take a look at what evidence-based approaches already exist, as reinventing the wheel by developing new programs was not the best use of time and resources. Having had experience in disseminating the adoption of parent-child feeding policies among various WIC clinics in the state, she shared with Hector that the most cost-effective approach that had the greatest potential for success was based on a theory that provides guidance in taking different innovations and diffusing them into program needs.

Hector contacted state and national offices on violence prevention, reviewed curricula and school bullying programs, surveyed the literature, and talked to school administrators, law enforcement personnel, parents, and students. In addition, he took part in a webcast sponsored by the state Department of Education on violence and bullying prevention. Hector had gathered a great deal of information, but the problem was how to select a curriculum that would most likely be adopted by the schools within the county. Having identified bullying, fighting, and threatening violence as the problems to be addressed and establishing related goals and objectives, they had to determine what approach along with what methods and materials to use.

He chose the Diffusion of Innovation Theory to help them with this task. In so doing, he applied the five criteria designed to select the best innovation. In particular, he identified what the schools were presently doing (relative advantage), used a focus group to determine the innovation's compatibility with schools and its degree of difficulty to use (compatibility and complexity), and conducted a pilot test to determine extent of experimentation before it was adopted and to see if there were tangible results (treatability and observability). He next looked at the characteristics of adopters to determine what to expect from administrators regarding their readiness to adopt or buy into the program. He planned the marketing approach, selecting methods and strategies addressing each level of adopter.

▶ Conclusion

This chapter presented a brief introduction to concepts and theories applicable to community health education methods. Health education theory is still in a stage of development and borrows from already established behavior change theories. Health education specialists need to stay abreast of new theories as they evolve and how they tie into the selection of intervention methods. At the same time, health education specialists need to ensure the methods they are applying are relevant to the problems at hand and focus on impacting the priority population's key determinants of health from a social ecological rather than only an individual perspective.

Key Terms

Action Stage of readiness to change in which an individual is actively engaging in behavior change.
Behavioral capability The capability of an individual to change a behavior by having the knowledge and skills necessary to enact a desired behavior.

Compatibility How consistent an innovation is with the values, habits, experiences, and needs of potential adopters.
Complexity How difficult an innovation is to understand.

Contemplation Stage of readiness to change in which an individual may consider changing a behavior.

Early adopters Individuals interested in adopting an innovation but who do not want to be the first to do so.

Early majority adopters Individuals who accept innovations once others they respect have done so.

Expectation What is expected as a result of modifying a behavior.

Innovators The first individuals to adopt an innovation.

Late adopters (laggards) The last individuals to get involved, if at all, in adopting an innovation.

Late majority adopters Individuals who are skeptical and late to adopt an innovation.

Maintenance Stage of readiness to change in which an individual has been sustaining the behavior change over time.

Observability The extent to which the innovation provides tangible or visible results.

Observational learning The ability to learn by observing others.

Precontemplation Stage of readiness to change in which an individual is not interested in changing behavior.

Preparation Stage of readiness to change in which an individual is ready to change behavior but lacks the self-efficacy to do so.

Reciprocal determinism The theory that behavior changes are determined by interactions between a person and his or her environment.

Reinforcement The response to an individual's behavior that will increase the continuance of the behavior.

Relapse Regressing to a previous stage of readiness to change.

Relative advantage The degree to which an innovation is seen as better than the idea, practice, program, or product it replaces.

Self-efficacy Believing that one has the ability to take action.

Theory Knowledge, assumptions, or a set of rules or principles for the study or practice of a discipline.

Treatability The extent to which an innovation can be experimented with before a commitment to adopt it is required.

References

1. McLeroy, K. R., Steckler, A., & Bibeau, D. (Eds.) (1988). The social ecology of health promotion interventions. *Health Education Quarterly, 15*(4), 351–377.

2. Cottrell, R., Girvan, J., & McKenzie, J. (2002). *Principles and foundations of health promotion and education* (2nd ed.). San Francisco, CA: Benjamin Cummings.

3. Rosenstock, I. M. (1966). Why people use health services? *Milbank Memorial Fund Quarterly, 44*, 94–124.

4. Ajzen, I. (1988). *Attitudes, personality, and behavior.* Chicago, IL: Dorsey Press.

5. Prochaska, J. O. (1979). *Systems of psychotherapy: A transtheoretical process.* Homewood, IL: Dorsey Press.

6. Bandura, A. (1977). *Social learning theory.* Englewood Cliffs, NJ: Prentice-Hall.

7. Rogers, E. M. (1983). *Diffusion of innovation* (3rd ed.). New York, NY: Free Press.

Additional Resources

Print

National Commission for Health Education Credentialing, Inc. (NCHEC), & Society for Public Health Education (SOPHE). (2015). *A Competency-Based Framework for Health Education Specialists-2015.* Whitehall, PA: National Commission for Health Education Credentialing, Inc. (NCHEC) and Society for Public Health Education (SOPHE).

CHAPTER 2

Becoming a Health Education Professional

M. Elaine Auld, MPH, MCHES
Kathleen J. Young, PhD, MPH
Mike Perko, PhD, MCHES

▶ Author Comments

This chapter is about becoming a health education professional. What does it mean to be a professional entering the workforce? When does it begin? Does the art and practice of professionalism ever end? This chapter provides the new and seasoned health education specialist with concepts and building blocks of professionalism. The authors are health education academics and practitioners who have (collectively) spent some 80 years honing the craft of professionalism both within their personal careers and as mentors for students and interns. We hope this chapter helps those entering the field of health education, as well as those with an established community health education career, plan and advance their lifelong journey as a health education professional.

⌕ CHES COMPETENCIES

7.4.1	Explain the major responsibilities of the health education specialist.
7.4.2	Explain the role of professional organizations in advancing g the profession.
7.4.3	Explain the benefits of participating in professional organizations.
7.4.4	Advocate for professional development of health education specialists.
7.4.5	Advocate for the profession.
7.4.7	Explain the role of credentialing (for example, individual, program) in the promotion of the profession.
7.4.8	Develop and implement a professional development plan.
7.4.9	Serve as a mentor to others in the profession.*
7.4.11	Engage in service to advance the profession.*

*Advanced level competency

▶ Introduction

This chapter defines and introduces professionalism as a fundamental concept for the health education specialist. It also addresses important questions about professionalism such as: Does one simply become a professional on the day after walking across the stage, diploma in hand? Can professionalism be taught or is it a gradual transformation on the job? How has health education professionalism been shaped by historical events? And, how are contemporary trends such as technology, global interconnectedness, and the recognition of social determinants influencing today's views of health education professionalism? This chapter also addresses how the health education profession helps guide its members to uphold professionalism through established standards and benchmarks and strategies for enhancing professionalism throughout one's career.

Defining Professionalism

Being a professional can be defined simply as upholding the standards and conduct expected of one who has been trained in a profession. The concept of professionalism, however, is more intricate and complex. Professionalism can be defined as professional character, spirit, or methods and the standing, practice, or methods of a professional, as distinguished from an amateur.[1] In addition, a profession has three features: (1) training that was intellectual and involved knowledge, as distinguished from skill; (2) work that was pursued primarily for others and not for oneself; and (3) success that was measured by more than the amount of financial return.[2]

The emergence of professions and the beginning of professionalism in the Anglo-American and European systems of professions occurred roughly in the 16th century, when society saw value in the practice of theology, law, medicine, and university teaching.[3] Professionalism as a systematic area of inquiry has been researched in diverse fields such as architecture, engineering, computer science, law, and the medical and allied health professions. The practice of professionalism also can vary by region, ethnicity, culture, and time period, and is closely related to ethics and boundaries.[3]

The medical profession is among the most studied field in terms of defining and operationalizing professionalism, and illustrates how principles of professionalism change over time. The Hippocratic Oath to "put the patient at the focus of practice" and to "do no wrong" has guided physicians' professional conduct for some 2,500 years. Sir William Osler, often referred to as the father of modern medicine, summarized professionalism in medicine as "an art, not a trade; a calling, not a business; a calling in which your heart will be exercised equally with your head."[4] Yet, at the turn of the current century, changes in healthcare delivery, increasing public expectations, corporate involvement, and the digital revolution led to the Medical Professionalism Project. Its resulting publication, *The Charter on Medical Professionalism*, ushered in medical professionalism standards for the 21st century.[5] Focusing on new medical and healthcare challenges in virtually all cultures and societies, this project highlighted three fundamental principles, which also are relevant to health education: principle of primacy of patient welfare; principle of patient autonomy; and principle of social justice.[5]

Throughout the years, extensive research has taken place to assess the meaning of professionalism.[3] From this vast body of work, however, terms have emerged that best represent the culture of professionalism and what it means to be a professional: altruism, accountability, advocacy, duty, ethical and moral standards, excellence, honor, integrity, respect, and service, to name a few.[6]

A Historical Look at Professionalism in Health Education

Although health education professionalism has not yet been defined, an overarching concept in the field of community and public health education is the professional edict to promote and safeguard the health of all people. Many aspects of human potential such as employment, social relationships, and political participation are contingent on health, making it a public good.[7] Health equity and social justice too are underlying values of the health education profession. So creating the conditions for people to be healthy should be a goal of health education professionalism.

Mayhew Derryberry was among the health education pioneers to advance professionalism in health education. In 1941, he was named the first chief of health education in the U.S. Public Health Service and engaged behavioral and social scientists in studying public health problems. In addition, he was elected the second president of the Society for Public Health Education (SOPHE)

in 1951. Derryberry valued principles of autonomy in health behavior and also recognized the influences of society on health. In terms of demonstrating professionalism, he has been cited as doing "more to develop and enhance the profession of public health education than any other single individual" and a person "with unflagging courage, vision, and leadership who made a profound difference in the history of public health."[8]

In more contemporary times, David Birch, president of SOPHE from 2016 to 2017, added his philosophy of health education professionalism. In addition to equity and respect, he cited passion, caring, and lifelong learning as characteristics of a true health education professional.[9] **TABLE 2.1** further highlights characteristics of a health education professional.

TABLE 2.1 Qualities That Bring Professionalism to Health Education

- *Be passionate for what you do.* Love what you do and believe in the importance and impact of your work if it is done with passion (it should be much more than a job).
- *Caring.* Genuinely care for the well-being of the individuals you work with—your colleagues, students, program participants, and so on.
- *Respect.* Treat others with respect—you might be older, more experienced, or more informed, but all should be equal in terms of respect.
- *Lifelong learning.* Realize that to be the "best you can be," you need to continue to learn about life and all those things that are important to your profession.
- *Honesty and transparency.* Little should be done in private (though at times there is a need for privacy).
- *Dependability.* If you make a commitment, follow through to the best of your ability. If you cannot uphold your duties, be honest and transparent about your inability to follow through.

Source: Birch, D. A. (2017). Qualities that bring professionalism to health education (personal communication, June 7, 2017).

Ethics in Health Education Professionalism

As cited earlier in this chapter, ethics and moral standards undergird the practice of every profession. The study of ethics or moral philosophy enables professionals to make personal and expert decisions based on basic principles that reflect the values and morals of a society and a chosen profession. The body of ethics typically centers on four principles:

- *Personal freedom or* **autonomy**. One should respect people's rights. People have the right to choose and act. Sometimes, freedom is overridden to prevent harm. When this occurs, it is called **paternalism**.
- *Avoiding harm or* **nonmaleficence**. One should not inflict harm on others.
- *Doing good or* **beneficence**. One should help others or, at the least, remove harm.
- **Justice**. One should treat others equally and fairly.

In addition, **professional accountability**—being accountable to oneself, clients, participants, employer, the profession, and society—has been generally considered as an essential ethical principle.

The Code of Ethics for the Health Education Profession reflects these basic principles and precepts for health education specialists' behavior; these also are reflected in the Health Education Specialist Practice Analysis (HESPA) 2015 Competencies and Sub-Competencies.[10,11] The preamble to the Code of Ethics for the Health Education Profession states:

> The Code of Ethics provides a framework of shared values within which health education is practiced. The Code of Ethics is grounded in fundamental ethical principles that underlie all health care services: respect for autonomy, promotion of social justice, active promotion of good, and avoidance of harm. . . . Regardless of job title, professional affiliation, work setting, or population served, health educators abide by these guidelines when making professional decisions.[10]

TABLE 2.2 provides further insight into the Health Education Code of Ethics and how these ethical standards intersect with the HESPA 2015 competencies.

Why are ethics important in health education? Health education specialists are in the position of helping or possibly harming others by the various methods and strategies used to influence their behaviors. Health education interventions influence people's decisions regarding their health and the health of their families, organizations, and communities. Thus, health education professionals must fulfill their responsibilities and apply their knowledge and skills ethically at all times.

As with all professions, however, it is not unusual for a conflict to exist between knowing what is ethical and behaving ethically. In health education, ethical dilemmas are a part of the job. Some controversial, intensely debated topics include school-based (K–12) sexuality education, reproductive rights, community fluoridation, genetically modified foods, and access to universal health care. When faced with decisions, some professionals may choose a less than optimal path because doing what may be considered correct could result in ridicule or termination of employment. These unpleasant consequences can overpower decision-making in favor of the ethical choice. Health educators who act unethically not only harm individuals but also damage their own professional reputation and integrity.

The critical connection between knowing what is ethical and behaving ethically is **character** or **virtue**. Character is based on personal traits such as loyalty, kindness, integrity, self-esteem, self-efficacy, and discipline. These traits provide courage and strength to "walk the talk" of ethical practice. Professional character, guided by the code of ethics and health education competencies, enable health education specialists to conduct themselves in an honorable and professional way. By so doing, professional standards are upheld as well as each person's integrity and respect.

TABLE 2.2 The Health Education Code of Ethics and HESPA 2015 Competencies

Health Education Code of Ethics	HESPA 2015 Competencies and Sub-Competencies (* Advanced level competency)
Article I: Responsibility to the Public A Health Educator's responsibilities are to educate, promote, maintain, and improve the health of individuals, families, groups, and communities. When a conflict of issues arises among individuals, groups, organizations, agencies, or institutions, health educators must consider all issues and give priority to those that promote the health and well-being of individuals and the public while respecting both the principles of individual autonomy, human rights, and equality.	*1.1.5* Apply ethical principles to the assessment process.* *2.3.11* Apply ethical principles in selecting strategies and designing interventions. *3.4.8* Monitor adherence to ethical principles in the implementation of health education/promotion.
Article II: Responsibility to the Profession Health Educators are responsible for their professional behavior, for the reputation of their profession, and for promoting ethical conduct among their colleagues.	*5.5.10* Adhere to ethical principles of the profession. *6.3.5* Apply ethical principles in consultative relationships.*
Article III: Responsibility to Employers Health Educators recognize the boundaries of their professional competence and are accountable for their professional activities and actions.	*5.1.13* Apply ethical principles when managing financial resources.* *5.2.2* Apply ethical principles in managing technology resources. *5.6.14* Apply ethical principles when managing human resources.*
Article IV: Responsibility in the Delivery of Health Education Health Educators deliver health education with integrity. They respect the rights, dignity, confidentiality, and worth of all people by adapting strategies and methods to the needs of diverse populations and communities.	*3.1.5* Apply ethical principles to the implementation process. *3.4.8* Monitor adherence to ethical principles in the implementation of health education/promotion.
Article V: Responsibility in Research and Evaluation Health Educators contribute to the health of the population and to the profession through research and evaluation activities. When planning and conducting research or evaluation, health educators do so in accordance with federal and state laws and regulations, organizational and institutional policies, and professional standards.	*4.1.10* Apply ethical principles to the evaluation process.* *4.2.14* Apply ethical principles to the research process.*
Article VI: Responsibility in Professional Preparation Those involved in the preparation and training of Health Educators have an obligation to accord benefits to the profession and the public.	*5.5.10* Adhere to ethical principles of the profession. *6.3.5* Apply ethical principles in consultative relationships.*

Reproduced from *A Competency-Based Framework for Health Education Specialists—2015*. Whitehall, PA: National Commission for Health Education Credentialing, Inc. (NCHEC) and Society for Public Health Education (SOPHE). Reprinted by permission of the National Commission for Health Education Credentialing, Inc. (NCHEC) and Society for Public Health Education (SOPHE).

Health Equity in Health Education Professionalism

Pursuing health equity is a central responsibility of all health education professionals. Despite many historical landmark reports and research, pervasive health inequities still exist among many vulnerable populations. In 1966, health education luminary Dorothy Nyswander provided a roadmap for health equity in her treatise on the Open Society. She characterized the Open Society as:

> One where justice is the same for every [person]; where dissent is taken seriously as an index of something wrong or something needed; where diversity is expected; . . . where the best of health care is available to all; where poverty is a community disgrace not an individual's weakness; [and] where desires for power over [people] become satisfaction with the use of power for people.[12]

Some 20 years later, U.S. Department of Health and Human Services Secretary Margaret Heckler's *Task Force Report on Black and Minority Health* (1985) provided a wake-up call to America with regard to pervasive health disparities among racial and ethnic minorities.[13] The report recommended sweeping changes in research, policies, programs, and legislation to advance health equity at the national, state, tribal, territorial, and local levels, because African Americans, Hispanic Americans, Native Americans, Asian Americans, and Native Hawaiians/Other Pacific Islanders were shown to have shorter life expectancies and higher rates of diabetes, cancer, heart disease, stroke, substance abuse, infant mortality, and low birth weight than non-Hispanic whites. Unfortunately, a follow-up report in 2002 by the National Academies of Medicine (*Unequal Treatment: Confronting Racial and Ethnic Disparities in Health Care*) showed little progress had been made in eliminating health disparities.[14] Racial and ethnic minorities were found to be less likely to receive even routine medical procedures and were provided a lower quality of health services than white Americans. For example, minorities were less likely than white populations to undergo lifesaving cardiac bypass surgeries or receive kidney dialysis treatment.[14]

While the latter report focused on health inequities in healthcare delivery, national and international researchers also began to document the impact of the broader social environment on health and health disparities. They reported that individuals' decisions about health behaviors were influenced by historic disadvantage and inequality conferred on the basis of race, ethnicity, and socioeconomic status and the social environment in which they are born, work, and play.[15] Even in high-income countries, differences of almost 20 years in life expectancy were evident depending on the collective influences of economics, housing, health care, transportation, and education. For example, one's opportunities for a healthy lifestyle are severely limited if there is no affordable low-income housing, no transportation infrastructure that allows individuals to pursue employment outside of their neighborhood, no supermarkets in the neighborhood with fresh produce, no safe parks in which to play or exercise, or no neighborhood schools that provide a quality education.

To promote health equity, today's health education specialists are called to help change policies, systems and environments to help make the healthy choice the easy choice. They must advocate for vulnerable populations so the right to "life, liberty, the pursuit of happiness"—and health—are available to all. Each individual, regardless of age, gender, race, ethnicity, sexual orientation, gender identity, or socioeconomic status should have access to high-quality health care, free from stigma and discrimination.[16]

▸ Steps for Building Professional Skills

If professionalism is indeed defined as professional character, spirit, or methods,[1] professionalism begins with one's involvement as a student and the ability to envision oneself as a practicing health education specialist. This might occur, for example, in the first core course in a professional preparation program or when declaring a major. Throughout a career, however, professionalism evolves; there is never any single event or time during which an individual can no longer learn or demonstrate health education competencies. The opportunities to progress as a health education professional are endless: developing and updating a health education philosophy statement and portfolio; participating as a mentor or protégé; contributing to a national or local health education professional organization; earning and maintaining certification in health education; advocating for policy change to an elected official; contributing new knowledge to the field by presenting at a health conference or submitting a manuscript for publication; and participating in service learning or volunteering.

---

⑦ DID YOU KNOW?

Everything you do reflects your professionalism. Your attire, social media pictorial and written remarks, public choice of words, advocacy for vulnerable populations, and blog all reflect on you and your image in the profession. Commit now to make these works and actions reflect the values of your chosen health education profession.

Develop a Health Education Philosophy and Portfolio

An important step in becoming a health education professional is developing a personal philosophy statement. The word philosophy roughly translates to "love of wisdom." In his 2005 SOPHE presidential address, Stephen Gambescia posed the following questions to help health education professionals develop their own philosophy (or mission, as some professionals prefer to call it) statement:[17]

- Who are we?
- What areas of the human condition do we choose to affect?
- Why do we do the things we do and the way we do them?
- What difference is it making?

Gambescia also posed three themes for consistent reflection that encourage professionalism:

- How do I know what I know?
- What should I do? How should I behave?
- How do I interact with others?

Answering these questions requires deep reflection, but is an important part of professionalism. A sample health education philosophy statement is provided in **FIGURE 2.1**. Both new and seasoned

---

COMMUNITY CONNECTIONS 2.1

Sureka is a recent community health education graduate of Springville University, who was hired by the Springville Department of Public Health to develop a health literacy campaign aimed at mostly rural residents of Springville County. Sureka earned excellent grades in her community health education classes, and was on point with her interview. She learned, however, that grades were just part of her professional development. In order to get experience in the field, she joined her university's chapter of Eta Sigma Gamma (ESG). As an active member, she participated in many research, service, education and advocacy activities. It was hard work! Coupled with her desire to maintain good grades, she often found that balance was difficult to find. Since she was hired, she knew that active participation in her academic career was worth every minute. In her first week on the job, Sureka was given three tasks regarding the health literacy campaign: (1) gather information about health literacy that would best show how residents benefit from the health literacy campaign, (2) attend meetings with a group of rural physicians invested in preventive care in the area, and (3) present the information to a local foundation known for funding Springville causes. Challenging, but her coursework, previous instructors, and ESG projects would help her figure out the best strategies to meet these objectives.

My Health Education Philosophy

The World Health Organization's definition of health education is defined as "any combination of learning experiences designed to help individuals and communities improve their health by increasing their knowledge or influencing their attitudes." In my eyes, health education is looked at as a broad topic that covers many areas of health. My definition of health is to have a positive health status in all five categories of health: spiritual, mental, emotional, physical, and social. An individual's mind, body, and soul all balance each other out and influence whether an individual will reach optimal wellness.

My philosophy on health education is that health behaviors can only be influenced by the knowledge, attitudes, values, and beliefs that an individual holds. As a health educator, one must understand these things about an individual before attempting to change their health behaviors. For health educators to understand human health behaviors, they must be motivated, obtain high self-efficacy, be culturally competent, and require a set of health counseling skills. I believe these skills listed are the most important ones a health educator should possess. As a professional in health education, I live by the words: *be the change you wish to see in the world*.

FIGURE 2.1 Sample Health Education Philosophy Statement.

Reproduced from Bland, Brianna. My health education philosophy. Retrieved June 10, 2017 from www.slideshare.net/BriannaBland/health-education-philosophy

health education professionals should revisit their philosophy statements throughout their careers, as it will evolve with different experiences, professional interactions, new research, and societal events.[17, 18]

A philosophy statement should also be part of a health educator's career **portfolio**. A career portfolio is a compilation of examples of one's work in academic and nonacademic settings. In addition to a current **resume**, the portfolio should include various items that demonstrate competencies in particular subject areas and samples of work created in the health education setting. A portfolio may be in a hard copy or electronic version. The main purpose of a professional portfolio is to be able to display a selection of work that demonstrates competency in different areas of health education. **TABLE 2.3** lists common components of a professional portfolio.

⑦ DID YOU KNOW?

Spelling and grammar errors are the most common mistakes on a resume and cover letter. As simple as this seems, these errors may tell a potential employer that you lack attention to detail. Take the time to proofread, or better yet, have someone else read your materials for clarity and any potential grammatical errors.

Participate in the Mentoring Process

One of the most satisfying and traditional ways in which young professionals begin learning about professionalism is to identify a mentor.[19] A

TABLE 2.3 Examples of a Health Educator's Portfolio Items

- Table of contents
- Letter of application or recommendation
- Resume
- Unofficial transcripts
- Philosophy statements
- Work and school example items such as a health brochure designed, 3–5-minute teaching or training video, training manuals developed, teaching lectures, research conducted (data loading and analysis), and much more
- Work performance appraisals and/or recommendations
- Photographs of work projects or "works in progress"
- Scholarships, honors, and awards
- Volunteer or elected leadership positions and professional memberships
- Types of certifications (e.g., CPR, CHES)

mentor may simultaneously serve as an advisor, coach, counselor, role model, and supporter. It is not too early during undergraduate studies, or even during a health education internship or clerkship, to identify a mentor and to seek such guidance throughout professional life. Some universities and professional associations have formal mentoring programs, which can be excellent places to start.

Whether the relationship is formal or informal, face-to-face or online, the best mentor and protégé relationships all share the same qualities: respect for each other, a shared vision to reach a common goal, trust, opportunities for reciprocal enlightenment and growth, and two-way listening and reflection.[19, 20] It should be expected that good health education mentors regularly meet with their protégés to impart wisdom, advice, and inspiration; provide constructive and timely feedback; help clarify career and research goals; provide challenges toward establishing independence; and use their established stature and experience to help the protégé develop a professional network. For the protégé, involvement with a professional mentor does not connote incompetence, but rather the conscientious commitment and aspiration for excellence in one's career. The mentor can become a lifelong friend and colleague, and model the way for the protégé to one-day mentor other young health education professionals.

Mentors have as much to gain from these relationships as their protégés.[19] The one-on-one exchange creates opportunities for senior professionals to reevaluate their progression, reflect on their philosophy of health education, and live up to the commitment of lifelong learning. It also can be personally rewarding to "pay it back" and feel pride in helping the next generation of health education professionals advance on their journey.[19,20]

In summary, mentoring is a well-established method of advancing professionalism and lifelong growth in health education. Benefits accrue to both the mentor and protégé throughout their careers and advance workforce development.

Participate in a Health Education Membership Association

Becoming a member of a health education organization introduces both the new and the seasoned professional to the values of being invested in the profession.[21,22] Although specific benefits in a membership society vary from group to group, they generally include receiving professional journals publishing the latest research, methods, best practices, and processes of health education; providing discounts for conference registration, publications, or continuing education fees; accessing distance education; receiving policy advocacy alerts and training; accessing job or internship opportunities; and networking with others who can help shape and support professional growth.[22]

Additionally, a national organization serves as an overarching representative, spokesperson, and advocate for the discipline. For example, SOPHE's leadership led to the first standard occupational definition of "health educator" by the U.S. Department of Labor in 2000[23]; Certified Health Education Specialist (CHES) credential being recognized as eligible for reimbursement as part of diabetes or asthma clinical teams; and health education being included as a core subject in the Every Student Achieves Act.

TABLE 2.4 lists several national and global health education organizations health education specialists might consider joining. Many of these organizations have state, regional, or campus chapters that provide continuing education and networking events; advertise internships or jobs; and provide awards and scholarships. Students and new professionals often are eligible for reduced membership fees, as their involvement is considered the future lifeblood of the profession.

Beyond joining a health education organization, health education professionals will benefit from volunteering and actively participating in achieving the organization's strategic plan. Examples of volunteer opportunities include serving on committees, reviewing abstracts or manuscripts for publication, planning annual conferences, moderating online forums, and evaluating applicants for awards or scholarships.[21] Following

TABLE 2.4 Selected Health Education Membership Organizations

Organization	Mission	Website
American Public Health Association, Public Health Education & Health Promotion Section (APHA, PHE&HP)	The mission of the APHA, PHE&HP Section is: 1. To be a strong advocate for health education and health promotion for individuals, groups, and communities, and systems and support efforts to achieve health equity in all activities of the association. 2. To set, maintain, and exemplify the highest ethical principles and standards of practice on the part of all professionals and disciplines whose primary purpose is health education, disease prevention, and/or health promotion.	http://www.apha.org/apha-communities/member-sections/public-health-education-and-health-promotion
American School Health Association (ASHA)	The mission of the ASHA is to transform all schools into places where every student learns and thrives. The ASHA envisions healthy students who learn and achieve in safe and healthy environments nurtured by caring adults functioning within coordinated school and community support systems.	http://www.ashaweb.org/
Eta Sigma Gamma (ESG)	Founded in 1967, the mission of ESG is to promote the discipline by elevating the stands, ideas, competence, and ethics of professionally prepared man and women in health education.	http://etasigmagamma.org
International Union for Health Promotion & Education (IUHPE)	The IUHPE's mission is to promote global health and well-being and to contribute to the achievement of equity in health between and within countries of the world. The IUHPE fulfills its mission by building and operating an independent, global, and professional network of people and institutions to encourage free exchange of ideas, knowledge, know-how, experiences, and the development of relevant collaborative projects, both at global and regional levels.	http://www.iuhpe.org
Society for Public Health Education (SOPHE)	Founded in 1950, the mission of the SOPHE is to provide global leadership to the profession of health education and health promotion and to promote the health of society. SOPHE is the only independent professional organization devoted to health education and health promotion.	http://www.sophe.org

initial service, health education volunteers may be eligible to run for office and directly shape the future of their professional home. As an added bonus, many employers view professional service favorably in hiring decisions.

Become a Certified Health Education Specialist

Health education was the first population-based profession to articulate areas of responsibility and competencies needed for professional practice.[24] This set of knowledge and skills was published in the 1985 landmark report *Framework for the Development of Competency-Based Curricula for Entry Level Health Educators.*[25] During the last several decades, three research studies have been conducted to update the knowledge and skills needed for contemporary health education practice.[26] Although the competencies have been modified slightly over the years, the seven overarching responsibilities of a health education specialist still remain the basis for both preservice and in-service programs in health education. Health education specialists interested in working internationally may also find it helpful to review the eight domains of core competencies required to engage in effective health promotion practice: catalyzing change, leadership, assessment, planning, implementation, evaluation, advocacy, and partnerships.[27] **TABLE 2.5** lists the current responsibilities of health education specialists.

The first U.S. health education competencies also led the way for establishing a voluntary certification system in health education to ensure a high level of competence in the health education

TABLE 2.5 Seven Areas of Responsibility for Health Education Specialists	
Area I:	Assess Needs, Resources, and Capacity for Health Education/Promotion
Area II:	Plan Health Education/Promotion
Area III:	Implement Health Education/Promotion
Area IV:	Conduct Evaluation and Research Related to Health Education/Promotion
Area V:	Administer and Manage Health Education/Promotion
Area VI:	Serve as a Health Education/Promotion Resource Person
Area VII:	Communicate, Promote, and Advocate for Health, Health Education/Promotion, and the Profession

Reproduced from *A Competency-Based Framework for Health Education Specialists—2015.* Whitehall, PA: National Commission for Health Education Credentialing, Inc. (NCHEC) and Society for Public Health Education (SOPHE). Reprinted by permission of the National Commission for Health Education Credentialing, Inc. (NCHEC) and Society for Public Health Education (SOPHE).

workforce. The National Commission for Health Education Credentialing, Inc. (NCHEC) was launched in 1988. CHES recognition is available through NCHEC for those health educators who wish to show they have proficiency in the *Seven Areas of Responsibility for Health Education Specialists* and pass a national examination. The CHES exam is open to new or seasoned health education professionals who possess a bachelor's, master's, or doctoral degree from an accredited institution of higher education; AND one of the following:

■ An official transcript (including course titles) that clearly shows a major in health education (e.g., health education, community health education, public health education, school health education). Degree/major must explicitly be in a discipline of health education.

OR

■ An official transcript that reflects at least 25 semester hours or 27 quarter hours of coursework (with a grade C or better) with specific preparation addressing the *Seven Areas of Responsibility and Competency for Health Education Specialists.*[28]

COMMUNITY CONNECTIONS 2.2

In an effort to develop her health literacy knowledge, Sureka spent much of her time at work on her computer searching for information about health literacy. She knew this research would help give her a sense of the overall picture of health literacy that would later come in handy when she interacted with her priority population. She joined a health education member organization that had a Special Interest Group devoted to health literacy, in order to interact and collaborate with other professionals who had more experience. This way, she could further assess best practices regarding health literacy and her community in Springville. She also got on the agenda for the rural physicians group because these doctors worked with her population on a consistent basis. Thank goodness for good coworkers—they provided advice when needed and took her to lunch a few times to give her breaks from her focused work.

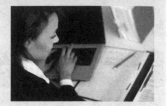
© Kzenon/Shutterstock.

In 2011, NCHEC introduced the Master Certified Health Education Specialist (MCHES), which is based on both academic requirements with courses in health education; at least five years of work experience as a health education specialist; and successfully passing a comprehensive examination based on the latest advanced-level competencies and sub-competencies verified in the most recent health education job analysis.[29] To maintain the designation of CHES or MCHES, an annual recertification fee must be paid and at least 75 hours of continuing education must be completed every five years, according to NCHEC guidelines. Beginning in fall 2018, computer-based testing will be available, enabling eligible individuals to select their test day and time, and get test results immediately after taking the exam.

Why be certified in health education? Health education certification demonstrates a health education specialist's unique knowledge and skills in the health education profession and distinguishes those who are certified from other job applicants. Some employers require CHES or provide preference to CHES/MCHES in hiring decisions. The certification also attests to a health education professional's commitment to continuing education and conveys a sense of pride and accomplishment in the profession.

⑦ DID YOU KNOW?

Both the CHES and the MCHES are fully accredited by the National Commission for Certifying Agencies (NCCA). The CHES and MCHES credentials of the NCHEC, Inc. are "recognized for demonstrating compliance with the NCCA Standards for the Accreditation of Certification Programs."

Advocate Health Education

Advocacy for health, health education/promotion, and the profession is among the *Seven Areas of Responsibility* of all health education professionals. An **advocate** is someone who defends or pleads the cause of another person or group or a specific proposal. Much of the work of today's health education specialist involves advocating for changes in policies or systems that affect the health of vulnerable and priority populations. Health education specialists must use their expertise and experience to promote national, state, or local legislation, regulations, and other policy decisions to support the public's health.

Health education specialists can advocate in many ways: writing letters, sending emails, or providing testimony to elected or appointed policymakers, including school board or local board of health officials; submitting a letter to the editor or op-ed of a local newspaper; developing a resolution or policy statement for an organization; signing up to receive action alerts on important public health issues and alerting others via social media; or organizing or marching in a peaceful demonstration to show support for an advocacy issue. Each fall, SOPHE sponsors an Annual Health Education Advocacy Summit in Washing-ton, D.C. to provide policy advocacy education and skill building for health professionals. The event culminates in opportunities for participants to meet with their elected officials.

In addition to enhancing political and social engagement for important issues affecting the public's health, advocacy improves civic development, communication, and leadership skills, and connections with other experts from whom one can learn and grow. Creating social change for the betterment of society and humanity at large is one of the most important ways to personally and professionally grow.

COMMUNITY CONNECTIONS 2.3

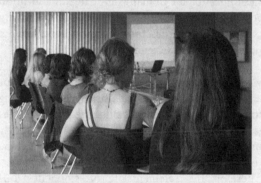

© Marc Dietrich/Shutterstock.

Sureka worked long hours and eventually pulled together all she could on health literacy and rural populations. When it came time to present her findings to the local foundation, she was punctual, professionally dressed, and prepared. She presented to the foundation board about how health literacy impacted the specific needs of the rural residents of Springville. She stated that other programs were very successful and would most likely work in the community with the modifications made based on the rural physicians group input. When Sureka was asked if she had been out in the rural areas of Springville, she replied she had spent time with leaders in the community who ensured the campaign's objectives were feasible and culturally appropriate. After all questions had been answered, Sureka was excused. She felt confident she would receive the funding based on her preparedness throughout the process.

Share Health Education Research and Practice

Still another important facet of professionalism that is specified in the *Seven Areas of Responsibility of Health Education Specialists* is contributing to the knowledge base of the field. Health education professionals can share the qualitative and quantitative results of health education interventions and evaluations with peers at national, state, or local conferences or in professional journals. Following a scientific approach to asking questions, carefully gathering and examining the evidence, and presenting the findings is vital to expanding the theoretical and evidence base of the health education profession. Most professional organizations that sponsor an annual meeting begin the conference planning process by issuing a call for abstracts. Formats can vary in terms of being accepted to present a poster, oral presentation, workshop, roundtable, or other type of sharing knowledge session. Meeting presentations also are excellent opportunities for students and young professionals to share their research or theses/dissertation papers.

Conference presentations or theses/dissertations also can serve as the basis for scientific publications. In addition to many professional health education journals, numerous specialty journals exist in fields such as HIV/AIDS, mental health, obesity, nutrition education, and adolescent health, to name a few. Journal specifications vary, including some that require author fees, so it is important to carefully consult the guidelines before beginning authorship. Serving as a journal peer reviewer is another opportunity to learn how to prepare and communicate health education findings.

Volunteer and Participate in Service Learning

In addition to volunteering in professional organizations, local community groups provide top-notch opportunities for new and seasoned health educators. By volunteering time and skills, the notion of professionalism is reinforced; that is, being a professional is not only about looking the part, but also about actually doing the job. All professionals have a social responsibility to the community in which they live.

Local organizations that welcome and rely on volunteers include, for example, the American Heart Association, American Cancer Society, and American Red Cross as well as many other nonprofit organizations, neighborhood councils, schools, and religious organizations. Ways to get involved can include organizing or participating in fundraising walks such as the American Foundation for Suicide Prevention's Out of the Darkness walks; organizing health fairs; serving in soup kitchens; assisting at domestic shelters; and participating in environmental cleanup campaigns. Such volunteerism is not driven by financial rewards but from one's own sense of purpose and motivation, and the desire to make a difference in the community and the lives of fellow citizens.

A central tenet of the health education profession involving service learning is emphasis on co-participatory collaboration. **Service learning** can be thought as a collaborative partnership between an institution and the community it serves.[30] The primary goal of service learning is to provide community member(s) with services that (in turn) create hands-on learning experiences for the volunteer.[29] Elements of service learning practice that aid health education specialists in professional development include problem-solving skills, teamwork, and research and training proficiencies.[30, 31] Service learning activities also

COMMUNITY CONNECTIONS 2.4

In looking back at her work behavior, Sureka could see her efforts had paid off, much like they did when she was a student. She showed up to her job on time, worked hard, dressed the part, and was pleasant. These were all very important attributes of being a professional, but she also learned that professionalism is much greater than looking the part; it is about following through using the competencies of the health education profession.

provide students and volunteers with opportunities to participate in many of the health education competencies in community settings, including community needs assessment, program planning development, and community health advocacy.[30]

Service learning has a broader effect, in that while the health education specialist develops a sense of professional identity, service learning involvement also provides all participating parties (i.e., student, supervising faculty, and community member) with a chance to independently reshape the direction of their professional practice.[30] Therefore, these elements of professional development become central to each member involved in the learning experience.[30, 31]

▶ Conclusion

One of the most significant benefits of taking an active role in one's professional growth is the opportunity to establish oneself as a community health education professional. Although professionalism is on a constant participatory continuum, it can be a positive endeavor with the assistance of other professionals who are committed to the excellence of the health education profession. Regardless of one's level of experience as a community health educator, there are many diverse professional building blocks for growth in professionalism, whether beginning the process (as a newcomer) or in continuing to refine one's practice as a seasoned careerist in the field of community and public health education.

Key Terms

Advocate A person, or entity, who publicly supports or recommends a particular cause or policy.

Autonomy Independence or freedom, as of the will or one's actions.

Beneficence The doing of good; active goodness or kindness; charity.

Character The mental and moral qualities distinctive to an individual.

Justice The quality of being just; righteousness, equitableness, or moral rightness.

Nonmaleficence The ethical principle of doing no harm.

Mentor A wise and trusted counselor or teacher.

Paternalism The attitude or policy of a government or other authority that manages the affairs of a country, company, community, and so on, in the manner of a father, for example, by usurping individual responsibility and the liberty of choice.

Portfolio A compilation of various pieces of one's best work in both academic and nonacademic settings.

Professional accountability Being accountable to oneself, clients, participants, employer, the profession, and society.

Resume Formal presentation of an individual's education, skills, and work experience.

Service learning A teaching and learning strategy that integrates meaningful community service with instruction and reflection to enrich the learning experience, teach civic responsibility, and strengthen communities.

Virtue Conformity of one's life and conduct to moral and ethical principles.

References

1. *Random House Webster's Unabridged Dictionary.* (2017). New York, NY: Random House Information Group. Retrieved June 11, 2017, from http://www.dictionary.com/browse/professionalism?s=t

2. Brandeis, L. D. (1922). *Business: A profession.* Boston, MA: Hole, Cushman, and Flint.

3. Lawson, W. D. (2004). Professionalism: The golden years. *Journal of Professional Issues in Engineering Education and Practice, 120*(1), 26–26. Retrieved June 28, 2017, from http://doi.org/10.1061/(ASCE)1052-3928(2004)130:1(26)#sthash.2VOXxvYK.dpuf

4. The Osler Symposia. *Sir William Osler & his inspirational words.* Retrieved June 25, 2017, from http://www.oslersymposia.org/about-Sir-William-Osler.html

5. Brennen, T. (2002). Medical professionalism in the new millennium: A physician charter. *Annals of Internal Medicine, 126,* 242–246.

6. University of Alabama School of Medicine. (2005). *Professionalism: By faculty and residents.* Retrieved August 1, 2017, from http://www.uab.edu/uasomume/ccadmin/general/proffac.htm

7. Institute of Medicine. (2003). *The future of the public's health in the 21st century* (p. 2). Washington, DC: The National Academies Press.

8. Allegrante, J. P., Sleet, D. A., & McGinnis, J. M. (2004). Mayhew Derryberry: Pioneer of health education. *American Journal of Public Health, 94*(2), 270–271.

9. Birch, D. A. (2017). Qualities that bring professionalism to health education. (personal communication, June 7, 2017).

10. Coalition of National Health Education Organizations. (2011). *Code of ethics for the health education profession.* Retrieved June 25, 2017, from http://www.cnheo.org/

11. National Commission for Health Education Credentialing, Inc. (2017). *Responsibilities and competencies for health education specialists.* Retrieved June 24, 2017, from http://www.nchec.org/responsibilities-and-competencies

12. Nyswander, D. B. (1982). The open society: Its implications for health educators. In *The SOPHE heritage collection of health education monographs* (Vol. 1, pp. 29–42). Oakland, CA: Third Party Publishing.

13. U.S. Department of Health and Human Services. (1985). *Report of the Secretary's task force on black and minority health.* Washington, DC: Author. Retrieved June 28, 2017, from http://archive.org/details/reportof secretar00usde

14. The National Academies of Sciences, Engineering, and Medicine. (2002). *Unequal treatment: Confronting racial and ethnic disparities in health care.* Washington, DC: Author. Retrieved June 29, 2017, from http://www .nationalacademies.org/hmd/Reports/2002 /Unequal-Treatment-Confronting-Racial -and-Ethnic-Disparities-in-Health-Care.aspx

15. World Health Organization. (2002). *The social determinants of health: The solid facts.* Retrieved June 28, 2017, from http://www .health-equity.lib.umd.edu/2812

16. Society for Public Health Education. (2016). *Resolution for achieving health equity.* Retrieved June 25, 2017, from http://sophe .ivygroup.com/wp-content/uploads/2017/01 /Resolution-to-Promote-Health-Equity.pdf

17. Gambescia, S. F. (2007). 2007 Presidential address: Developing a philosophy of health education. *Health Education and Behavior*, *24*(5).

18. Goltz, H. H., & Smith, M. L. (2015). Forming and developing your professional identity: Easy as PI. In *Health education tools of the trade 3* (pp. 138–143). Washington, DC: Society for Public Health Education.

19. Wagner. R. (2001). Why you'll want a mentor outside the ivory tower, too. *The Chronicle of Higher Education.* Retrieved June 25, 2017, from http://www.chronicle.com/article /why-youll-want-a-mentor/45513

20. Goldman, K. D., & Schmalz, K. (2005). Follow the leader: Mentoring. In *Health education tools of the trade* (pp. 138–143). Washington, DC: Society for Public Health Education.

21. Escoffery, C., Kenig, M., & Hyden, C. (2015). Getting the most out of professional associations. *Health Promotion Practice*, *16*(3), 309–312.

22. Young, K., & Boling, W. (2004). Improving the quality of professional life: Benefits of health education and promotion association membership. *California Journal of Health Promotion*, *2*(1), 29–44.

23. Bureau of Labor Statistics, U.S. Department of Labor, Occupational Outlook Handbook, 2014–2015 Edition, Health Educators and Community Health Workers. Retrieved June 25, 2017, from http://www.bls.gov/ooh /community-and-social-service/health -educators.htm

24. Livingood, W., & Auld, M. E. (2001). The credentialing of a population-based health profession: Lessons learned from health education certification. *Journal of Public Health Management and Practice*, *7*(4), 28–45.

25. Cottrell, R. R., Girvan, J. T., & McKenzie, J. F. (2005). *Principles and foundations of health promotion and education* (2nd ed.). San Francisco, CA: Pearson Benjamin Cummings.

26. McKenzie, J. F., Dennis, D., Auld, M. E., Lysoby, L., Doyle, E., Muenzen, P. M., … Kusorgbor-Narh, C. S. (2016). Health Education Specialist Practice Analysis 2015 (HESPA 2015): Process and outcomes. *Health Education and Behavior*, *42*(2), 286–295.

27. Allegrante, J. P., Barry, M. M., Airhihenbuwa, C. O., Auld, M. E., Collins, J. L., Lamarre M. C., … Mittelmark M. B. (2009). Domains of core competency, standards, and quality assurance for building global capacity in health promotion: The Galway Consensus Conference statement. Galway Consensus Conference. *Health Education and Behavior*, *26*(2), 476–482.

28. National Commission for Health Education Credentialing, Inc. (2017). *CHES exam eligibility.* Retrieved June 25, 2017, from http:// www.nchec.org/ches-exam-eligibility

29. National Commission for Health Education Credentialing, Inc. (2017). *MCHES exam eligibility.* Retrieved June 25, 2017, from http:// www.nchec.org/mches-exam-eligibility

30. Young, K., & Spear, C. (2005). Addressing health education responsibilities and competencies through service learning. *California Journal of Health Promotion, 2*(2), 17–22.

31. Clark, P. (1999). Service-learning education in community-academic partnerships: Implications for interdisciplinary geriatric training in the health professions. *Educational Gerontology, 25*, 641–660.

Additional Resources

Print

Bull, S. S., Domek, G., & Thomas, D. (2016). eHealth and Global Health Promotion. In R. Zimmerman, R. J. DiClemente, J. K. Andrus, & E. N. Hosein (Eds.). *Introduction to global health promotion.* San Francisco: Jossey-Bass.

National Commission for Health Education Credentialing, Inc. (NCHEC), & Society for Public Health Education (SOPHE). (2015).

A Competency-Based Framework for Health Education Specialists-2015. Whitehall, PA: National Commission for Health Education Credentialing, Inc. (NCHEC) and Society for Public Health Education (SOPHE).

The National Academies of Sciences, Engineering, and Medicine. (2017). *Communities in action: Pathways to health equity.* Washington, DC: The National Academies Press.

Internet

American Public Health Association Advocacy Public Health Action Campaign (PHACT). Retrieved from http://www.apha.org/policies-and-advocacy/advocacy-for-public-health/phact-campaign

CDC Health Equity Resource Toolkit for State Practitioners Addressing Obesity Disparities. Retrieved from http://www.cdc.gov/nccdphp/dnpao/state-local-programs/health-equity/pdf/toolkit.pdf

National Commission on Health Education Credentialing, Inc. Retrieved from http://www.nchec.org

SOPHE Annual Health Education Advocacy Summit. Retrieved from http://www.sophe.org/advocacy/advocacy-summit/

The Goals Institute. Retrieved from http://www.goalpower.com/

World Health Organization. Health Equity Assessment Toolkit (HEAT). Retrieved from http://www.who.int/gho/health_equity/assessment_toolkit/en/

CHAPTER 3

Promoting Health Education in a Multicultural Society

Jodi Brookins-Fisher, PhD, MCHES
Liliana Rojas-Guyler, PhD, CHES

▸ Author Comments

When professionals act with human dignity toward one another, we can more effectively reach each other. In today's multicultural society and with the charged sociopolitical climate, it is even more imperative that health education professionals are equipped to understand our communities, their expectations, their needs, and their struggles. How are we to develop and implement effective programs if we do not know the people with whom we are working? Although there has been an increased interest and emphasis in cultural competence and diversity in recent years, it is vital we continue to consider and validate the important similarities and differences in our communities. Our neighbors should not have to be members of a majority group in order to receive services in this country. Unfortunately, just the opposite is often true.

This chapter addresses our growing diversity from a practical perspective. But beyond that, we need to constantly consider the impact of diversity in the practice of health education because it is the *human* thing to do. We should all be able to enjoy our health because we are citizens of a great country—not because of our skin color, sexual orientation, country of familial origin, or even age. Health education specialists can make the world a better place, and we can begin by acknowledging all the people that make up its uniqueness.

🔍 CHES COMPETENCIES

2.1.1	Identify priority populations, partners, and other stakeholders.
2.1.3	Facilitate collaborative efforts among priority populations, partners, and other stakeholders.
2.3.4	Apply principles of cultural competence in selecting and/or designing strategies/interventions.
2.3.5	Address diversity within priority populations in selecting and/or designing strategies/interventions.
2.3.7	Tailor strategies/interventions for priority populations.
3.3.4	Apply principles of diversity and cultural competence in implementing health education/promotion plan.
4.3.10	Ensure fairness of data collection instruments (e.g., reduce bias, use language appropriate to priority population).*
7.1.2	Identify level of literacy of intended audience.
7.1.3	Tailor messages for intended audience.
7.2.1	Identify current and emerging issues requiring advocacy.

*Advanced level competency

Reprinted by permission of the National Commission for Health Education Credentialing, Inc. (NCHEC) and Society for Public Health Education (SOPHE).

▶ Introduction

For the last several years, an increased emphasis on the recognition of underserved populations in the United States has played a major role in health education efforts. Community-based efforts have been initiated in response to increases in disease among particular populations (e.g., stroke among African Americans and diabetes among Latinos). In addition, an understanding of concepts such as cultural awareness, cultural sensitivity, cultural competence, and multiculturalism has become necessary for a health education specialist to be effective. More recently, concepts such as cross-cultural communication, cultural responsiveness, and cultural pluralism have been explored. It is easy to give terminology lip service, but what do these terms really mean? What must health education specialists do to effectively address the issues of diversity in the many settings in which they are expected to play their professional roles? How does an individual health education specialist become better prepared to work with diverse populations? This chapter addresses the need for a multicultural focus in health education and presents ideas on how to facilitate the development of a multiculturally competent community health setting as well as lists diversity resources available to health education specialists.

▶ Increasing Diversity in the United States: The Need for Multicultural Awareness in Health Education

From an ethnic and racial standpoint, the U.S. population has changed from one that was largely White to one that is now more diverse. This change in demographics will continue. It has been projected that by the year 2044, more than 50% of Americans will belong to a racial/ethnic group other than non-Hispanic White, and in 2016 nearly one in five of the total U.S. population was foreign born.[1] The fastest growing population group over the next four decades will be that of people who identify as having 'two or more' races (225% increase), and the second fastest growing is projected among people who identify as Asian only.[1] In contrast, an 8.2% decrease will occur among the White population during this same time period, so that "**minority**" ethnic groups, collectively, will surpass the white population in numbers in 2044, accounting for 56.4% of the population.[1] This shift will result in the United States being more in line with global statistics, in which people of color comprise the majority.

Other demographic indicators also demonstrate growing diversity in the United States. For instance, lesbian, gay, bisexual, transgender, and queer (LGBTQ) persons are part of diversity conversations and continue to secure human rights. Gay and lesbian persons have been estimated to represent between 2% and 10% of the U.S. population, respectively.[2] A more recent review reports that 3.5% of the U.S. population is LGBTQ.[3] With health **disparities** being a primary focus of public health efforts, it is essential that health education specialists, in both the present and the future, continue to be aware of and respond to demographic changes. Growing "minority" and other hitherto **underserved** populations will need services that are appropriately delivered to them and meet their specific needs. Regardless of the specific priority population, the development of health education services must take into consideration the population's **culture**. This requires the priority population's input in community health assessment and improvement, program planning, implementation, and evaluation.

Some U.S. populations have continued to experience problems with certain health issues. Poverty, lack of proper immunizations, heart disease, cancer, stroke, chronic obstructive pulmonary disease, pneumonia, and diabetes have continued to unequally affect some ethnic groups, while older adults continue to experience chronic diseases such as arthritis, hypertension, osteoporosis, and dementing illnesses. As the country's demographics change, it is imperative health education specialists provide programming that addresses the dynamic health concerns of their diverse populations. An additional factor as to why certain health problems occur more in certain populations can also be attributed to the many social determinants of health.

Social Determinants of Health

For health education specialists to truly be multiculturally competent, social determinants of health should be central to all program and policy planning, implementation, and evaluation. For example, if a statistic is stated that "African American women have higher obesity rates than their White counterparts," a competent health education specialist will ask "Why?" Many health professionals would say that these women should "lose weight" or "eat healthier food." What is missing is the root problem as to what causes the obesity. Could it be food insecurity due to a scarcity of fresh fruits and vegetables (i.e., "food deserts") in their neighborhoods? Is a contributing factor then the lack of transportation to get to fresh food? Is it the plethora of fast food chains (i.e., "food swamps") in these same neighborhoods? It is simplistic to look and work on the behaviors of an individual and blame them for health issues, the idea of "lifestyle drift."[4] Looking beyond lifestyle to potential root causes of obesity allows the health education specialist to truly transform a community. By looking deeper, there could be systemic issues that require health and economic policy changes versus, for example, simply conducting a program for African American women that focuses on exercise and healthy foods.

As defined by the World Health Organization, the **social determinants of health** are the "conditions in which people are born, grow, live, work and age. These circumstances are shaped by the distribution of money, power and resources at the global, national and local levels." They include "poverty, lack of access to high-quality education or employment, unhealthy housing, unfavorable work and neighborhood conditions, and exposure to neighborhood violence."[5] These factors lead to inequities and disparities among and between groups of people.

The realization of the social determinants of health and their implications on a community's health lead to the need to monitor the structural determinants of health—policies, programs, decision-making/governance, economics,[6] and health care. Health care will not be able to adequately address the social determinants of health unless public health is integrated into the picture.[7] Furthermore, research findings have suggested that interventions target social structures and policies including "education and early childhood education, urban planning and community development, housing, income enhancements and supplements, and employment."[8] Multiculturally competent health education specialists need to broadly envision what is happening in a community and how to best make its unhealthy conditions better. They must be part of an interprofessional team that assesses the impact of their programs and policies on these various determinants of health. Multidimensional programming is required to deal with complicated health issues, as demonstrated through the *Health Impact Pyramid*.[9]

Of course, each social determinant of health is not a standalone issue, making multidimensional health education programs mandatory. Additionally, **intersectionality** must be considered in all well-rounded programs and policies. Intersectionality is a concept used to explain that individuals are not simply defined by one part of their culture (e.g., race/ethnicity, sexual orientation, gender identity). These combine to provide circumstances of advantage, disadvantage, and privilege in society. So, an individual could be both advantaged (e.g., as a White American) and disadvantaged (e.g., as a woman) at the same time. Intersectionalities complicate the social determinants of health by adding another unique layer to the overall picture of the health status of the individuals in a community.

When addressing the "big picture," these social determinants of health are political in nature. Therefore, health education specialists can no longer think in a nonpolitical manner to be effective—public health is truly a profession of **social justice** (i.e., social, economic, and political equality).[10]

? DID YOU KNOW?

The CDC reports that compared to their heterosexual peers, lesbian, gay, and bisexual students were nearly two times more likely to be bullied at school and electronically bullied. They were more than twice as likely to be victims of sexual violence and dating violence. LGBTQ youth from the 7th to the 12th grade also are more than twice as likely to attempt suicide as their heterosexual peers.

Data from Centers for Disease Control and Prevention. Personal Communication. June 7, 2017.

The Language of Diversity

Terminology pertaining to multiculturalism abounds. At times, the meaning of a particular word or how that word differs from another can be confusing. Although the following is an attempt to define the language of diversity, a well-trained health education specialist should always consider the source, as words may be used interchangeably in some circumstances or settings.

- *Diversity* refers to divergence among people, rooted in age, culture, health status and condition, race, ethnicity, experience, gender, sexual orientation, and various combinations of these traits.
- *Cultural awareness* is the consciousness of cultural similarities and differences.[11]
- *Cultural sensitivity* is the knowledge that cultural differences exist. It is the ability to apply the understanding that stems from that knowledge in different settings and situations to ensure or facilitate a useful interaction for all parties concerned.
- *Cultural intelligence* is the capability to function effectively across a variety of cultural contexts and the ability to communicate, network, and lead in cultural diverse workplaces and a globalized world.[12]
- *Cultural competence* is a "characteristic of those individuals who hold academic and interpersonal skills which allow an increased understanding and appreciation of another group's differences and similiarities."[13]

Culturally competent individuals have made an effort to learn about other cultures and have incorporated the information to the point where assumptions about others are not made. Additionally, it is "a developmental process defined as a set of values, principles, behaviors, attitudes, and policies that enable health professionals to work effectively across racial, ethnic, and linguistically diverse populations."[14]

- *Cultural humility* is a process of openness, self-awareness, being egoless, and incorporating self-reflection and critique after willingly interacting with diverse individuals.[15]
- *Cultural confidence* is a lifelong process based upon individuals' self-reflection about their personal biases and prejudices as evidenced by being flexible and humble enough to admit ignorance and willing to be uncomfortable addressing complex racialized issues.[14]
- *Multiculturalism* has been defined as a recognition of racial and cultural diversity, respect for the beliefs and culture of others, and a recognition that all members of a society have contributions to make for its betterment.[16] It includes the concept of equality among people regardless of such factors as race, ethnicity, gender identity, sexual orientation, age, or ability. In addition, multiculturalism can be both a vocabulary term and a phenomenon at the individual or institutional level, inclusive of cultures outside of the majority.[17]

Multiculturalism has been an integral component in expanding the notion of education. The term *multicultural education* has been developed to refer to "the process of gaining an enhanced knowledge, understanding, and acceptance of the methods of constructive interactions among people of differing cultural backgrounds."[17] Within the health education profession, multicultural health education has been defined as learning opportunities that are carried out in relevant languages and are designed with sensitivity to culture, values, beliefs, and practices. These education activities are developed and implemented with the active participation of people reflective of the priority population and take into account their cultural diversity.[18]

While society has become trapped in the muddied waters of "political correctness," the present and future of the health education profession require an understanding of multicultural issues beyond "correctness." For health education specialists, the importance lies deeper than that of learning the language—it lies in equalizing the playing field for all players; the concept of **health equity**. Health education specialists should strive for fairness (i.e., equity) instead of sameness (i.e., **equality**).[19]

In addition to knowing the terminology, health education specialists should contribute to change in societal structure for the betterment of all people in order not to miss a critical component in the development of the profession in the 21st century.

---

⑦ DID YOU KNOW?

The United States has the worst inequality of any of the rich nations, and among the worst health outcomes.

▶ Being Multiculturally Competent In Health Education

In order to provide culturally appropriate services to diverse populations, several competency areas should be addressed. First, it is imperative that a health education specialist become aware of diversity and their role in ensuring diversity issues are addressed in the professional setting. Next, being culturally competent results in health education specialists going the extra mile to ensure their workplaces and the services they provide are inclusive of the diverse needs of the population being served. Last, building skills in creating an inclusive environment, using inclusive language, understanding culture, establishing discussion guidelines, developing facilitation skills, choosing materials that reflect diverse peoples and viewpoints, and diversifying teaching techniques and learning styles will increase the health education specialist's ability to meet the needs of others. Although these are not easy tasks, this section provides further ideas about how to incorporate each into one's personal and professional interactions.

Heighten Personal Awareness

Before developing and implementing programs for diverse populations, health education specialists must first understand their own belief systems regarding issues of diversity (e.g., race, ethnicity, religion, gender identity, sexual orientation, age, ability). The first step in this process involves becoming familiar with personal biases. Health education specialists need to be in touch with their personal biases so that they do not disrupt services and education provided in cross-cultural or transcultural (i.e., experiences with others different from oneself) settings. People have had different experiences and they naturally bring biases to interactions with others who differ from themselves. Previous social experiences and political interactions, as well as the communication and problem-solving capabilities of individuals, affect interactions with others and may lead to stereotyping or misunderstanding.[16] With an understanding of personal biases, health education specialists have a clearer understanding of their limitations in communicating with focus populations. Health education specialists also must exhibit professionalism, separating their personal biases from their professional interactions, especially as they are called on more frequently to work with diverse populations. This is a difficult task, and one that should be carefully analyzed prior to programming at any level.

To continue this ongoing process of becoming and being multiculturally competent, known and unknown biases should be addressed. For example, **microaggressions** that are used without knowing they can be very harmful to others should be identified. *Racial microaggressions* are brief and commonplace daily verbal, behavioral,

or environmental indignities that, whether intentional or unintentional, communicate hostile, derogatory, or negative racial slights and insults toward people of color.[20] Even well-meaning individuals commit microaggressions while trying to make conversation. For example, if an individual asks someone who looks Asian "Where are you from?," this is naively based on the assumption that if one is Asian he or she is not from the United States. Imagine how a third or fourth generation Asian American would feel. Imagine how she or he would feel after being asked things like these repeatedly. Image further how one would feel after being asked not only where he or she is from, but also hears how well English is spoken? The cumulative effect of being "othered" or seen as an outsider based on looks can be very frustrating, to say the least. Other examples would be attending a college or university where all of the statues of prominent scholars and all the buildings reflect White men; or an African American student who excels in a course is being told by the professor that they are a "credit to their race"; or hearing that he or she is "articulate" for an African American. How would these experiences affect a person's well-being overtime? How would they affect the person's confidence? Microaggressions like this occur over time and in different places and situations. There are many examples and excellent dialogue on this topic for further exploration (see Additional Resources).

---

⑦ DID YOU KNOW?

Not all health disparities have a negative effect on "minority" populations. For example, the recent opioid epidemic disproportionately affects the White population. White Americans account for 65% of the population, yet they represented 82% of the opioid-related deaths in 2015.

Data from The Commonwealth Fund, http://www.commonwealthfund.org.

Along with careful evaluation of personal biases, listening, watching, reading, and participating are important in becoming a more culturally competent professional. Health education specialists can learn the most about other cultures

Gabe, a new health education specialist with the local health department, was asked to give a talk to a local high school group about tobacco product use prevention. This emerging health topic was becoming increasingly relevant with 15%–17% of high school students reporting hookah use. This particular community high school had a diverse student population, with many diverse immigrant communities represented. Many youth came from India and the Middle East, where hookah use is prevalent. Although he felt confident in the subject matter to be presented, he realized he had very limited knowledge of and past interaction with those of differing ethnic backgrounds from himself. Additionally, many of the students in his audience had a long cultural and family tradition of hookah use. He wanted to make sure the information presented helped the young people but did not alienate them because of his lack of knowledge about them as both a population and individuals.

Over the next several weeks, Gabe obtained a lot of background information for his presentation. He felt comfortable with hookah use prevention and control messages, but still uneasy as to his ability to deliver the information within the context of the group. He decided he needed to further research smoking prevention programs and messages in the literature focusing on diverse youth in general, and would ask the high school group if he could attend a couple of its meetings. There, he would listen to the group, observe their interactions, and interview willing individuals.

is written. Establishing relationships with people from different cultures is perhaps the most beneficial way to learn about other cultures. These relationships will allow free discussion and provide opportunities to listen and learn from other points of view.

? DID YOU KNOW?

Hispanic as a group identifier can include individuals from all races and includes people with ancestry from Spain and Latin and Central American Spanish-speaking countries. Most Latin and Central American Hispanics prefer the term Latino or Latina American. But, even more important, many Latinos identify their cultural background with their country of familial origin rather than their ethnicity. For example, they might prefer to identify as coming from a Colombian family and identify as Colombian American. This national identity can be a better way for Latinos to relate to their ancestors and familial roots versus the Latino or Hispanic label.

Data from The Henry J. Kaiser Family Foundation. Opiod overdose deaths by race/ethnicity—2015. *KFF.org.* Retrieved from http://kff.org/other/state-indicator/opioid-overdose-deaths-by-raceethnicity

Transfer Personal Knowledge into Professional Settings

The resulting knowledge associated with becoming aware of personal biases and learning about other cultures should be transferred into professional practice and the workplace. At a broader professional level, the following strategies can enhance a health education specialist's ability to understand diversity and help ensure it is incorporated into professional practice and workplace interactions[16]:

■ Determine whether current expertise addresses both regional and worldwide diversity and responsibility for human and international interactions.

■ Determine whether programs enhance people's skills and knowledge about the diverse world around them so that people better understand themselves and the values of other cultures.

when they immerse themselves in those cultures. Learning about other cultures and increasing comfort level around others can be accomplished by attending cultural events such as *Pride Day, Cinco de Mayo*, powwows, healing ceremonies, Martin Luther King Jr. events, or other ethnic celebrations; participating in workshops or lectures about topics on different cultures; being involved in neighborhood activities in the community; and reading materials on and from people of different cultural backgrounds, especially those materials verified by the people about whom the material

- Determine whether materials, curricula, services, and resources benefit all priority populations. Materials should reflect gender, racial, and other cultural differences (e.g., gender-neutral language).
- Determine whether an action plan has been developed relating to special information for underserved populations such as migrant farm workers, immigrants, homeless persons, and people with differing sexual orientation.
- Determine whether plans incorporating *Healthy People 2020*[21] into programming have also included the needs of diverse populations.
- Tailor an evaluation mechanism to suit the needs of the particular organization that measures the extent to which the health education workplace is meeting its responsibilities of responding to the diversity of its clientele, with input from the population or populations being served.

The process of becoming culturally competent is not a single-time event, but one that needs constant reevaluation and reappraisal both at individual and organizational levels. A culturally competent health education specialist is in a position to determine the extent of the cultural competence of the professional setting, assess and document the strengths and weaknesses of the organization, and focus on areas for improvement in both the workplace and programming.

Create an Inclusive Environment

Creating an educational environment inclusive of the diversity among participants can be one of the greatest challenges in health education programming. In doing so, several areas of concern should be addressed, including: (1) language and verbiage, (2) the priority population culture, (3) discussion guidelines, (4) facilitation skills, (5) materials, and (6) techniques and learning styles. These ideas will help to infuse culture into the educational environment and will help ensure that method selection has taken culture into account.

COMMUNITY CONNECTIONS 3.2

Upon completing his research regarding Indian and Middle Eastern youth, Gabe discovered youths often thrive in educational environments that facilitate cooperation rather than competition and that allow for group work. As far as hookah and tobacco use prevention and control messages, there were a few ideas, but not many focused on immigrant youth. He decided he would incorporate a group activity into the presentation after consulting with the youth group.

From interviewing young Indian and Middle Eastern students from the high school group, he discovered very few could identify services or resources available to them for tobacco use prevention. He decided to explore his own agency's ability to meet immigrant youth needs and its response to youth as they utilized health department services. He found that although the health department was often empathetic to people with diverse cultures and backgrounds, they did not have specific resources available to youth about hookah use, and that the pamphlets that were available were really directed to White and African American populations. He decided to further explore the resources in the community in order to develop a resource list. That way, when young people utilized health department services, the providers could have a referral sheet for existing resources upon request. He also decided to revise the smoking prevention information available to Indian and Middle Eastern youth with the youth group's input, to make it more appropriate, attractive, and applicable.

Use Inclusive Language

Health education specialists need to consider the importance of **inclusive language** when presenting information to individuals and community groups. Language is one of the most important methods for communicating, yet can be the hardest to change for inclusiveness. Both oral and written communication must be clearly understood by diverse populations. Strategies for ensuring inclusiveness include oral and written communication that is gender neutral (e.g., using words such as *partner* and *spokesperson*), in the appropriate language, and at the appropriate literacy level. Reading level analysis programs and learner verification procedures should be used with written materials. Members of the priority population should be involved in developing materials in different languages. Translation and back translation should be carried out to ensure the appropriate message is conveyed. Pictures and words conveying health messages should be used as much as possible and where appropriate. If language issues are not considered, health education specialists risk not connecting with the priority population at the most basic level.

Understand the Priority Population Culture

Another area of challenge is becoming aware of the culture, beliefs (especially health beliefs), and values of the priority population. It is very difficult for someone living outside the cultural parameters of a community to understand that population's culture if it has not been personally experienced. Culture in itself is diverse, and generalizations from past experiences will not necessarily hold true for any particular population or help a health education specialist with a current program or event. Even when the health education specialist is properly prepared, cross-cultural interaction may include participants' previous experiences that may impede the educational process. Further, the more diverse perspectives within the same culture one can include, the more well-rounded the discussion. This is important because within any culture, there is also diversity (e.g., not all Latinos are the same, not all people who have a disability are the same). No individual can represent his or her entire racial or ethnic group. Culture is a collective that requires time and effort to explore and which is constantly dynamic and adapting to the environment in which it exists. Although this may be frustrating, the health education specialist should remain motivated and interested in the participants' points of view. If needed, community resources and organizations that are culture specific can be utilized for troubleshooting problematic areas. Additionally, it is recommended to include cultural brokers (e.g., members of the priority population who assist the health education specialist) in all stages of program design, planning, implementation, and evaluation.

Establish Discussion Guidelines

Group discussion guidelines (e.g., for use with focus groups or classes) should be determined and stated at the beginning of any program or event, and should be maintained by the facilitator and group members. Discussions among groups should be sensitive to diversity. Guidelines for inclusiveness may include any or all of the following: (1) respecting the confidentiality of all participants' comments and actions, (2) being sensitive to different personal experiences of group members, (3) being sensitive to different levels of expertise among the group, (4) avoiding assumptions about the cultural or ethnic backgrounds of other group members, (5) allowing privacy (i.e., the right to pass in any discussion or activity), and (6) other guidelines the group deems important in order to facilitate tolerance and respect for each person's point of view.

Develop Facilitation Skills

Health education specialists should be facilitators of acceptance and respect in any setting. Good facilitation skills require negotiation; the ability to deal with controversy; and being approachable, open, objective, and impartial. If proper facilitation occurs, a health education specialist can be a role model for inclusiveness.

Choose Materials Wisely

Efforts should be made to select pieces from many perspectives when determining which materials to include in programming. For instance, articles written by women and people of color can culturalize a curriculum. By remembering there is diversity among participants, health education specialists will utilize materials from more than one viewpoint. It may also be necessary to use focus group discussions to determine what materials and methods are appropriate and acceptable for the population at hand.

Diversify Presentation Techniques for Learning Styles

It is always easiest to teach how one prefers to be taught, but this may not reach all participants. Presentations should include various methods (e.g., lectures, small groups, role plays, computer exercises) to be inclusive of the various learning styles among participants. Because learners may be visual, tactile, or audio oriented, a variety of teaching methods should be incorporated to accommodate different preferences. Values clarification exercises are also beneficial in heightening cultural sensitivity because they help further participant awareness of personal values, while allowing others to state their values. As stated by the late Noreen Clark, former Dean of the School of Public Health at the University of Michigan:

> As a society we have to get agreements on what is important, what we value. . . . It's not a matter of your values being better than mine . . . it's a matter of creating a society where both our values coexist.[22]

COMMUNITY CONNECTIONS 3.3

Feeling more prepared for his presentation because he had learned more about his focus population and its culture, Gabe began to gather materials for the presentation. Although he prided himself in his ability to adapt to different presentations, he knew if he was to be truly effective with his group he would need to ensure he was attentive to cultural considerations. After learning about the collective nature of their culture and the importance of harmonious group dynamics, he thought a collaborative learning environment with a group activity and culturally appropriate materials (i.e., materials correctly translated into Hindi, Arabic, Turkish, and Hebrew in appropriate readability level and with images that were appealing and relatable to the group) were crucial. These ideas, some easier than others to infuse into the presentation, might make all the difference in helping his population relate to him and connect with his hookah use prevention and control messages.

▶ Tips and Techniques for Incorporating Cultural Competence into Professional Practice

As health education specialists attempt to positively change themselves and the environments in which they work, they should be aware of a few issues that will aid in the process of establishing multicultural competence in the heart of professional practice.

Take Small Steps toward Change

Being a culturally competent health education specialist takes time and effort, and is an ongoing process. Old habits are hard to break, so effort must be made to institute change over time. It is important to remain oneself throughout the process, as humanness in the effort of trying to be culturally sensitive is an admirable quality. People will be aware of a fake persona anyway, so truthfulness is the best policy. Additionally, as small steps are taken toward inclusiveness, a trust in others must be established. Each client or participant is a unique individual, so care should be taken to not judge based on past experiences. With each successful venture at attaining cultural sensitivity, the health education specialist will become more culturally competent (**TABLE 3.1**).

Infuse Cultural Issues into Facilitation

Although the information presented in Table 3.1 will help equip the health education specialist with facilitation skills, other tips are also important.[16] Cultural differences can be brought into the discussion through a planned activity regarding a health topic. For example, special remedies for dealing with common illnesses might be discussed, or ethnic or more readily available or obtainable foods might be evaluated for nutritional content. By providing these types of opportunities, health education specialists are encouraging expression

TABLE 3.1 Characteristics of a Multiculturally Competent Health Education Specialist

- Is aware that no one person can represent or understand a whole group or culture, even his or her own, for all cultures/groups are heterogeneous within themselves.
- Acquires knowledge about individuals and groups of people different than oneself.
- Participates in diverse cultural events.
- Empathizes with humankind and the human experience.
- Is competent in process and content areas of health education.
- Facilitates discussion about the importance of culture among varying individuals and groups.
- Provides a safe environment for exploring the meaning of culture.
- Provides an inclusive environment.
- Speaks in gender-neutral and inclusive language.
- Promotes not only inclusion, but also respect and acceptance.
- Strives to reduce health disparities by promoting equity.
- Encourages diverse populations to empower and help themselves.
- Models the importance of diversity in personal and professional settings.
- Includes cultural considerations in all programming and activities.
- Understands the importance of linguistic competence.
- Includes cultural brokers from focus population whenever possible.

of and acceptance for differences in culture, food or other preferences, and socioeconomic class, while allowing for an exchange of ideas and even the fostering of relationships between people in a nonthreatening environment.

Participants may disagree on a concept being presented. As the facilitator, the health education specialist should be careful to not support or oppose one view. By being open in discussions, the health education specialist establishes a climate of caring and acceptance. Inclusive language

and use of variety in examples will also improve facilitation skills.

Know Your Limits

Health education specialists may find at times that their personal values intrude in professional settings. If this is a continual problem, clients should be referred to another competent professional who is better able to deal with the issue. This is not to say the health education specialist should avoid all potential clients that cause internal struggle, because continued effort at working with others may help to sort through conflicting personal values and professional obligations.

▶ Overcoming Challenges to Becoming Multiculturally Competent

There are many challenges to becoming a multiculturally competent professional and ensuring a multiculturally competent workplace. Both personal and professional barriers as well as outside opposition may impede a well-intended effort. Following are ideas for reducing barriers and lessening community resistance.

Reduce Personal Barriers

Perhaps, the biggest barrier to attaining cultural competence at the personal level is a lack of awareness. Getting beyond one's paradigm and life focus is difficult and occurs best when awareness is first heightened. Awareness at a global level encourages sharing of wealth, prosperity, and economic development among all U.S. citizens. It is a difficult process that is still expressed very eloquently in the following sentiments:

> Simply put, at a time when the economy is weak and many politicians are employing old strategies of blaming minorities for getting more than their fair share, it is not difficult to understand the resistance that many people express

towards texts and programs that, in their minds, merely "rewrite" history. For these people, all this talk about multiculturalism is little more than an attempt to create a narrative that makes them less than heroic by virtue of acknowledging the significance of others, others who have been oppressed and who have been hitherto viewed not as important but rather as problematic. Because of this, educators cannot underestimate the importance of the reevaluation of the status of individuals and groups of people; many will be compelled to see their own significance challenged, if not threatened with erasure, as others gain a new place in both texts and the nation.[23]

Health education specialists should adhere to the *Unified Code of Ethics for the Health Education Profession* when dealing with personal barriers.[24] Article IV, Section 1, specifically addresses the need to be sensitive to social and cultural diversity: "Health Educators are sensitive to social and cultural diversity and are in accord with the law, when planning and implementing programs." By following the Unified Code of Ethics, health education specialists will ensure they are abiding by professional expectations rather than personal beliefs when conflict arises. Reviewing literature in related disciplines may also help a health education specialist increase cultural awareness. Health education specialists should avail of the various opportunities that present themselves to become more educated on cultural awareness and the provision of culturally appropriate care such as attending conferences and symposia and reading the growing body of literature available. The reader is referred to Marin and colleagues,[13] Buckner,[16] and Perez and Luquis[25] for more information on the importance of cultural diversity in health education programming. Finally, the health education specialist can combat personal resistance by referring to several organizations and resources that can help professionals become more culturally aware and competent (**TABLE 3.2** and Additional Resources).

TABLE 3.2 Sampling of Organizations Promoting Multicultural Health Education

American Public Health Association
Policy statements, publications and professional development resources (e.g., "Better Health Through Equity: Case Studies in Reframing Public Health Work" 2015) http://www.apha.org/topics-and-issues/health-equity

Centers for Disease Control & Prevention
Tools, programs and policy resources. Specialty pages on health disparities and health equity (e.g., "Social Determinants of Health: Know What Affects Health"; "Promoting Health Equity: A Resource to Help Communities Address Social Determinants of Health") http://www.cdc.gov/socialdeterminants/

The National Center for Cultural Competence
Distance learning, publications, resources, and more (e.g., "Engaging Ethnic Media to Inform Communities about Safe Infant Sleep." Toolkit for providers) http://nccc.georgetown.edu/

National Commission for Health Education Credentialing, Inc.
Continuing Education opportunities (e.g., "The Meaning of Food in Our Lives: A Cross-cultural Perspective on Eating and Well-Being") http://www.nchec.org/

National Partnership to End Health Disparities
Community-driven, cross-sector and partnership-based approaches. Resources. http://minorityhealth.hhs.gov/npa/

Society for Public Health Education
Publications, professional development continuing education (e.g., "Improving Health Outcomes for Culturally Diverse Populations Through Cultural Competency" webinar). http://www.sophe.org/

Data from American Public Health Association. www.apha.org /topics-and-issues/health-equity; Centers for Disease Control and Prevention. www.cdc.gov/socialdeterminants; National Center for Cultural Competence. www.nccc.georgetown.edu; National Commission for Health Education Credentialing. www.nchec.org; U.S. Department of Health and Human Services. www.minorityhealth.hhs.gov/npa; Society for Public Health Education. www.sophe.org.

Lessen Professional Barriers

Professionally, the greatest barriers to multiculturalism confronting health education specialists include a lack of research, available health education programming specifically targeting diverse populations, and preprofessional training. Much of the research in health-related fields, up until a few years ago, has predominantly used White males as the point of reference. Additionally, research has shown traditional health education approaches are not as effective with underserved groups of people as with the rest of the population.[13] In more recent years, there has been an increase in research with **vulnerable populations** and **marginalized groups**, inclusive and specific to women's health needs, and identifying disparities by race and ethnicity in health outcomes and healthcare access.[26] A lack of research specific to the health education field, health promotion programs, and effective public health education strategies to address health education needs of diverse and disenfranchised populations still exists. Increasingly, professional preparation courses address health disparities as population health issues, but there is still a need to increase the understanding and preparation of what makes programs more effective and how to tailor them for diverse priority populations. These barriers may affect a health education specialist's ability to effectively work with the many diverse populations for which programs are designed. Professional conferences are one way to access cutting edge research and program evaluation outcomes.

Even in a profession in which most individuals consider themselves open-minded, the road to cultural competence has been slow. Many organizations and agencies still face barriers that impede their ability to effectively incorporate culture into programming, method selection, and material development. At the institutional level, health education agencies can avoid barriers by (1) being aware and accepting of cultural differences and similarities; (2) having the ability for cultural self-assessment (i.e., assessing the cultural competence of the organization); (3) having the required awareness, understanding, and knowledge of focus populations; (4) developing skills that facilitate diversity; and (5) being sensitive to dynamics inherent with cultural interaction.[13]

To improve the status of research regarding multicultural issues in health education, researchers need to see cultural diversity as important. Previous studies have identified a need for more emphasis on multicultural issues related to health education. For instance, one study found only 78 titles of 774 articles that appeared in prominent health education journals over a four-year period alluded to a multicultural emphasis.[27] More recently, as ethnic minority populations have grown, their growth has not been reflected in our professional literature. For example, a 2016 analysis of Latino health issues in health education journal publications found a disproportionately low number of articles addressing Latino health. Out of the 2,646 total articles published between 2010 and 2015, only 102 (nearly 4%) had a Latino population primary focus.[28] More research projects will need to be specific to priority populations and must be conducted by adequately trained health education specialists. To avoid barriers to multiculturalism, professional research should adhere to a number of guidelines, including the following[13]:

- Demographic information must be collected on all priority populations.
- Better means of reaching underserved populations through interventions must be developed and implemented.
- Peer education must be utilized.
- Studies need to include not only health problems, but also social and contextual indicators of their incidence and prevalence.
- Evaluation components should address both process as well as impact indicators.

Approaches that can be more useful than traditional health education programs in helping underserved populations include trained community health workers, peer education, lay health workers (e.g., family members, significant others in the communities), interaction with healthcare providers, self-help groups, and school-based interventions. When implementing any of these approaches, cultural issues should be addressed by taking into account the values, expectancies, norms, beliefs, and behavioral preferences of the focus group.[13]

Along with a multicultural focus, a mindset of advocacy must be instilled in professionally prepared health education specialists, because they will be in positions to work with people (e.g., administrators, legislators) who have a profound impact on other groups' causes. Colleges and universities training future health education specialists should incorporate skill building and training in areas of community organization and empowerment, advocacy, volunteerism, and diversity, in order to prepare students for the realities of changing demographics and the various social determinants of health. Developing culturally sensitive programs will increase the level of culturally competent health education specialists.

Plan for and Dissipate Community Resistance

Community resistance may also be a barrier to incorporating cultural diversity at the agency level, especially when dealing with multicultural issues that ignite debates among those with different value systems. For example, inclusion of a LGBTQ youth support program in a school district may initiate controversy because of differing belief systems among educators, administrators, parents, and students. Religious values and lack of information about an issue may also contribute to the resistance.

It is important to be able to handle community opposition to multicultural programming. Opposition to multicultural programming may even include the priority population itself. For example, Native American populations who have had negative past experiences with health education programs may not be supportive of additional programming. Finding out why the priority population or populations feel as they do, and making sure the program is developed incorporating their perspectives, will increase the likelihood of program success.

Overcoming community opposition can be accomplished by developing relationships with key individuals associated with the priority population. These key individuals and groups will provide insight into community norms, values, and belief systems. By believing in what the agency is trying to accomplish and by the agency seeking goals that are relevant to the priority populations, they will help the health education specialist create a successful plan to reduce or eliminate opposition.

Whenever possible and appropriate, broad-based coalitions or partnerships concerning a particular health issue should be developed. By beginning with a common point of interest (i.e., the health issue), individuals will focus on the issue at hand rather than individual biases about the focus population. For example, if a coalition is organized to promote comprehensive sexuality education, including gay youth, the group should focus on the issue at hand instead of personal views about homosexuality.

It is always better for a program to work with the opposition than to exclude them. By finding a common concept for agreement (e.g., reducing risks for a specific disease), barriers such as conflicting values and personal stereotypes will begin to break down. An attempt at working together shows empathy and concern on the health education specialist's part. Once the opposition is heard, they may be satisfied and no longer be a threat to the program. Some groups, however, will refuse to agree with other positions and will not be willing to compromise. When this occurs, partnerships will not likely work for either party involved.

▶ Expected Outcomes

By following the suggestions described earlier, health education specialists can expect to enhance their cultural competency. This, in turn, will lead to more culturally competent institutions, organizations, programs, and research. By including priority populations throughout program development, materials and resources will be inclusive of their point of view and more likely to be utilized in the future.

Another outcome is mutual trust and respect between groups that traditionally have had turbulent relationships. Many minority groups distrust the

COMMUNITY CONNECTIONS 3.4

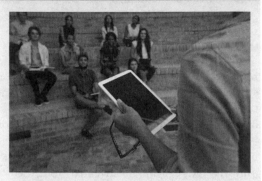

© Klaus Vedfelt/DigitalVision/Getty.

After the presentation about hookah use and health consequences, many young people stayed to ask Gabe further questions. His preparation had paid off. By carefully selecting methods for the presentation that incorporated the unique cultural considerations of the diverse and largely immigrant youth group, his messages were well received. Besides imparting information on an important risk factor for disease prevention to a group of young people, he also had increased his comfort level regarding different populations. The youth knew he was open and respectful, and in turn, they encouraged his continued involvement in the health lecture series at their group meetings. Indirectly, he had also established a trusting bond between the health department and a group of traditionally disenfranchised youth.

more dominant or **majority** populations (i.e., those populations with power in the social structure) and their services. Ensuring cultural diversity in programming can build relationships with mutual understanding. The power of reestablishing trust relationships is not to be underestimated in the context of relationships between individuals and the institutions represented by other individuals.

A very important outcome of obtaining cultural competence at individual and professional levels is the development of health education programs including method selection that are embraced by the community to the extent they are institutionalized by the priority population. They are more likely to take ownership because they have been empowered and involved in the process.

The goal of all the aforementioned is to pave the way for the elimination of disparities in health outcomes across populations within the United States. Clearly, barriers to continuous quality care are very important reasons for the continued disparities in health status and outcomes of members of underserved populations. Thus, at the personal, professional, and community levels, greater awareness of diversity issues must be achieved, paving the way for new directions in programming for diverse populations. The goal of multicultural diversity can best be summarized by the following:

> We [health educators] have to begin with developing an awareness and knowledge of culture which implies a non-judgmental acceptance of the worth of all ethnic groups—a willingness to see people as much as human beings as members of a particular group. . . . The final stage is to be able to perform a specific task while taking culture into account such that the outcome is better than it would have been had the role of the client's culture not been considered.[22]

▶ Conclusion

Society demographics are changing, which directly affects the practice of health education specialists. New and evolving strategies need to be inclusive of cultural diversity and should be implemented by culturally competent health education specialists. The health education profession must continue to examine its professional preparation programs, research, literature, programming and curricula, methods, and evaluation strategies to ensure the inclusion of cultural diversity.

The goal of attaining a multiculturally competent profession begins with the health education specialist. By each individual examining his or her own biases, beliefs, and values, and determining how these transfer into the professional setting, he or she can devise more inclusive ideas and activities, if needed. Once all health education specialists are responsive to the diverse needs of their focus populations, workplaces can then be transformed into respectful and inclusive settings. Above all, the health education profession can be responsive to Buckner's challenge[16] to be at the forefront of meeting the needs of our ever-changing American population.

Key Terms

Culture Similar ideas, beliefs, values, and perceptions among people of a particular group.

Disparity The vast differences that exist between populations in terms of access to services, morbidity, and mortality statistics, availability of resources, and the like.

Equality The idea of everyone having access to the same resources and enjoying the same benefits from the community in which they live.

Health equity A fair distribution of health outcomes for everyone in a community. The lack of health disparities.

Inclusive language Using language that does not leave out a particular group or population. For example, referring to the top position in a local agency as the *chairperson* rather than *chairman*.

Intersectionality When categories of culture overlap and potential advantages, disadvantages, and privileges change according to the situation.

Majority The group that holds the power in a population. This may or may not mean they have the greatest number of individuals in the community (e.g., White men hold the power in American political arenas, although they may not account for most people in the community).

Marginalized group A group of people who is seen and or treated as outsiders or not belonging to the larger predominant group.

Microaggression Daily forms of discrimination (which may be subtle and unintentional) that an individual in a marginalized group experiences.

Minority A government-invented word used to categorize people. This term is often seen as inferring to "lesser than" or somehow inferior; therefore, its use is on the decline.

Social determinants of health Factors that affect an individual's health outside personal behavior. These are often societal, structural and environmental such as poverty, education levels, and access to health care.

Social justice Having social, economic, and political equality.

Underserved Populations that do not have the same amount of services, resources, and so forth needed to deal with individual and community health issues compared with other populations.

Vulnerable population Any population for which a set of characteristics or circumstances place it at a disadvantage for services, resources, and positive outcomes.

References

1. Colby, S. L., & Ortman, J. M. (2015). *Projections of the size and composition of the U.S. population: 2014 to 2060.* Retrieved May 19, 2017, from http://www.census.gov/content/dam/Census/library/publications/2015/demo/p25-1143.pdf

2. Greenberg, J. S., Bruess, C. E., & Conklin, S. C. (2007). *Exploring the dimensions of human sexuality* (3rd ed.). Sudbury, MA: Jones and Bartlett.

3. Gates, G. J. (2011). *How many people are lesbian, gay, bisexual, and transgender?* Retrieved May 19, 2017 from http://williamsinstitute.law.ucla.edu/wp-content/uploads/Gates-How-Many-People-LGBT-Apr-2011.pdf

4. Marmot, M., & Allen, J. J. (2014). Social determinants of health equity. *American Journal of Public Health, 104*(Suppl 4), S517–S519.

5. Braveman, P., Egerter, S., & Williams, D. R. (2011). The social determinants of health: Coming of age. *Annual Reviews in Public Health, 32*, 381–398.

6. Penman-Aguilar, A., Talih, M., Huang, D., Moonesignhe, R., Bouye, K., & Buckles, G. (2016). Measurement of health disparities, health inequities, and social determinants of health to support the advancement of health equity. *Journal of Public Health Management & Practice, 22,* S33–S42.

7. American Academy of Family Physicians. (2015). *Integration of primary care and public health.* Retrieved May 19, 2017, from http://www.aafp.org/about/policies/all/integprimarycareandpublichealth.html

8. Thornton, R. L. J, Glover, C. M., Cene, C. W., Glik, D. C., Henderson, J. A., & Williams D. R. (2015). Evaluating strategies for reducing health disparities by addressing the social determinants of health. *Health Affairs, 35*(8), 1416–1423.

9. Frieden, T. R. (2010). A framework for public health action: The Health Impact Pyramid. *American Journal of Public Health, 100*(4), 590–595.

10. National Center for Cultural Competence. (n.d.). *Public health in a multicultural environment.* Retrieved from http://nccc.georgetown.edu/curricula/public/C10.html

11. Redican, K., Stewart, S. H., Johnson, L. E., & Frazee, A. M. (1994). Professional preparation in cultural awareness and sensitivity in health education: A national survey. *Journal of Health Education, 25,* 215–217.

12. Livermore, D. A. (2011). *The cultural intelligence difference: Master the one skill you can't do without in today's global economy.* New York, NY: American Management Association.

13. Marin, G., Burhannsstipanov, L., Connell, C. M., Gielen, A. C., Helitzer-Allen, D., Lorig, K., … Thomas, S. (1995). A research agenda for health education among underserved populations. *Health Education Quarterly, 22,* 346–363.

14. Report of the 2011 Joint Committee on Health Education and Promotion Terminology. (2012). *American Journal of Health Education, 43* (Suppl 2).

15. Foronda, C., Baptiste, D., Reinholdt, M. M., & Ousman, K. (2016). Cultural humility: A concept analysis. *Journal of Transcultural Nursing, 27*(3), 210–217.

16. Buckner, W. P., Jr. (1994). Promoting multicultural sensitivity among educators. In P. Cortese & K. Middleton (Eds.), *The comprehensive school health challenge: Vol. 2* (pp. 661–686). Santa Cruz, CA: ETR Associates.

17. Staddon, D. T. (1992). *Multicultural resource manual.* Mt. Pleasant, MI: Central Michigan University Printing Services.

18. MacDonald, J. L., Thompson, P. R., & DeSouza, H. (1998). Multicultural health education: An emerging reality in Canada. *Hygiene, 7,* 12–16.

19. Centers for Disease Control and Prevention. (2016). *Reaching for health equity.* Retrieved June 6, 2017, from http://www.cdc.gov/minorityhealth/strategies2016/

20. Sue, D. W., Capodilupo, C. M., Torino, G. C., Bucceri, J. M., Holder, A., Nadal, K. L., & Esquilin, M. (2007). Racial microaggressions in everyday life: Implications for clinical practice. *American Psychologist, 62*(4), 271.

21. U.S. Department of Health and Human Services. (2014). *Healthy People 2020.* Retrieved June 6, 2017, from http://www.healthypeople.gov/2020/topics-objectives

22. Clark, N. M. (1994). Health educators and the future: Lead, follow, or get out of the way. *Journal of Health Education, 25,* 136–141.

23. Scapp, R. (1993). Feeling the weight of the world (studies) on my shoulders. *The Social Studies, 84,* 67–70, Taylor & Francis Ltd., reprinted by permission of the publisher.

24. Coalition of National Health Organizations. (2011). *The code of ethics for the health education profession.* Retrieved from http://cnheo.org/files/coe_full_2011.pdf

25. Miguel, A. P., & Luquis, R. R. (2013). *Cultural competence in health education and health promotion.* New York, NY: John Wiley & Sons.

26. Department of Health & Human Services. (2015). *Action plan to reduce racial and ethnic health disparities: implementation progress report 2011–2014.* Retrieved May 19, 2017, from http://www.minorityhealth.hhs.gov/assets/pdf/FINAL_HHS_Action_Plan_Progress_Report_11_2_2015.pdf

27. Brookins-Fisher, J., & Rieckmann, T. (1996). The presence of multiculturalism in titles of selected health education journal articles. *The Health Educator, 28*, 3–7.

28. Price, J. H., & Khubchandani, J. (2016). Health education research and practice literature on Hispanic health issues: Have we lost sight of the largest minority population? *Health Promotion Practice, 17*(2), 172–176.

Additional Resources

Print

Airhihenbuwa, C. O., Ford, C. L., & Iwelunmor, J. I. (2014). Why culture matters in health interventions: Lessons from HIV/AIDS stigma and NCDs. *Health Education & Behavior, 41*(1), 78–84.

Arousell, J., & Carlbom, A. (2016). Culture and religious beliefs in relation to reproductive health. *Best Practice & Research Clinical Obstetrics & Gynecology, 32*, 77–87.

Betancourt, J. R., Green, A. R., Carrillo, J. E., & Owusu Ananeh-Firempong, I. I. (2003). Defining cultural competence: A practical framework for addressing racial/ethnic disparities in health and health care. *Public Health Reports, 118*, 293–302.

Eldredge, L. K. B., Markham, C. M., Kok, G., Ruiter, R. A., & Parcel, G. S. (2016). *Planning health promotion programs: An intervention mapping approach.* New York, NY: John Wiley & Sons.

Fredriksen-Goldsen, K. I., Simoni, J. M., Kim, H. J., Lehavot, K., Walters, K. L., Yang, J., & Muraco, A. (2014). The health equity promotion model: Reconceptualization of lesbian, gay, bisexual, and transgender (LGBT) health disparities. *American Journal of Orthopsychiatry, 84*(6), 653.

Heilman, E. E. (2004). Hoosiers, hicks, and hayseeds: The controversial place of marginalized ethnic whites in multicultural education. *Equity and Excellence in Education, 37*, 67–79.

Herrick, A. L., Egan, J. E., Coulter, R. W., Friedman, M. R., & Stall, R. (2014). Raising sexual minority youths' health levels by incorporating resiliencies into health promotion efforts. *American Journal of Public Health, 104*(2), 206–210.

Huff, R. M., Kline, M. V., & Peterson, D. V. (Eds.). (2014). *Health promotion in multicultural populations: A handbook for practitioners and students.* Thousand Oaks, CA: SAGE publications.

Koh, H. K., Gracia, J. N., & Alvarez, M. E. (2014). Culturally and linguistically appropriate services—advancing health with CLAS. *The New England Journal of Medicine, 371*(3), 198.

Lecca, P. J., Quervalu, I., Nunes, J. V., & Gonzales, H. F. (2014). *Cultural competency in health, social & human services: Directions for the 21st century.* New York, NY: Routledge.

Marmot, M. & Allen, J. J. (2014). Social determinants of health equity. *American Journal of Public Health, 104*(Suppl 4), S517–S519.

Mendes, R., Plaza, V., & Wallerstein, N. (2016). Sustainability and power in health promotion: Community-based participatory research in a reproductive health policy case study in New Mexico. *Global Health Promotion, 23*(1), 61–74.

Munn, S. K., & Ryan, T. G. (2016). An examination of mental health promotion within international schools and current reform practices that can benefit third culture kids. *International Journal of Educational Reform 25*(N2), 170.

National Commission for Health Education Credentialing, Inc. (NCHEC), & Society for Public Health Education (SOPHE). (2015). *A Competency-Based Framework for Health Education Specialists-2015.* Whitehall, PA: National Commission for Health Education Credentialing, Inc. (NCHEC) and Society for Public Health Education (SOPHE).

Penman-Aguilar, A., Talih, M., Huang, D., Moonesinghe, R., Bouye, K., & Beckles, G. (2016). Measurement of health disparities, health inequities, and social determinants of health to support the advancement of health equity. *Journal of Public Health Management and Practice, 22,* S33–S42.

Perez, M. A., & Luquis, R. R. (2013). *Cultural competence in health education and health promotion.* New York, NY: John Wiley & Sons.

Simmons, R., Bennett, E., Ling Schwartz, M., Tung Sharify, D., & Short, E. (2002). Health education and cultural diversity in the health care setting: Tips for the practitioner. *Health Promotion Practice, 3,* 8–11.

Spector, R. E. (2004). *Cultural diversity in health and illness* (6th ed.). Upper Saddle River, NJ: Pearson Prentice Hall.

Trevino, R. P. (2005). Social capital and health: Implications for working with minority and underserved populations. *The Health Education Monograph Series, 22,* 12–18.

U.S. Department of Health and Human Services, Substance Abuse and Mental Health Services Administration, Center for Mental Health Services. (2001). *Cultural competence standards in managed mental health care services: Four underserved/underrepresented racial/ethnic groups.* Washington, DC: Author.

Woolf, S. H., Purnell, J. Q., Simon, S. M., Zimmerman, E. B., Camberos, G. J., Haley, A., & Fields, R. P. (2015). Translating evidence into population health improvement: Strategies and barriers. *Annual Review of Public Health, 36,* 463–482.

Internet

American Journal of Public Health Supplement, Beyond health equity. Retrieved from http://ajph.aphapublications.org/toc/ajph/105/S3

Camara Jones: *Achieving health equity: Tools for a national conversation on racism.* Video retrieved from http://www.youtube.com/watch?v=VroNBw8gaBE

Center for Disease Control & Prevention. *Strategies for reducing health disparities.* Retrieved from http://www.cdc.gov/minorityhealth/strategies2016/

Commission for a healthier America. Retrieved from http://www.commissiononhealth.org/

Cross cultural health care program. Retrieved from http://xculture.org/

Healthy People 2020: Social determinants of health. Retrieved from http://www.healthypeople.gov/2020/topics-objectives/topic/social-determinants-of-health

Immigration data & statistics. Retrieved from http://www.dhs.gov/immigration-statistics

Minority population profiles. Office of Minority Health. Retrieved from http://minorityhealth.hhs.gov/omh/browse.aspx?lvl=2&lvlid=26

National Institute on Minority Health and Health Equality. Retrieved from http://www.nimhd.nih.gov/

Race: The power of an illusion. Video retrieved from http://www.pbs.org/racc/000_General/000_00-Home.htm

Unnatural causes. Video retrieved from http://www.unnaturalcauses.org/resources.php

CHAPTER 4

Exploring Social Marketing Concepts

Mike Newton-Ward, MSW, MPH
Karen Denard Goldman, PhD, MCHES

▶ Author Comments

Mike: I have practiced social marketing for 20 years. I believe it is the best approach we have to create the conditions to support behavior change and social change to improve the health of individuals and communities. I still remember where I was sitting at the conference when "the key went in" for me about social marketing. I realized it provided me with a way to understand all the factors that determine health behavior and a way to create multiple interventions to support healthy behavior change. Whether public health practitioners decide to do social marketing full time or use it as one of several approaches in their toolbox, a marketing mindset can help them ask questions, gain insights, and create effective interventions that they would not have thought of before.

Karen: Years ago, Karen attended a continuing education course on marketing and her approach to health education changed forever. The use and promotion of social marketing became an integral part of her career as a health education practitioner and college professor.

According to Karen, "Both health education and social marketing are about planning, implementing, and evaluating offerings to voluntarily change behavior. Social marketing principles and practices complement health education priorities and processes. Their interaction is synergistic."

⌕ *CHES COMPETENCIES*

2.3.3	Apply principles of evidence-based practice in selecting and/or designing strategies/interventions.*
2.3.5	Address diversity within priority populations in selecting and/or designing strategies/interventions.
2.3.7	Tailor strategies/interventions for priority populations.
2.4.1	Use theories and/or models to guide the delivery plan.
2.4.6	Select methods and/or channels for reaching priority populations.
3.3.7	Use a variety of strategies to deliver plan.
6.1.4	Adapt information for consumer.
6.1.5	Convey health-related information to consumer.
7.1.1	Create messages using communication theories and/or models.
7.1.3	Tailor messages for intended audience.
7.1.7	Deliver messages using media and communication strategies.

*Advanced level competency

Reprinted by permission of the National Commission for Health Education Credentialing, Inc. (NCHEC) and Society for Public Health Education (SOPHE).

▸ **Introduction**

Social marketing. People in public health seem to either like it or dislike it. Those who dislike marketing claim it is expensive, manipulative, time intensive, or staff intensive. With equal passion, those who believe in the importance of social marketing praise its ability to provide a 360 degree view[1] of the determinants and solutions to problems; make behavior change fun, easy and popular[2]; increase the satisfaction of the target audience; and allow more efficient use of limited resources. What is the difference between these two groups? Usually, it is the fact that those who like social marketing understand what it *really* entails. Those who dislike it tend to think marketing means selling.

Regardless of one's views, a niche exists for social marketing in health education. Social marketing is defined as "a process that uses marketing principles and techniques to change target audience behaviors to benefit society as well as the individual. This strategically-oriented discipline relies on creating, communicating, delivering, and exchanging offerings that have positive value for individuals, clients, partners, and society at large."[3] It can be said that when there is only a hammer, every problem is treated as if it were a nail. The wide variety of

problems with which health education specialists are faced requires the use of an equally broad array of tools and techniques. Expanding the repertoire of problem-solving, intervention-designing, and program-planning strategies to include marketing orientation, marketing concepts, and marketing tools can help health education specialists achieve their health education goals.

Marketing is a deliberately planned, orchestrated, and implemented *process* of providing mutually satisfying exchanges between the customer or client and the business or public health agency. In commercial marketing, a company succeeds (makes money) by accurately identifying the needs and wants of target markets and offering products or services that more effectively and efficiently satisfy those needs and wants than competitors' offerings.[3] Marketing cannot be successful if potential consumers do not attach greater value to what a company has to offer than what they—the consumers—already have or do.

Marketing first became popular in the mid-1950s among consumer packaged goods businesses such as General Electric, Procter & Gamble, and Coca-Cola. Its orientation toward satisfying consumers' needs differed from other commercial approaches that focused on getting a consumer's business either by offering low prices (made possible by low production costs), making the best possible product, or focusing on product promotion.[4] Marketing's appeal and success spread from packaged goods firms to companies producing durable goods (furniture, automobiles) for individual consumers and to industrial equipment companies. Soon after, service organizations such as airlines, banks, insurance companies, stock brokerage firms, colleges and universities, and hospitals were adopting a marketing approach—or at least claiming to adopt it. Next, business professionals, including lawyers, accountants, and physicians, became interested in marketing their services and professions. In time, more professions began applying marketing principles to their organizational development plans and program and service strategies. Eventually, marketing experts began to see the value of using commercial principles and strategies to address social issues.[5]

Social marketing "is a distinct marketing discipline [that] refers primarily to efforts focused on influencing behaviors that will improve health, prevent injuries, protect the environment, contribute to communities, and, more recently, enhance financial well-being."[6] Social marketing was first conceptualized in 1971 by two marketing professors at Northwestern University (Philip Kotler and Gerald Zaltman), who considered whether marketing concepts and techniques could be effectively applied to the promotion of social objectives.[7] During its 45-year history, social marketing has been used globally to ameliorate problems as diverse as handwashing, breastfeeding, responsible drinking, topping off gas tanks, composting, managing backyard woodlands, domestic violence treatment, encouraging savings accounts, and volunteer recruitment. Governmental organizations as diverse as state and local health departments—the Centers for Disease Control and Prevention (CDC), the National Institutes of Health, the U.S. Department of Agriculture, and the National Highway Transportation Safety Administration—have used social marketing. Nonprofit organizations and foundations have also been noteworthy users of social marketing, including the Bill and Melinda Gates Foundation, the Robert Wood Johnson Foundation, American Association of Retired Persons, church

denominations, Boys and Girls Clubs of America, United Way, Planned Parenthood, Rock the Vote, and American Red Cross, to name a few.

This chapter is not designed to teach the reader how to develop, implement, and evaluate a social marketing plan (see Additional Resources for guidance in this). Rather, it introduces the social marketing process, emphasizing concepts associated with a social marketing approach.

▶ The Social Marketing Process

The social marketing process is a program planning process with some major similarities and differences when compared with traditional health education program planning models (**TABLE 4.1**).[8] Though the jargon is different, the planning processes of health education and social marketing are similar. Both include assessing potential consumers and the intervening organization(s); setting clear goals and objectives; and planning, implementing, evaluating, and modifying offerings. There are several key differences. Marketers gather information about the groups they are working with through formative research activities in order to gain insight into the causes of the problem and the determinants of behavior. Using these insights, they segment the market of potential customers into smaller groups. Social marketers develop separate interventions for each segment using the marketing strategies. They pretest or pilot test the interventions, then monitor them along the way, making changes if an intervention is not having the desired impact.

Because success in marketing depends on achieving desired exchanges by satisfying the needs and wants of members of priority populations, social marketers begin with formative research. The first step is to identify the problem, which often begins with epidemiological and health services utilization data. Marketers then want to understand the barriers and benefits populations associate with the healthy actions. They also want to be able to understand the daily lives of the members of the populations of interest and

TABLE 4.1 Social Marketing Process

1. **Describe the social issue, background, purpose, and focus related to the problem or issue**
   - State the issue or problem you are addressing.
   - Provide background information establishing that the problem needs to be addressed.
   - State the campaign purpose (i.e., the intended impact, e.g., to reduce infant mortality).
   - State the campaign focus (i.e., the intervention focus you intend to take, e.g., improving access to prenatal care, providing preconception counseling, supporting effective contraceptive use to control timing, and spacing births).

2. **Conduct a situation analysis**
   - Perform a SWOT analysis.
   - Review similar interventions.
   - Perform additional audience research to fill in knowledge gaps.

3. **Select and describe the priority populations**
   - Use insights from your audience research to segment the population on key variables.
   - Describe the population in terms of factors such as demographics, psychographics, and behavioral variables.

4. **Decide on behavioral objectives and target goals**
   - Describe what, specifically, the behavior you want to support your population to do.
   - Use SMART goals to quantify the amount of behavior change.

5. **Describe the barriers and benefits for the priority population, competing forces**
   - List the barriers and benefits the population perceives related to doing the healthy behavior.
   - Describe any competing services, programs, or behaviors.

6. **Develop a positioning statement**
   - Describe the "personality" you want the population to associate with your service, program, or behavior that differentiates it from other similar offerings.

7. **Develop the marketing mix**
   - Develop the product, price, place, and promotion interventions that will lower the barriers and increase the facilitators for doing the desired behavior among your population.

8. **Develop a monitoring and evaluation plan**
   - State why you are doing evaluation (e.g., to track health indicators, for accountability to decision-makers, for increased program funding).
   - State to whom you present your evaluation findings.
   - State what you will measure (e.g., program and resource inputs, behavioral outcomes, impact on health status).
   - Describe the methods you will use, who will perform the evaluation, and when it will be done.
   - Describe the ways in which you might communicate your findings to different stakeholders (e.g., formal written report, PowerPoint presentation, social media posts).

9. **Develop a budget**
   - Note: A budget may already be provided.
   - Consider how much you will spend on each 4P intervention and on evaluation.
   - Consider other sources of funding you might access if expenditures exceed the available budget.

10. **Develop an implementation plan for the interventions**
    - Describe who will do what, when, using which resources.

Modified from Lee, L. R. & Kotler, P. (2016). Social marketing planning primer. *Social marketing: Changing behaviors for good* (5th ed.). Los Angeles: Sage. (pp. 51-52). Permission conveyed through Copyright Clearance Center, Inc.

what is important to them. Marketers often first turn to secondary sources such as journal articles and social marketing case studies. This can be easily done through social marketing literature, email Listserv, and professional online discussion groups. To obtain a more granular understanding of their local population, social marketers can use observations in the community, interviews, focus groups, and surveys of the affected groups of people already doing the healthy behavior as well as discussions with organizations providing similar services and topical experts.

Second, social marketers set an overall goal for their interventions (e.g., increase participation in diabetes self-management programs by 30% over two years). They may also set objectives for awareness, knowledge, and beliefs, but behavior change is the bottom line for social marketers. At this point, market segmentation occurs. **Market segmentation** is the process of dividing a heterogeneous population into homogeneous target groups by demographic, psychographic (e.g., attitudes, interests, values, lifestyles, opinions, fears, life goals), behavioral variables (e.g., benefits, barriers, use rate, readiness to change), and factors such as communication preferences or access to services. Commercial and social marketers often speak in terms of knowing the audience well enough to paint a picture of them. The goal is to know potential audiences so well that services, products, and programs are developed, priced, promoted, and distributed in ways specifically designed to meet their preferences.

The goal of all up-front research is for health education specialists to know and understand members of each key market segment to the point where they are able, in the next phase, to develop a **marketing mix** for each key market segment that meets or satisfies their needs. Developing interventions in the marketing mix involves the traditional marketing strategies of product, price, place, and promotion (the four Ps). Developing the interventions basically is a two-step process of initial design and test marketing. To make certain the marketing mix is appropriate, a pilot test (pretest) is essential. Pilot testing reduces the risk of product failure, agency embarrassment, and financial loss if any of the marketing mix

components are off target. The final steps in the marketing process are generic to all good program planning: program (marketing mix) implementation, evaluation, and modification.

▶ Marketing Concepts

A thorough understanding of how social marketing can be used requires an understanding of how traditional marketing concepts such as consumer orientation, exchange, market segmentation, formative research, demand, competition, marketing mix, positioning, and consumer satisfaction can be applied to health-related issues.

Consumer Orientation

To be a consumer-driven health education specialist, one should adopt a mindset of "the customer is king." **Consumer orientation** is the basic concept that an organization's mission is to bring about behavior change by meeting the priority market's needs and wants. It is recognizing that customers have unique perceptions, needs, and wants in which marketers must learn about and to which they must adapt. It means conducting formative research, because the most important activity in marketing oriented health education is learning as much as possible about the people whose behavior is to be influenced. It means recognizing consumers have their choice among competing services, products, and behaviors and, for whatever reasons, are more satisfied by the current offering or behavior. Last, it means believing the organization most knowledgeable about and responsive to consumer needs will "win."

Exchange

The concept of **exchange** is at the heart of marketing. It is the idea that people are willing to give up something of value or to experience costs (e.g., time, money, embarrassment, the discomfort of changing habits), in order to receive something they value (e.g., tangible products, confirmation of their identity, more energy to do a hobby, or

COMMUNITY CONNECTIONS 4.1

Marko, a health education specialist working at a local health department, was asked to design a childhood lead poisoning prevention program for families living in older homes likely contaminated with peeling lead paint and dust. An effective health education specialist, Marko has always been sensitive to the needs and interests of many stakeholders: his supervisors, staff, the agency, program funders, community members, local political leaders, and other actual and potential supporters. Thinking like a marketer, Marko realized he must also approach his latest challenge from the perspective of his potential clients. He realized that in order to design a program that would help reduce lead poisoning among children in the community, he needed to know all he could about the people whose behavior he would be trying to change. He realized that before he could jump in and announce any initiatives, he needed to see his clients as consumers whose wants and needs need to be satisfied if he wanted to be successful.

COMMUNITY CONNECTIONS 4.2

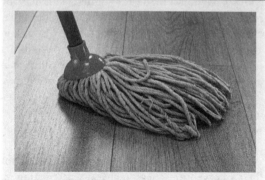

© taviphoto/Shutterstock.

While thinking about devising a home cleaning campaign to reduce lead poisoning, Marko asked himself, "What benefits can I build into my program that my clients would value and be willing and able to pay for in terms of their time, energy, and money? If I want parents to more thoroughly clean their homes to reduce their children's exposure to lead, what kind of a cleanup system are they able and willing to engage in that will reduce their children's exposure?" In thinking about his parental population, Marko realized these parents were young, juggling both childrearing and a job. They did not have much time and money to invest in the cleaning process. Given who they were, Marko contemplated what would be the least time-consuming cleanup he could ask them to do that would reduce their children's exposure to lead. Marko's question became "What can I ask them to do that they can and will do?"

living long enough to see a child graduate). The health education specialist and health agency also receive a benefit in the exchange such as professional recognition, improved health indicators, or, for example, additional funding from national agencies such as CDC. The exchange is voluntary on the part of the client because more benefits than barriers are experienced.

The essence of marketing-oriented health education is thinking "How can I lower the barriers and increase the benefits and facilitators for doing the healthy behavior for my population of interest, so that they voluntarily exchange what they are currently doing for the new behavior?" In short, "How can I make the healthy behavior 'fun, easy, and popular' to do?"

Market Segmentation

Because no single offering will please everyone, offerings are designed for and promoted to subgroups of the universe of all the people to be reached (the market). These subgroups or market segments are composed of members of the population united by a group of distinctive features, which become the focus of the marketing plan. For example, the market for smoking cessation offerings might be segmented by (1) a demographic characteristic (e.g., age, gender, education level, occupation, ethnicity, or religion), (2) a behavior (e.g., experimenting with smoking, social smoking only, smoking one pack a day every day), (3) an attitude (e.g., "my health is my business," "I wouldn't do anything to hurt anyone else," "I need to set a good example for my children"), (4) an opinion (e.g., smoking is not harmful, smoking can be harmful in some ways, smoking kills), (5) a value (e.g., family, excitement, professional development, control, independence, looking good), (6) barriers to the new behavior (e.g., access, time, lack of knowledge or skills, policy constraints), or (7) desired benefits (e.g., sex appeal, fitness level, pleasure, image, or social connection).

Formative Research

The point of **formative research** is to deepen an understanding into the determinants of healthy and unhealthy behavior and to answer the question, "Why do people do the things they do?" The insights gained help in developing specific interventions for specific groups of people that help them begin to do healthier behaviors. Traditional formative research techniques include interviews, surveys, and focus groups. Behavioral scientists and social marketing practitioners have come to appreciate that people cannot always explain verbally why they do what they do.[9,10] In recent years, social marketers have employed formative research approaches such as direct observation, journey mapping, drawings, and storytelling by the people to be served, and development of group personas to create deeper understanding.

Demand

Though the goal of marketing is to facilitate exchanges through the satisfaction of client needs, the frequency with which these exchanges or transactions occur varies depending on the market segment. In short, **demand** for services varies; everyone in a given market does not desire a particular service, program, or product all the time and at the same level. It would be ideal to have full demand for one's products, meaning that an organization or company has precisely the amount of business it wants. However, they vary because demands are human needs shaped by culture and personality and backed by purchasing power.

COMMUNITY CONNECTIONS 4.3

Marko knew he did not have much money to work with, but needed to find a way to divide his potential clients into categories based on some key defining characteristics. Based on his past experiences, he knew there were at least two types of families in his community—households with more than one adult working and living at home and single-parent households with limited income. He knew he would need to modify his initiatives based on whether or not they were designed for people with economic means and shared support at home. Marko planned to use what he learned about these two different groups to design different interventions for each, as he knew each group would respond best to the strategy specifically designed for it.

In considering how to design his different interventions for the different market segments, Marko realized that for each of the market segments he identified, he was going to have to determine the level of demand for a home cleaning program. When he discovered parents were interested in cleaning, but more so in the winter when the children were in the house, he used his knowledge of this seasonal demand to change what he asked parents to do at different times of the year. In the winter, he would stress cleaning and in the summer he would stress other activities like running the water before using it for drinking, cooking, or washing children's hands.

Competition

No matter what the topic or who is in the market segment, competition must be expected and addressed. **Competition** is any alternative to an offering. Sometimes, it is the same program or product offered by someone else (but who, perhaps, has more credibility) such as two smoking cessation programs offered by two different organizations. Sometimes, it is another (somehow more appealing) version of what is being offered—a prettier nicotine patch, a shorter series of cessation classes, or a more user-friendly self-help website. Often, it is a different and more appealing way of achieving the same benefits sought—a smoking cessation gum versus a nicotine patch. And, sometimes, it is something more compelling the consumer wants to accomplish before engaging in an activity such as losing 20 pounds before trying to quit smoking. Continuing the same unhealthy behavior—maintaining the status quo—is also a form of competition. The health education specialist thinking like a marketer will want to understand what the benefits are that the population receives from the competition.

The Marketing Mix

The marketing mix refers to the use of the four Ps—product, price, place, and promotion—of traditional marketing strategies, to create the conditions that support the population doing the healthy behavior. These strategies constitute the interventions the marketing-minded health education specialist develops to lower the barriers that prevent people from engaging in the healthy behavior. They work together, synergistically, so the impact of the sum is greater than the whole of the parts.

- *Product* is the "physical goods, a service, an experience, an event, a person, a place, a property, an organization, information, or an idea"[11] that satisfies a need for the population. Products have three dimensions: (1) the *core* product is the intangible benefit one receives from performing a behavior (e.g., getting a blood test for lead poisoning for a two-year-old child should give parents peace of mind or equal opportunity for their child, who may now escape a major handicap), (2) the *actual* product is the good or service one receives and special features of the good or service (e.g., physical components of the blood lead test clients can see such as a kind person drawing blood, clean equipment, and attractive bandages to place on the child's arm), and (3) the *augmented* product, which is additional elements that provide encouragement, lower barriers, or sustain a behavior (e.g., having a parent who has already had their child tested accompany the client, follow-up counseling support, and referral to other services).[12]
- *Price* interventions include anything that reduces barriers (e.g., financial, temporal, emotional, or energy) that the population perceives is a cost for performing the healthy behavior. Example barriers to receiving prenatal care and potential price interventions a marketing-minded health education specialist could help put into place include:
  - Lack of transportation (e.g., use health department van, provide vouchers for taxis or public transportation).
  - Financial cost of babysitters (e.g., provide child care at the clinic).

- Financial cost of prenatal care service (e.g., offer services free or on a sliding scale).
- Emotional cost of undressing before a health care provider and answering personal questions (e.g., offer a provider of the same gender).
- Time cost of taking an afternoon or day off from work (e.g., provide appointments after hours and on the weekends or arrange to provide appointments at the workplace).
- Worrying about what will be learned from the provider (e.g., allow the client to have a support person in the room or provide a patient navigator).

■ *Place* has both a geographical and a temporal aspect. It can refer to the physical location where the population is expected to perform a behavior or the location where a service is offered (e.g., buy fruits and vegetables at a farmer's market, drop off materials at a recycling center, nurse or pump breast milk at the worksite). Physical locations should be convenient and comfortable, have available important tangible items (e.g., recycling bins for plastic, glass, paper, and cardboard), or have staff prepared to respond to clients (if offering a service). A setting that is dirty, in an unfamiliar neighborhood, hard to reach, staffed with untrained or culturally insensitive personnel, not properly setup, or located "too close to home for comfort" among the people to be reached will jeopardize the exchange. The temporal aspect of place refers to whether there are particular times clients will be thinking about the health issue. For instance, people may be especially attuned to their stress level after work or at family holidays. This can provide an opening, for example, to promote physical activity or hints on how to meditate. Health education specialists should be aware of events occurring in local, state, or national news related to a health problem and prepared to capitalize on the extra attention provided. For example, news of flu deaths offers an opportunity to provide vaccinations. As another example, every

month highlights a variety of health issues (e.g., October breast cancer awareness). The national promotions associated with these provide an opportunity to highlight services an agency already offers.

■ *Promotion* includes both the health messages being provided and the communication channels used to provide them. The marketing-savvy health education specialist should always ask the people they are serving their preferred channels of communication, and then strive to utilize these as much is possible. It is appropriate that promotion is the last of the four Ps, because the marketer first needs to identify the product and have price and place strategies set up in order to have something to promote. Some authors have identified a fifth P, focusing on the people in which the marketing effort is being directed.[13]

COMMUNITY CONNECTIONS 4.5

Marko designed a separate offering for each of the major market segments he identified (i.e., young single parents and households with two parents). Each offering differed in terms of product, price, place, and promotion. However, Marko was always careful to make sure that from the client's perspective (1) the offering provided valued benefits, (2) there were few financial, temporal, emotional, and energy costs or barriers to the offering, (3) the offering was easy and convenient in terms of location, and (4) the strategies used to let people know about the offering were appealing, easy to remember, and credible.

When one of Marko's market segments did not respond to its marketing mix, Marko knew he had to examine all four components of the marketing mix—the product, price, place, and promotion—to see what needed to be changed. Marko, as a marketer, had to assume the exchange did not happen because he did not identify, understand, or respond to that particular market segment's needs. Marko then went back to the drawing board, studied his clients more closely, and, based on what he learned, revised the marketing mix.

Positioning

Positioning refers to how a behavior, product, or service stacks up against competing behaviors, products, or services. A well-positioned offering holds a unique place or niche in the consumer's mind. For example, imagine a consumer considering the purchase of an over-the-counter medication. One medication is designed to be and is promoted as "strong on pain, but soft on your stomach." This product was created for people who want something that fixes the problem but does not cause uncomfortable gastric side effects. It differs from a second medication for the same purpose that was designed for people who need to know their medication is actively working on their problem. Each medication has a different personality and was designed to meet the needs of consumers with different needs. From a social marketing perspective, a public health clinic may position itself as the place with the warm, helpful staff who know the community and who really care about their clients. It is important that an organization have in place the services, physical facility, location, and trained staff to enable it to uphold the positioning or personality it wants to put forth to the public.

Consumer Satisfaction

The goal of marketing is **consumer satisfaction**—giving people either what they expect or more than they expected. Some dissatisfied customers will do nothing about being dissatisfied, some will quietly defect from the service or organization, and some will tell people in their network about their dissatisfaction, creating negative advertising for the program. Conversely, satisfied consumers can become a key part of advertising. Marketing-savvy health education specialists should encourage satisfied clients to tell others about their experiences in order to enhance promotion efforts. Recent research in neuromarketing (using learning from neuroscience to understand how a brain processes experiences and emotions) has demonstrated the importance of providing a positive client experience to the acceptance of new information and the uptake of new behaviors.[14] Maintaining a client focus and utilizing insights from formative research helps ensure consumer satisfaction with delivered services.

COMMUNITY CONNECTIONS 4.6

Marko discovered that when it came to reducing children's exposure to lead in the home, single-parent households with lower incomes wanted a strategy that would not take much time and was not unnecessarily burdensome or costly (e.g., involving a lot of equipment and using products that had strong odors and were expensive). He realized he might get more people to adopt cleaning if he dropped his earlier push for the use of a special HEPA vacuum cleaner and focused on damp mopping. When that still did not work in a few cases, he realized he was going to have to sit down and devise an approach with those individuals' input, to determine what they would be willing and able to do. He had to change the product rather than hammer away at new promotion strategies for an unsatisfying product.

COMMUNITY CONNECTIONS 4.7

Marko knew people would be satisfied with their home cleaning experience if it met their expectations. Therefore, Marko's job was to control client expectations by giving them information about home cleaning that would lead to realistic expectations and a reduced sense of risk and uncertainty. He then had to make sure the home cleaning solution—the method and the people who taught it—met client expectations. Marko focused on the tangible aspects of the cleaning services he would offer, including an initial house cleaning and a demonstration of routine (twice a week) cleaning and exposure control (damp mopping and dusting). He put time and energy into allaying client anxieties by providing testimonials about the service from past users. He prepared the priority population for the service by thoroughly describing it and he developed a mechanism for feedback. He informed his staff to observe reactions and empowered them to do all they could within the guidelines of the agency to satisfy the population being reached. Before launching the cleaning services, Marko double-checked to make sure his services, procedures, and materials were user friendly, reliable, and culturally appropriate. He knew how important it was to try to see everything his agency offered through the intended audience's eyes. He learned a key marketing principle: The more he anticipated and satisfied the population's needs, the more loyal they became, resulting in the reduced risk of lead exposure.

▶ Overcoming Challenges to Social Marketing

Even with the many positive rewards to the social marketing process, a number of barriers may exist. Following is a list of common barriers health education specialists have encountered and suggestions for addressing them.

⊘ DID YOU KNOW?

The Social Marketing Association of North America (http://www.smana.org) offers free continuing education webinars, an email Listserv, and live Q&A sessions with experienced social marketers.

Dispel the Belief that Social Marketing is Cost and Labor Intensive

This perception originates from people equating marketing with promotion. As should now be evident, marketing is much more than just communication alone. Marketing is as much a

mindset—a set of different questions to ask—as it is a set of activities to be done. The social marketing mindset is very low cost and consists of thinking behavior change, knowing what is important to the population, thinking barriers and benefits for the healthy behavior, asking when and where is the audience is in the right frame of mind to be thinking about the health issue and open to doing something different, and asking when and where is the right place and time to conduct the interventions.

Other actions can be taken to minimize labor and financial costs. The social marketing email Listserv offered by the Social Marketing Association of North America (see Additional Resources) can be used to query other marketing-minded public health professionals. In addition, partner organizations could lend assistance, or, if located near a university, public health or marketing graduate students might be able to provide assistance.

Differentiate Social Marketing from Social Media

Since the rise of social media, some have begun to equate social media with social marketing rather than social media marketing. Helping others understand definitions of social marketing can help in differentiating the two concepts. Using images also might help. For example, social marketing can be described as the whole blueprint for a house, whereas social media is just one tool, like a hammer. Another image is social marketing is like a whole "salad of interventions," whereas social media is only one ingredient.

Differentiate Social Marketing from Advertisements and PSAs

This differentiation could be addressed by explaining social marketing uses the four Ps strategy, not just advertising. Sharing an example that differentiates the two can help others better understand the process. For example, asking someone to think of their favorite beverage refreshment and ask if it tasted bad was hard to find and cost $10 per cup, would they still buy it even if it had excellent advertising.

Address Agency Decision-Makers' Concerns

If resistance to using a social marketing-based approach comes from agency supervisors or decision-makers, it is best to be a good marketer and ask questions to determine the sources of their reticence! Resistance can be addressed by finding out what their goals are for the agency and see if the use of social marketing-based health education ties into it. For example, if the health director is interested in cost savings, it can be shared with her that a marketing mindset helps to focus interventions on the determinants of problems that are most likely to "move the needle" on remediating the problem. If questions arise as to whether or not social marketing is a vetted best practice, refer to CDC's *Gateway to Health Communication & Social Marketing Practice* and to other items listed under Additional Resources in this chapter. If decision-makers have a lack of knowledge about marketing approaches, a copy of *The Manager's Guide to Social Marketing* can help educate about the process (see Additional Resources). The Robert Wood Johnson Foundation's *Social Marketing National Excellence Collaborative* (see Additional Resources) was developed to help public health decision-makers understand

marketing and to support their staff's use of social marketing.

Address Concerns About the Ethics of Social Marketing

Possibly, the most often voiced concern about marketing (both commercial and social) is that marketing manipulates people into buying something they do not want to buy or doing actions they do not want to do. The image that comes to mind is of the unscrupulous used car salesman haranguing people into purchasing a clunker of a car. On the contrary, the experience of one of the primary authors of this chapter is that best practice social marketing honors the dignity and right to the self-determination of others. Well-done formative research ensures interventions are client-centered by allowing the practitioner to understand what is important to individuals— their hopes, dreams, fears, aspirations—and the circumstances of their daily lives. The concept of exchange then guides the marketing-minded health education specialist to look for ways that engaging in a healthier behavior will help people achieve something they want in their lives.

Issue is sometimes taken with the assertion that marketing approaches focus on reaching the "low hanging fruit"[15]—those who are most ready to change or who are easiest to intervene with— neglecting others who are affected by a health issue. For the social marketer, the low hanging fruit is the place to begin, not the place to end. Public health programs, by default rather than by design, seem to continually face resource constraints that cause them to limit their reach into affected populations. The social marketing planning process allows health education specialists to make these decisions thoughtfully, intentionally, and with compassion rather than allowing the decision to just happen. The agency then can look for other resources and means by which to reach more of the affected populations.

Social marketers may look for guidance to the American Marketing Association's Statement of Ethics.[16] As Lee and Kotler pointed out: "Many of the principles apply to social marketing environments...including do no harm, be fair, provide full disclosure, be good stewards, own the problem, be responsible, and tell the truth."[17] In addition, with any intervention approach, health education specialists should always consider the Health Education Unified Code of Ethics, especially articles I (Responsibility to the public) and IV (Responsibility in the delivery of health education).[18]

Keep Abreast of Emerging Influences and Tools

A strength of social marketing is that the field continues to grow based on advances in commercial marketing, communication, and other approaches for understanding behavior and influencing change, including social media and human-centered design. **Social media** platforms offer the marketing-savvy health education specialist numerous channels with which to engage populations of interest. The power of social media lies in its ability to allow health education specialists to follow, and then join, conversations people are having about issues that are important to them. Therefore, it can be used as a method of formative research. Social marketers can use social media platforms as part of their promotion strategies, but not as a "cyber brochure" to push out information to people. A more powerful use of social media is to engage the population in conversations and questions and answers about a health issue to elicit their ideas for solutions to health problems. CDC was an early adopter of social media channels to address public health issues, and provides a rich source of best practice guidance and case examples on the *Social Media at CDC* page on their website (see Additional Resources).

Human-centered design (also known as **design thinking**) borrows from the problem-solving process designers use to develop a deep understanding about problems in daily living and to generate creative solutions. There is an emphasis on understanding the experiences of users or individuals firsthand through ethnographic methods like direct observation, using cameras to record their daily life related to a problem, and telling stories about experiences.[19,20] Design thinkers focus on the experiences of those they call extreme doers and non-doers of a behavior. Focusing on these segments highlights the thoughts and feelings of people in the middle and provides insights into the emotions people associate with a behavior, product, program, or service. This approach exposes disparities between how consumers describe what they do and their actions in daily life. The approach also provides insight into environmental cues that prompt behavior (e.g., painted lines in a parking lot), thoughtless acts (e.g., looping the teabag string around the teacup handle), workarounds (e.g., labeling the plugs on an extension cord), and other surprising product uses.[21] From these observations, design thinkers create a journey map that graphically illustrates what people have to go through to perform a behavior. They focus on pain points, which are the barriers people encounter. Then, they use a system of brainstorming that generates creative interventions that can be rapidly tested and implemented.

▶ Expected Outcomes

Health education specialists can expect many benefits from using social marketing. Social marketing is an established, systematic approach in public health for creating the conditions to support social change and health behavior change. Health education specialists can draw on the 45-plus years history of social marketing that has been used globally to remediate public health, environmental, and safety problems, and used to address public health systems-level issues of funding and legislation.[2,8,22-25] Social marketing enables a health education specialist to get a 360-degree view of the problem as well as a 360-degree view of potential solutions. It allows for focusing on the determinants of behavior that are most germane, allowing interventions to be cost-effective. A social marketing approach opens up the intervention landscape, allowing the ability to use a variety of interventions by virtue of focusing on lowering the behaviors and increasing the facilitators related to the desired healthy behavior. Furthermore, the social marketing process enables one to tie the various interventions together, so they support each other and provide an effect that is greater than the individual parts. A marketing approach can improve buy-in to interventions and increase program effectiveness, because formative research can generate insights into what is important to the priority population and engage them to be cocreators of solutions. Social marketing brings together the expertise of public health professionals with the expertise of people living their daily lives.[26] Additionally, it is an approach that can be used downstream with affected populations, upstream with policy and decision-makers, and side stream with partnering organizations. Finally, because the science and practice of social marketing is always evolving, it allows the health education specialist to continue to develop.

---

⑦ DID YOU KNOW?

The government of the United Kingdom selected social marketing as its "go-to" strategy for addressing public health issues.

▶ Conclusion

Social marketing utilizes marketing principles and processes to create the conditions favorable for social change and behavior change to improve the health of individuals and communities. It provides a systematic, strategic planning process to create interventions that mesh well with traditional health education program-planning models.

Social marketing goes beyond promotion-only tactics, such as PSAs and advertisements. Rather, it utilizes the traditional marketing strategies of product, price, place, and promotion to create interventions that satisfy the needs of priority populations and meet organizational goals. The power of a marketing approach is grounded in understanding the wants, needs, fears, and daily lives of the people it seeks to serve as well as the barriers and benefits people associate with behaviors. Marketing-savvy health education specialists then use these insights to create interventions that lower the barriers and increase the benefits people want.

Social marketing has a history of addressing numerous health, environmental, safety, and civil issues. Health education specialists can draw on this experience and on the resources listed in this chapter, to create interventions for the health issues they face that will make behavior change fun, easy, and popular.

Key Terms

Competition Alternatives to a behavior, product, program, or service that have desirable qualities.

Consumer orientation The basic concept that an organization's mission is to bring about behavior change by meeting the priority market's needs and wants.

Consumer satisfaction The extent to which consumers' expectations of a product, program, or service are met.

Demand The degree to which a behavior, product, program, or service is desired by consumers.

Exchange A concept—central to marketing—that consumers must perceive that a behavior has more benefits than costs in order to perform the behavior.

Formative research An investigative method used to deepen an understanding into the determinants of healthy and unhealthy behavior.

Human-centered design (also known as **design thinking**) The problem-solving process designers use to develop a deep understanding about problems in daily living and to generate creative solutions.

Market segmentation The process of dividing a large, diverse population into subgroups based on shared factors that are key to influencing a behavior.

Marketing mix The combination of product, price, place, and promotion strategies created to support consumers performing a behavior.

Positioning Creating a personality for a product, program, or service that differentiates similar offerings.

Social marketing The systematic application of marketing principles to create the conditions for social and behavior changes that improve the quality life for individuals and for the community.

Social media Electronic communication channels that allow users to create and engage in online communities to collaborate and to share and comment on ideas and experiences.

References

1. Newton-Ward, M. (2012). Issues in the marketing and promotion of social enterprises. In T. Lyons (Ed.). *Social Entrepreneurship*. Santa Barbara, CA: Praeger/ABC-CLIO.
2. Smith, B. (1999). Marketing with no budget. *Social Marketing Quarterly, 5*(2), 6–11.
3. Lee, L. R., & Kotler, P. (2016). *Social marketing: Changing behaviors for good* (5th ed.). Los Angeles, CA: Sage.
4. Kotler, P., & Armstrong, G. (1998). *Principles of marketing* (8th ed.). Englewood Cliffs, NJ: Prentice-Hall.
5. Fine, S. (1981). *The marketing of ideas and social issues*. New York, NY: Praeger.
6. Lee, L. R., & Kotler, P. (2016). *Social marketing: Changing behaviors for good* (5th ed.). Los Angeles, CA: Sage.
7. Kotler, P., & Zaltman, G. (1971). Social marketing: An approach to planned social change. *The Journal of Marketing, 35*(3), 3–12.
8. Lee, L. R., & Kotler, P. (2016). *Social marketing: Changing behaviors for good* (5th ed., pp. 51–52). Los Angeles, CA: Sage.
9. Zaltman, G. (2003). *How customers think: Essential insights into the mind of the market*. Boston, MA: Harvard Business School Press.
10. Lefebvre, R. C. (2013). *Social marketing and social change: Strategies and tools for improving health, well-being, and the environment*. San Francisco, CA: John Wiley & Sons.
11. Kotler, P., & Keller, K. L. (2005). *Marketing management* (12th ed.). Upper Saddle River, NJ: Prentice Hall.
12. Lee, L. R., & Kotler, P. (2016). *Social marketing: Changing behaviors for good* (5th ed., p. 270.). Los Angeles, CA: Sage.
13. McKenzie, J. F., Neiger, B. L., & Thackeray, R. (2016). *Planning, implementing, & evaluating health promotion programs: A primer* (7th ed.). New York, NY: Pearson.
14. Shaw, C., Dibeehi, Q., & Walden, S. (2010). *Customer experience: Future trends and insights*. New York, NY: Palgrave Macmillan.
15. Hastings, G., Angus, K., & Bryant, C. (Eds.). (2011). *The Sage handbook of social marketing*. London, UK: Sage.
16. The American Marketing Association. (2017). Statement of ethics. Retrieved May 1, 2017, from https://www.ama.org/AboutAMA/Pages/Statement-of-Ethics.aspx
17. Lee, L. R. & Kotler, P. (2016). *Social marketing: Changing behaviors for good* (5th ed., pp. 493–496) Los Angeles, CA: Sage.
18. Society for Public Health Education. *Code of ethics for the health education profession*. Retrieved May 1, 2017, from http://www.sophe.org/careers/ethics/
19. Brunner, S., Waugh, C., & Kretschmar, H. (2007). Human-centered design, innovation, and social marketing. *Social Marketing Quarterly, 13*(3), 26–30.
20. Berger, W. (2009). *Glimmer: How design can transform your life, your business, and maybe even the world*. Canada: Random House.
21. Brunner, S., Waugh, C., & Kretschmar, H. (2007). Human-centered design, innovation, and social marketing. *Social Marketing Quarterly, 13*(3), 27.
22. Cheng, H., Kotler, P., & Lee, N. (2011). *Social marketing for public health: Global trends and success stories*. Burlington, MA: Jones & Bartlett Learning.
23. McKenzie-Mohr, D., Lee, N. R., & Kotler, P. (2011). *Social marketing to protect the environment: What works*. Thousand Oaks, CA: Sage Publications.

24. French, J., & Blair-Stevens, C. (2010). Key concepts and principles of social marketing. In A. Truss, J. French, C. Blair-Stevens, D. McVey, & R. Merritt (Eds.), *Social marketing and public Health: Theory and practice* (pp. 29–44). Oxford, UK: Oxford University Press.

25. Resnick, E. A. & Siegel, M. (2013). *Marketing public health: Strategies to promote social change.* J. French, C. Blair-Stevens, D. McVey, & R. Merritt (Eds.). Oxford, UK: Oxford University Press.

26. Newton-Ward, M. (2017). Social marketing in public health [Class notes]. Public Health Leadership Program, Gillings School of Global Public Health, University of North Carolina, Chapel Hill, NC.

Additional Resources

Print

Berger, W. (2010). *Glimmer: How design can transform your world.* Toronto: Vintage Canada.

Heath, C. & Heath, D. (2011). *Switch: How to change things when change is hard.* New York, NY: Broadway Books.

Journal of Social Marketing. Emerald Group Publishing Limited. Retrieved from http://www.emeraldgrouppublishing.com/products/journals/journals.htm?id=JSOCM

Lefebvre, C. (2013). *Social marketing and social change: Strategies and tools for improving health, well-being, and the environment.* San Francisco: Jossey-Bass.

National Commission for Health Education Credentialing, Inc. (NCHEC), & Society for Public Health Education (SOPHE). (2015). *A Competency-Based Framework for Health Education Specialists-2015.* Whitehall, PA: National Commission for Health Education Credentialing, Inc. (NCHEC) and Society for Public Health Education (SOPHE).

Weinreich, N. K. (2010). *Hands-on social marketing: A step-by-step guide to designing change for good.* Thousand Oaks, CA: Sage Publications.

Internet

Centers for Disease Control and Prevention, Gateway to Health Communication and Social Marketing Practice. Retrieved from www.cdc.gov/healthcommunication/index.html

Health Education Code of Ethics. Retrieved from http://www.nchec.org/assets/2251/coe_full_2011.pdf

International Social Marketing Association. Retrieved from http://i-socialmarketing.org/

National Conference on Health Communication, Marketing, and Media. Retrieved from http://www.cdc.gov/nchcmm/

On social marketing and social change. Retrieved from http://socialmarketing.blogs.com/

Rescue blog. Retrieved from http://rescueagency.com/blog/

Social marketing and public health: Lessons from the Field. Retrieved from http://socialmarketingcollaborative.org/smc/pdf/Lessons_from_field.pdf

Social Marketing Quarterly. Sage Publishing. Retrieved from http://smq.sagepub.com

Social Marketing Association of North America. Retrieved from http://smana.org/

Social marketing conference. Retrieved from http://thesocialmarketingconference.org/

Social marketing exchange. Retrieved from http://socialchange.ogilvypr.com/about/

Social Marketing National Excellence Collaborative (Turning Point). Retrieved from http://socialmarketingcollaborative.org/smc/

Social media at CDC. Retrieved from http://www.cdc.gov/socialmedia/

The basics of social marketing. Retrieved from http://socialmarketingcollaborative.org/smc/pdf/Social_Marketing_Basics.pdf

The manager's guide to social marketing. Retrieved from http://socialmarketingcollaborative.org/smc/pdf/Managers_guide.pdf

CHAPTER 5

Building a Health Communication Framework

Gary L. Kreps, PhD
Rosemary Thackeray, PhD, MPH
Michael D. Barnes, PhD, MCHES

▶ Author Comments

Having worked on health communication campaigns in community health education settings for a collective 90 years, we have found the work to be both exciting and challenging. We know that when health communication interventions are properly developed and implemented, they can influence health knowledge, attitudes, awareness, norms, and values, which are instrumental to changing health behaviors to improve health and reduce both chronic and infectious diseases. But properly developing and implementing health communication interventions is surprisingly complex. Effective health communication is so much more than writing a press release or a pamphlet. It involves careful planning; strategic analysis; thoughtful selection of strategies, settings, channels, and communication methods; and continual return to the consumers to ensure they receive the intended messages, understand them, positively respond to them, and adopt the intended health behaviors.

Accordingly, this chapter presents health communication interventions as a consumer-based health promotion process composed of several interrelated stages. We believe that if you understand the health communication process presented in this chapter, you will soon realize how powerful health communication is for any health education method you select for implementation. You will soon begin to strategically think about health interventions and apply sound communication principles to all your health education methods. This chapter has been written to reflect the best thinking that health communication has produced in the past 20 years. It will help you gain an appreciation for how intricate a process it really is.

Remember, success in health communication intervention begins with the consumer. The more you invest in your priority audience before, during, and after your interventions, the more effective you become in influencing change. Combine this investment in your audience with a willingness to think about health communication and a daringness to be creative, and you will soon realize how influential your work can become. Good luck in your efforts!

🔍 CHES COMPETENCIES

1.1.1	Define the priority population to be assessed.
1.4.1	Identify and analyze factors that influence health behaviors.
1.4.2	Identify and analyze factors that impact health.
2.2.1	Identify desired outcomes using the needs assessment results.
2.3.1	Select planning model(s) for health education/promotion.*
2.3.3	Apply principles of evidence-based practice in selecting and/or designing strategies/interventions.*
2.3.4	Apply principles of cultural competence in selecting and/or designing strategies/interventions.
2.3.6	Identify delivery methods and settings to facilitate learning.
2.3.7	Tailor strategies/interventions for priority populations.
2.4.1	Use theories and/or models to guide the delivery plan.
2.4.6	Select methods and/or channels for reaching priority populations.
3.3.2	Apply theories and/or models of implementation.*
3.3.7	Use a variety of strategies to deliver plan.
6.1.5	Convey health-related information to consumer.
7.1.1	Create messages using communication theories and/or models.
7.1.3	Tailor messages for intended audience.

*Advanced level competency

Reprinted by permission of the National Commission for Health Education Credentialing, Inc. (NCHEC) and Society for Public Health Education (SOPHE).

▶ Introduction

Health communication has become increasingly central to health promotion efforts during the last 20 years. For example, health communication plays a primary or contributing role in *Healthy People*, which in the 2010 version introduced a chapter dedicated to the role of health communication in promoting public health.[1] Yet, health communication is a very broad field of study that includes analysis of the interactions between healthcare providers and consumers in the delivery of care, the ways consumers seek relevant health information, the provision of social support, the preserving and sharing of health information using different media and information technologies, the sharing of health information for informed healthcare decision-making, the use of communication to coordinate interdependent activities between healthcare providers, the administration of personnel and resources within complex healthcare systems, and the development of health communication campaign interventions for health education and

health promotion. This chapter examines the role of health communication campaign interventions for promoting public health. When appropriately used, **health communication interventions** can influence attitudes, perceptions, awareness, knowledge, and social norms, which all act as precursors to behavior change.[2] Strategic health communication efforts can be effective at influencing relevant health behaviors and health outcomes because they draw on social psychology, health education, communication studies, digital information systems, and marketing to develop and deliver influential health promotion and prevention messages that appeal to unique audience capabilities and orientations.[3]

An early work that influenced the development of health communication interventions produced by the Office of Communications at the National Cancer Institute (NCI) was titled *Making Health Communication Programs Work: A Planner's Guide* (known as *The Pink Book* due to the pink color of the book's cover).[4] This guide stated that disciplines such as health education, social marketing, and communication studies all were important parts of health communication. It is not uncommon to hear it proposed that health communication may even be a better name for the profession than health promotion or health education—that everything done in health promotion involves communicating for health.[5] In fact, health communication has been defined by Everett Rogers, a pioneer in the communication field, as any type of human communication concerned with health.[6] The health communication field has been described as an interdisciplinary area of study concerned with the powerful roles performed by human and mediated communication in healthcare delivery and health promotion.[7]

Health communication intervention specialists examine the ways health issues are perceived by select audiences, how different audiences access health information, and what message strategies (campaigns) are likely to be most salient for these audiences.[8,9] For example, *Healthy People 2020* states, "Health communication and health information technology (IT) are central to health care, public health, and the way our society views health. These processes make up the context and the ways professionals and the public search for, understand, and use health information, significantly impacting their health decisions and actions."[10] The NCI and the Centers for Disease Control and Prevention (CDC) define health communication as "the study and use of communication strategies to inform and influence individual and community decisions that enhance health."[11] Still others speak of the concept by emphasizing the various forms of its applications, including media advocacy, risk communication, entertainment education, print materials, digital information systems, and interactive communication.[12]

It is a mistake to think about a health communication intervention as only a narrow strategy or activity, such as a press release or the type of interpersonal communication that might occur between a health education specialist and a client.[13] These are just a couple of the communication methods or tools that are used in health communication interventions. In effective health promotion efforts, a great deal of communication strategy and research lies behind the use of different interrelated communication tools, media,

and channels. Health communication campaign interventions must be guided by evidence-based strategies if they are going to be effective.[3] It is best to view health communication campaigns as a comprehensive process that frames the implementation of health promotion interventions in accord with the key information demands related to the specific health issues being addressed and the unique background factors that influence the audiences for whom the campaigns are designed. The way health communication interventions are viewed has a major influence on the ways they are used and the impact they will have. Because of the complexities of health promotion, it is best to develop strategic health communication intervention processes that actively adapt to the unique communication demands inherent in each health promotion campaign.[9] This chapter presents health communication interventions as a situational, consumer-based, strategic communication process with several sequential and interrelated phases. In this sense, health communication intervention is a process that can help guide the development of a wide variety of unique and strategic intervention methods used in community health education.

Health Communication as a Process

Experts in health communication confirm the need to define health communication as a systematic and strategic process.[3] This means that the mere presentation of health information or data does not equal effective communication. To the contrary, those who plan and implement health communication campaigns must recognize the complexities of disseminating relevant information to different audiences and the unique ways that different audiences may interpret and respond to messages sent. Savvy campaign planners use strategic communication design grounded in established communication and behavioral theories, strong evaluation research data, and active audience feedback to design, refine, and implement campaign communication strategies.[13]

Three well-respected and influential institutions that have assumed leadership roles in health communication have very similar outlooks regarding what health communication interventions are and how they should be applied to health promotion. The Office of Communication at CDC first introduced a digital training tool in 1999 called *CDCynergy,* which was updated and re-released in 2001, and then again updated in 2004.[14] *CDCynergy* is a six-phase tool—delivered in print and digital formats—that can be used to systematically plan health communication interventions within a public health framework.[15] Before the introduction of *CDCynergy,* CDC used a 10-step framework for developing and implementing health communication campaigns.[16] A health communication campaign model presented in the NCI planner's guide involves six similar steps.[4] Finally, a health communication campaign model developed by the Center for Communication Programs in the Bloomberg School of Public Health at Johns Hopkins University also promotes a six-step process.[17] All these models or approaches present health communication as a comprehensive and strategic process.

Although these health communication campaign models vary in terminology and sequence, they share several common features. All three models involve analysis of the health problem as well as consumer characteristics that contribute to the problem. They include strategic design of communication based on analyses of consumers themselves, market factors, and communication settings, channels, and methods that are most consistent with the needs of the priority audience and most likely to result in accomplishing predetermined goals and objectives. They also involve **pretesting** communication components with intended priority audiences before full-scale implementation occurs. These models involve managing the implementation process and performing adequate evaluation to ensure the quality of communication methods is acceptable and to measure the impact of communication methods with respect to behavior change and disease outcomes. In essence, this means health communicators must carefully analyze an audience and develop appropriate methods to bring about desired outcomes.[3,18]

Rarely is a community health problem solved by using only one method or solution. Rather, a multicomponent approach is most useful in finding answers to public health issues. Therefore, health education specialists can use health communication interventions to support a variety of other methods presented in this text, such as legislative advocacy, media advocacy, community empowerment, media tools, and building and sustaining coalitions. For example, health education specialists can use health communication methods such as press conferences or one-on-one interactions with legislators to gain support for enacting policies (e.g., a mandatory motorcycle helmet law).

Health Communication Campaigns

Promoting public health and preventing the spread of dangerous health risks are integral functions of communication in modern society. Whether focusing on the prevention and control of HIV/AIDS, cancer, heart disease, or violence in neighborhoods, a fusion of theory and practice in communication is needed to guide effective health communication promotion efforts. Health communication campaigns involve a broad set of communication strategies and activities that health education specialists engage in to disseminate relevant and persuasive health information to groups of people who need such information to help them lead healthy lives.

Health communication campaigns are organized and conducted information dissemination efforts designed to help groups of people resist impending health threats and adopt health-promoting behaviors. Typically, health communication campaigns are designed to educate specific groups (priority audiences) about imminent health threats and risky behaviors that are potential hazards that might harm them, raising public consciousness about important health issues. Health campaigns are designed to both increase awareness of health threats and to move priority audiences to action by making informed decisions in support of public health. For example, health communication campaigns often encourage priority audience members to make informed choices about engaging in healthy behaviors to resist serious health threats such as adopting healthy lifestyles (concerning exercise, nutrition, stress reduction, and other behaviors), avoiding dangerous substances (such as poisons, carcinogens, tobacco, dangerous drugs, or other toxic substances), seeking opportunities for early screening and diagnosis for serious health problems (such as blood sugar with diabetes and cholesterol with heart disease), and availing themselves of the best available healthcare services, when appropriate, to minimize harm.

Campaigns are designed to influence public knowledge, attitudes, and behaviors. Yet, achieving these goals and influencing the public is no simple matter. There is no direct relationship between the messages sent to people and the reactions these people have to campaign messages. Individuals' responses to messages are mediated by their unique cultural backgrounds, beliefs, attitudes, and experiences. Not only do people interpret messages in unique ways, but also they idiosyncratically respond to the messages sent to them. For example, it might seem like a very straightforward health promotion goal to ask drivers to use their seat belts when they drive. A very simple communication campaign might develop the message "Wear your seat belt when you drive!" For this message to influence drivers' beliefs, attitudes, and values, the campaign planner must take many different communication variables into account. Is this message clear and compelling for its intended audience? How likely are audience members to respond to this message? Will they pay attention to it? Will they understand the message? Will they agree with the suggestions made? Will they adjust their behaviors in response to the message? Campaign planners must do quite a bit of background research and planning to answer these questions. Effective communication campaigns use messages that match the interests and abilities of the audience for which they are designed, and convey these messages via the communication channels that priority audience members trust and can easily access.

▶ The Strategic Health Communication Campaign Model

Health communication is a process with several sequential and interrelated stages. Each stage aids in properly selecting and implementing health communication methods. The *Strategic Health Communication Campaign Model* developed by Maibach, Kreps, and Bonaguro (**FIGURE 5.1**) is a synthesis of models, principles, and theories that have been presented over the last 20 years and

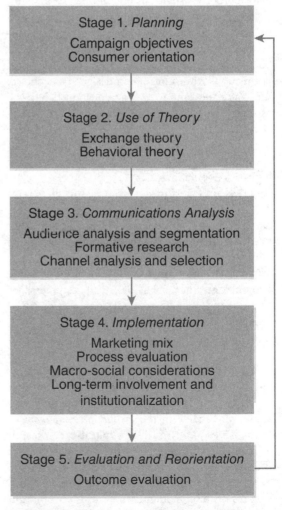

FIGURE 5.1 The Strategic Health Communication Campaign Model

represents the best of health communication's collective thought.[3,18] The *Strategic Health Communication Campaign Model* identifies communication strategies that incorporate multiple levels and channels of human communication. The model suggests that a wide range of different prevention messages and campaign strategies directed at several audiences will have to be employed to influence health knowledge, beliefs, values, and behaviors.

Effective health communication campaigns often employ a wide range of message strategies and communication channels (such as interpersonal counseling, support groups, lectures, workshops, newspaper and magazine articles, pamphlets, self-help approaches, digital health information systems, social media, mobile health programs, school- and primary care–based educational programs, billboards, posters, radio/television programs, and public service announcements) to focus on high-risk populations with information designed to educate, motivate, and empower risk reduction behaviors. Modern campaigns have become increasingly dependent upon integrating interpersonal, group, organizational, and mediated communication to disseminate relevant health information to specific high-risk populations.

Research performs a central role in strategic health communication campaigns. Data are gathered in the *planning stage* through **formative evaluation** research to identify consumer needs and orientations and in the communication analysis stage to focus on specific audiences, evaluate audience message behaviors, field test messages to guide message conceptualization and development, and identify communication channels with high audience reach, specificity, and influence. In the *implementation stage*, **process evaluation** research is used to monitor the progress of campaign messages and products and to determine the extent to which campaign objectives are being achieved. Finally, in the *evaluation and reorientation stage*, **summative evaluation** research is conducted to determine the overall effects of the campaign on priority audiences and public health. Note that the results of outcome evaluation research often identify new health promotion objectives and may initiate the planning of new health communication campaigns. This model

suggests that to maximize the effectiveness of health promotion efforts, health communication research must be used to guide the development, implementation, and evaluation of strategic health communication campaigns.[19]

Developing and implementing effective health communication campaigns is a deceptively simple enterprise. Health promotion campaign planners must recognize that mere exposure to relevant health information will rarely lead directly to desired health behavior changes. The *Strategic Health Communication Campaign Model* identifies five major stages and numerous key issues health promotion campaign planners should consider in developing and implementing health promotion programs.

Stage 1: Planning

The planning stage of the *Strategic Health Communication Campaign Model* addresses two major issues: setting clear and realistic campaign objectives; and establishing a clear consumer orientation to make sure the campaign reflects the priority audience's specific concerns and cultural perspectives. In setting clear and realistic campaign objectives, the campaign planner evaluates community health needs and deficits as well as examines the opportunity to introduce specific health promotion programs to improve public health. What are the objectives of the campaign? Is it to raise consciousness about a health issue, promote health education, change entrenched health behaviors, or maintain behavioral changes over time? Based on the campaign goals, different communication strategies will be needed. How realistic is it to introduce different health promotion programs within specific communities? What strategies are likely to be most effective within these communities? What is known about the health issues to be addressed? These are important planning questions that must be addressed before developing health promotion interventions. Campaign planners gather this information through **needs analysis**, often by examining available epidemiological data and reports about the health problems being addressed in the campaign. A **consumer orientation** means the whole campaign is designed from the unique cultural perspective of the priority audience and that members of the audience are involved, as much as possible, in campaign planning and implementation. It is important for campaign planners to understand the unique characteristics and needs of priority audiences as well as the best strategies for helping these audiences live healthy and fulfilling lives. Campaign planners gather information about the audiences they want to reach through a research process known as **audience analysis** that often involves conducting interviews and surveys of at-risk populations.

A crucial first step in the development of effective health communication campaigns is the identification and clear conceptualization of an important public health threat or issue that can be addressed by a communication effort. This means the threat addressed is genuine and of significant danger to warrant communication intervention. It also means the campaign planner understands the potential causes and solutions to these threats. There must be clearly identified and proven strategies for addressing these health threats that can be promoted with the campaign.

A primary goal of the campaign is to influence the way the audience thinks about the health threat. If the priority audience already believes this issue is very serious and of great relevance to their lives, this will lead the campaign planner to craft health promotion messages to support these preconceptions. If, on the other hand, members of the priority audience barely recognize this health threat and are not at all concerned about it, the campaign planner must design communication strategies to raise the audience's consciousness and concern about the threat.

Generally, campaign planners want to convince priority audiences to recognize and seriously consider the identified health threat. They want to influence the audience's beliefs, values, and attitudes about this issue to support the goals of the campaign. Only after a communication campaign raises audience consciousness and concern about the threat can it begin to influence (persuade) the priority audience to adopt specific recommendations for resisting and treating the identified health threat. The communication strategies used to raise consciousness and the strategies used to motivate action may be quite different. It is imperative the campaign planner understands the orientation and predispositions of the intended campaign audience to the focused health threats to craft the most appropriate and effective health promotion messages for this audience (audience analysis).

In this stage, the campaign planner evaluates the nature of the health problem (needs analysis) and considers possible messages and techniques that will influence the affected audience(s). Identifying the health problem involves articulating the health problem and identifying why it is a problem. There are many ways to approach this task. For example, it is possible to describe the death and disability associated with the health problem (e.g., health indicators, health behaviors), past and projected trends associated with the problem, costs associated with the problem (e.g., economic, social, environmental), or how the problem compares with other important health problems (e.g., why it is a priority health problem). Defining and describing the problem also requires identifying factors that directly or indirectly contribute to the problem. A direct cause is a behavioral, biological, or psychological factor that directly leads to the health problem. An indirect cause is a social, environmental, or political factor that exerts an effect on a direct cause (e.g., poverty, crime, lack of education).[10]

Stage 2: Theory

The second stage of the *Strategic Health Communication Campaign Model* uses relevant theories and models to direct health promotion efforts. Theories provide campaign planners with strategies for designing, implementing, and evaluating communication campaigns. It is recommended that a wide range of different theories be used to direct health promotion campaigns. Exchange theories,[20] behavioral theories,[21,22] and readiness-to-change theories (such as the Transtheoretical Model)[23] have been used in directing health promotion efforts at multiple levels (individual, network, organizational, and societal). For example, the Transtheoretical Model[23] assesses the readiness for change of priority audience members, and based on the members' current stage of readiness for change on any given campaign topic, the campaign planner can design the most effective campaign messages to influence movement through the stages of change to the adoption and maintenance of recommended health behaviors. This theoretical model provides campaign planners with important information about the most effective communication strategies to use with different audiences to influence their adoption of specific campaign recommendations.

Stage 3: Communication Analysis

The third stage of the *Strategic Health Communication Campaign Model* examines three critical communication issues in designing health promotion campaigns: (1) audience segmentation, (2) formative research, and (3) channel analysis and selection.

After the problem has been defined and described, it is important to identify a primary or specific **priority audience** that will receive the health communication. An analogy to define this process of narrowing a large population is the "shotgun and rifle" comparison. The shotgun approach represents a strategy that is widely implemented to everyone in a population. The hope is that enough of the population will become engaged in interventions and make the desired changes. In contrast, a rifle approach involves being more focused on a specific target. The term used to describe this approach in health communication is **segmentation**, which is the task of breaking a large population into manageable segments. Segmentation has been defined as a process of dividing a population into distinct segments based on characteristics that influence their responsiveness to interventions such as the product benefits they find most attractive or the spokespersons they trust the most. Programs that directly focus on a population segment are generally more effective because program efforts and resources can be focused on the specific wants and needs of that particular segment.

⑦ DID YOU KNOW?

Health communication played a primary or contributing role in the completion of 219 of 300 objectives in *Healthy People 2010*.

COMMUNITY CONNECTIONS 5.1

Olivia, the director of health education at an urban county health department, was assigned by her supervisor to assess the major health problems in her county and establish a priority health problem and focus. She and her staff began the task by reviewing all available mortality and morbidity data from the county. They collected and examined Behavioral Risk Factor Surveillance System data, Youth Risk Behavior Surveillance System, and other lifestyle risk factor data provided by the state health department, gathered data available from the county health department and visited the five primary care clinics and hospitals in the county and collected service, referral, and discharge data. After isolating what Olivia and her staff believed were the 10 most significant health problems in the county, they calculated several epidemiological rates, including years of potential life lost. They also assessed total economic costs and evaluated the general level of suffering, pain, and disability associated with each problem.

After analyzing and prioritizing the data, oral health was identified as the most important preventive measure among the county's vulnerable populations. Olivia proceeded to write a problem statement that defined and described the oral health problem in her county. It was determined that children aged 0–12 years are most at risk for missing school (Head Start, preschool or K-6) and that at least one parent is at risk for missing work hours. She found that low-income and minority parents had children who suffered twice the number of decayed teeth that had not been treated as compared to others in the county. Factors that directly led to the problem is an acknowledgment among parents and caregivers that oral health is important but that it is hard to help their children learn to brush twice per day. In this case, both parents and their children became the primary audience. Indirect factors included a lack of political and public health commitment to address the root causes of the health problem due to other more prominent diseases affecting adults.

Audience segmentation involves breaking down large, culturally heterogeneous populations into smaller, more manageable and more homogenous priority audiences for health promotion campaigns.[24–26] Segmentation requires the identification of a primary priority audience that shares common characteristics (e.g., levels of readiness for change, health beliefs) and that seems to be at highest risk for the health problem. Generally, demographics (e.g., age, sex, race, education, income), geographics (e.g., residence, place of work, cultural characteristics), or psychographics (e.g., attitudes, opinions, intentions, beliefs, values) are used to make initial decisions. Segmenting a population also requires identifying the following:

- The size of the subgroup or segment within the population.
- Where members of the segment live, work, or go to school.
- How the health problem affects the segment.
- The level of involvement the segment has with risk factors related to the health problem.

Gathering this information will allow a health education specialist to compare the relative merits of focusing on different segments and to decide on a final priority audience. The priority audience should be large enough and different enough from the general population to justify exclusive attention. The greater the cultural homogeneity of a priority audience (i.e., the more they share cultural attributes and backgrounds), the better the campaign planners are able to design health promotion messages for them.[27]

Campaign planners must identify specific (well segmented) focus populations who are most at risk for the identified health threats to be addressed in the health campaign. These populations of individuals become the primary audiences to receive strategic campaign messages. Too often, health promotion campaigns are used with audiences that are too broad and have different segments of people with very different attitudes and beliefs about the topic of the campaign. When this occurs, it is very difficult to generate uniform reactions to campaign messages. In fact, the campaign messages may work well with some segments of the population, but have negative ("boomerang") effects on other segments of the audience. This can result in negative campaign effects, where the campaign actually increases the negative health attitudes and behaviors it is designed to curtail. Sometimes, the health promotion messages are so broad they are not very effective at influencing segments of the population. It may be better to focus campaigns on a smaller and more homogenous (similar) audience with messages that are more likely to have influence.

Health communication campaign research focuses on the effective dissemination of relevant health information to promote public health. To develop and design persuasive health promotion messages that will be most influential with the specific priority audiences, campaign planners must conduct audience analysis research to gather relevant information about the health behaviors and orientations of priority audiences. Audience analysis also helps campaign planners learn about the communication characteristics and predispositions of priority audiences.

After segmenting the priority audience into the most culturally homogenous group possible, the campaign planner should gather as much information as possible about the group's relevant cultural norms, beliefs, values, and attitudes to guide the design of the campaign.[28] The more complete the audience analysis process, the more prepared the campaign planner is to tailor the health promotion messages to the specific needs and predilections of the priority audience.

It is necessary to gather input from the audience and perform assessments to better understand that audience. This process is known as **formative research**, which involves identifying the wants and needs of an audience as well as factors that influence their behaviors, including benefits, barriers, and readiness to change. Only after a priority audience has been segmented does the bulk of formative research really occur. Common formative research assessments include surveys, focus groups, in-depth interviews, expert interviews, opinion polls, and case studies. Formative research is used to guide the design and development of the campaign by gathering relevant information about the priority audience and their reactions to campaign messages. Formative research should also help campaign planners make knowledgeable choices about which communication channels to use in the campaign because they are most likely to reach and influence specific priority audiences.

Audience analysis is conducted to identify priority audiences' unique information needs, cultural characteristics, communication preferences and competencies, and any social/environmental factors that can either support or inhibit campaign implementation and success. It focuses on the distinct characteristics of the priority audience, including wants; needs; motivational and resistance points; general attitudes, behaviors, and preferences related to the health problem; what they know; what they fear; and how they will likely react to specific methods related to the health problem. Audience analysis is an attempt to get inside the head and heart of the priority audience and understand how they think and feel. Health education efforts that routinely include audience analysis as

part of formative research are generally more likely to develop interventions that ring true with consumers and produce the intended effects.[19,29]

The data gathered through audience analysis are crucial to identifying the most relevant priority audiences for communication campaigns as well as the most appropriate and effective communication media, messages, and delivery strategies to use with these audiences.

Formative research also involves market and channel analysis. **Market analysis** examines the fit between the focus of interest (e.g., desired behavior change) and important market variables within the priority audience. The term used in consumer-oriented communication and marketing for these variables is **marketing mix**. Marketing mix is composed of four components: product, price, place, and promotion, also known as the "four Ps." The *product* may be a behavior, a service, or product desired for priority audience use (e.g., a mammogram), or even an idea to be adopted. *Price* is the cost the consumer must pay

COMMUNITY CONNECTIONS 5.2

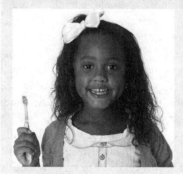

© Brocreative/Shutterstock.

Once Olivia had identified the priority health problem, priority audiences, and direct and indirect contributing factors, she and her staff became aware of a national communication campaign, *Two Minutes Twice a Day* (2Min2X) that could be tailored and implemented for her county. Several of the organizing principles of the 2Min2X campaign involved seeking audience input through formative research. After consulting with her supervisor and marketing specialists at the state health department, Olivia decided that in order to collect information from parents of children aged 0–12 years, particularly among low-income minority populations, she would contract with a local market research firm to conduct focus groups at six elementary schools in the county. It was decided her staff would also perform intercept surveys at local WIC clinic waiting rooms. Olivia also discovered that the oral health unit of the state health department recently conducted a statewide telephone survey of parents to determine the preventive and treatment actions needed for oral hygiene services. Because the survey report presented data by county, Olivia decided many of the findings could be used to assist her and her staff in their formative research process.

The focus groups and intercept surveys were designed to help Olivia and her staff understand the barriers, challenges, and concerns as well as the wants, needs, hopes, and aspirations of the priority audience related to factors associated with oral health. Formative research also addressed issues related to the marketing mix that would be helpful in sharing and effectively launching the 2Min2X campaign at the local level. With this information, Olivia and her staff were positioned to launch interventions for the priority audiences.

Source: http://2MIN2X.org

to adopt the new behavior. It may include money, time, energy, or convenience, to name a few. For example, exercise requires that a person exert a certain amount of energy and time to correctly perform the behavior. If those costs are too high for a consumer, the behavior will not be performed. *Place* is where the product is accessed or obtained. It is important to determine if the product is best provided in a setting that allows for social support (e.g., a class or group process) or if it is more appropriately distributed over the Internet, through the mail, via social media, or some other channel. Finally, *promotion* involves the methods used to communicate with the priority audience and is very similar to channel analysis. All the factors in the market mix are analyzed in the context of the priority audience and provide additional information to be incorporated in the development of settings, channels, and methods.

Channel analysis is a process that helps determine which communication settings, channels, and methods will most likely appeal to the priority audience. This includes an analysis of where the priority audience is most easily reached (settings), how they receive most of their information (channels), and their preferences for communication methods. **Setting** refers to the place or places where messages are best received or preferred to be received by the audience. It also refers to places where the audience can be reached and influenced to think about the message. Common settings for message delivery include homes, schools, workplaces, healthcare centers, retail businesses, community sites, churches, government agencies, libraries, malls, health fairs, coalitions, transportation devices, PTA meetings, and neighborhoods.

Channel analysis is concerned with television, radio, social media, and newspaper usage patterns; perceptions of who the priority audience sees as credible spokespersons; and computer literacy. For example, if the priority audience is young males aged 12–17 years, channel analysis may reveal that a significant percentage uses a particular form of social media multiple times throughout the day. It may be suitable to direct a portion of available communication resources

to this particular communication channel. In most cases, using multiple channels and methods increases the likelihood that the message will be heard and acted upon. If, however, the message is not consumer oriented and is not adequately supported by an effective market mix, the channel itself is relatively unimportant. That is why all these factors are analyzed in unison.[20]

⑦ DID YOU KNOW?

Health communication and health information technology constitutes a separate major chapter in *Healthy People 2020.*

COMMUNITY CONNECTIONS 5.3

Among other things, formative research indicated that although members of the priority audience understood the value of oral health, they did not know how to teach brushing skills nor was there consistent understanding about the need to brush twice per day for at least two minutes each. Furthermore, parents were generally willing to find a fun and easy way to help their children engage in the new behavior, especially for the "problem areas" of their children's mouths. It was discovered that the priority audience would make changes if they could find a new approach their children would like. They felt that brushing for two minutes, twice a day, could save children from severe tooth pain later. Their preferred communication channel was using the campaign videos to help their children mimic brushing behavior using fun and interactive video segments that could be easily displayed on hand-held devices.

With formative research in the forefront, Olivia and her staff studied the 2Min2X campaign materials and resources to assure the campaign was consistent with what they had learned about the priority audience. For example, Olivia found that media channels including television, radio, and print ads in English and Spanish along with social media banners were directed toward the main audience. With this in mind, Olivia decided to begin her campaign with health communication as the primary strategy.

Using the audience perspectives obtained through formative research, the health communication process focuses on identifying the messages, settings, channels, and methods that will compose the intervention strategy. Despite the additional work and resources necessary to obtain inputs such as proper segmentation and formative research, the payoff in terms of quality of interventions and successful outcomes is worth the investment. Note, however, circumstances exist in which identifying audience inputs is not feasible because of time or resources. In those rare cases, health professionals should consider all that is known about the audience as well as theoretical and best-practice perspectives to select the best combination of intervention strategies.

Stage 4: Implementation

The fourth stage of the *Strategic Health Communication Campaign Model* involves establishing effective strategies for implementing health promotion interventions. Successful health education practice involves much more than simple health fairs, media campaigns, and educational seminars. Although these techniques are valuable and widely used, leading health promotion experts have long advocated the use of strategies that encompass education and awareness along with other key activities. **Strategy** may be defined as a general plan of action that may encompass several activities and considers the characteristics of the focus population.[10] Strategy options help shape the selection of methods.

Strategic communication interventions often use **social marketing** principles to guide implementation of campaigns. The social marketing mix for the campaign involves evaluating the campaign process, identifying macrosocial conditions that may influence accomplishment of the campaign goals, and designing strategies for promoting long-term involvement and institutionalization of campaign activities with the priority audience.[28] Applying the marketing mix involves establishing a clear set of campaign activities and media (products) that promote objectives audience members can adopt with minimal economic or psychological costs (price) that are presented in an attractive manner likely to reach the priority audience (placement) and provide audience members with information about how, when, and where they can access campaign information and programs (promotion).[27]

Campaign planners identify appropriate intervention strategies (education, policy, health services, engineering, community mobilization) needed to modify the health problem. This includes determining whether communication is a primary or supporting strategy. For example, a media campaign intended to raise awareness about breast cancer (primary strategy) will use different methods from a health communication strategy designed to support passage of tobacco legislation (supporting strategy). It also involves creating messages necessary to support the selected intervention strategies. Selecting the appropriate setting—the place where the priority audience can be reached—is also very important. The best communication channels are selected (such as interpersonal, small group, organizational, mass media, social media, community, technology) to reach the audience. The best health communication media (such as press releases or conferences, presentations, counseling, web pages, social media apps, print material, or films) are also selected.

Once a strategy option (or options) is selected, messages to communicate to the priority audience need to be considered. The strategy selected will influence the type of message the priority audience will receive. For example, a water fluoridation campaign that focuses on building awareness through health communication may have the following message: "Water fluoridation is safe and effective for all, and will reduce dental decay by 38 percent. Contact your legislators and tell them you support improved dental health through water fluoridation." A policy/enforcement message could be as follows: "Water fluoridation is the most cost-effective approach to improve dental health among all citizens." A message to support engineering may be: "The monitoring and regulation of water fluoride in culinary water systems is the most sure way to decrease dental disease." A message supporting community mobilization may be: "Your elected legislator chooses not to support water fluoridation, despite the fact that his or her constituents overwhelmingly support this essential community priority. Your voice counts in making your elected official listen. Call 555-2222 to join your voice with others." Clearly, a well-designed health communication message is an important component of any type of strategy.

Effective messages are based on how the method will bring about change and appeal to its intended audience. Messages involve key points that will prompt the audience to an intended reaction. A message is more likely to be effective if it possesses specific characteristics that appeal and relate to its audience. Four characteristics should be considered when designing a message. The first characteristic is *quality*, which is often measured through appeals to emotion. Common emotional appeals include messages that are sad, funny, fear inducing, foreboding, one or two sided, fact or evidence based, implicit, or explicit. The second characteristic is *source*. A well-contrived message may be disregarded if it is not disseminated through an appropriate or credible source. Example message sources include celebrities, peers, government officials, physicians, counselors, nurses, scientists, news broadcasters, parents, teachers, religious leaders, administrators, and politicians. The third characteristic involves *internal factors* related to the audience such as attitudes, knowledge, values, behavioral intentions, behaviors, literacy level, race or ethnicity, psychological disposition, experience with recommended actions, skills, perceived susceptibility to and severity of health problems, readiness to change, concerns about approval of others, life goals, and self-standards. The final characteristic involves

external factors such as social support from family and friends, support from institutions, local media, social norms, socioeconomic status, political climate, laws, worksite policies, and access to health-relevant community services.

The implementation of many health communication messages includes the development of **supportive material**, which is defined as tangible items needed to support the health communication methods or messages. This supportive material helps enhance the message, improve its acceptance, strengthen its appeal, summarize its main points, and complement a message communicated through a channel within a given setting. Examples include media press kits, videos, posters, advertisements, thank you notes, fact sheets, social media posts, webinars, placemats, curricula, and program coordinator's guides (**TABLE 5.1**).

An essential component of any health communication activity is selecting the setting for communicating the message from those previously identified in the analysis conducted during Stage 3. Setting selection is related to both the message to be communicated and the strategy selected. The setting influences the types of ways or channels that can be used to reach a given audience. **Channel** refers to the means through which a message is communicated to a given audience. Selecting appropriate channels for an audience is often related to, or in some cases limited by, the setting or settings selected. The selection of appropriate channels is also based on audience feedback through the formative research activities described earlier. For example, if the home is identified as the prime setting, appropriate channels could include one-on-one home visits, technology

TABLE 5.1 Supportive Materials for Health Communication Methods

Brochures	Handouts	Curricula
Fact sheets	Public service announcements	Media press kits
Videos	Posters	Thank-you notes
Placemats	Program coordinator kits	Moderator guides
Advertisements	Bookmarks and stickers	Photovoice
Banners	T-shirts	Pens/pencils with inscriptions
Log books	"How To" handbooks	Scripts for oral presentations
Talking points	Hotline telephone numbers	Answers to frequently asked questions
Storyboards for television	Billboard layouts	Activities calendars
Bus/vehicle wraps	Health information websites	Computer health information portals
Mobile health programs	Electronic health records	Webinars
Health-related digital games	Infographics	Social media posts

via the telephone or Internet, or mass media via television or radio. The settings in which messages are to be delivered influence the types of channels needed to reach the priority audience. Many channel options exist, including:

- *Interpersonal channels*: Face-to-face or one-on-one interactions. For example, provider-to-patient sessions, peer counseling, and professional counseling are common ways to communicate health messages.
- *Small group channels*: Small numbers of persons often organized to receive educational messages or to interact with other members within that small group. Examples of specific channels include support groups, seminars, and classes.
- *Organizational channels*: Institutions or agencies that communicate messages to their members or that collaborate or communicate with each other and professional associations.
- *Mass media channels*: Mass reach media, including messages communicated via radio, television, school cable networks, newspapers, magazines, billboards, public transportation displays, and community newsletters.
- *Community channels*: A catchall category for channels that are not organizational in nature such as community messengers; community events; services or activities sponsored through malls, schools, hospitals, churches, libraries, or worksites; and open houses.
- *Digital channels*: The Internet, social media, interactive web pages, kiosks, videos, smartphone apps, and email.

Most health communication campaigns utilize mass communication channels (e.g., newspapers, radio, television) to convey health

COMMUNITY CONNECTIONS 5.4

Based on the process that had unfolded to this point, Olivia and her staff were now faced with promoting the media-based campaign throughout the county with particular focus on those with most risk. As Olivia and her staff reviewed data, they realized that several issues needed to be addressed in the design of messages. The main issues were that members of the priority audience felt the need for help in having brushing become fun and long lasting for their children. With that in mind, Olivia and her team identified a free gaming app from 2Min2X called *Toothsavers Brushing Game*. The app emphasizes specific behaviors that show how brushing removes food from their teeth and kills bacteria. Olivia's team felt the gaming app would be an effective way to meet the parent's desire for easily accessed and fun resources to be accessed at home.

In considering the quality of messages, it was determined the campaign's central messages reflect similar attitudes expressed in the formative research. Messages would be simple and would be enhanced by using the video demonstrations and allowing their children to play the interactive tooth brushing game. The campaign messages reflected vulnerable population characteristics deemed appropriate for the priority audience and their children. The campaign's internal factors were appropriate, because brushing was being made enjoyable and not a dreaded routine for parents or their children. Finally, external factors of the campaign messages were reflected in the social aspect of brushing through the interactive game app, thus reinforcing the value of the routine and the intrigue for unlocking more game characters as the children advanced along a map that helped overcome the curse that only brushing could end.

With the targeted resources available, Olivia and her team decided to pretest the campaign with the priority audience. Again, focus groups were conducted at six of the local elementary schools. Several videos were shown from the campaign website and screenshots of the Toothsavers Brushing Game app were presented. At the WIC clinics, intercept interviews were conducted that presented the same videos and screenshots. Based on feedback received from the priority audience, several videos were emphasized as being most appealing to the audience and the game app was recognized as a useful tool because the app was free and could be downloaded on Android and Apple mobile devices.

promotion messages to large and sometimes diverse audiences. These channels for communication often have the ability to reach many people over vast geographic distances. There is a trade-off, however, with the use of different communication channels. Some channels are more personal and dramatic than other channels, resulting in some more likely to be trusted than others. It is important for campaigns to match the use of communication channels and messages to the demands of the campaign and the message/channel preferences of priority audiences.

Stage 5: Evaluation and Reorientation

The fifth and final stage of the *Strategic Health Communication Campaign Model* is when a

summative evaluation (evaluation of campaign outcomes) is conducted to determine the relative success of the campaign in achieving its goals at an acceptable cost as well as to identify areas for future health promotion interventions. The information gathered through such outcome

COMMUNITY CONNECTIONS 5.5

With successful pretesting results, Olivia and her colleagues were able to promote the campaign. Easily accessed material in the convenience of their home was particularly meaningful to the audience and would be central to making the video and game app useful and sustainable. Olivia's next task was to determine how and through whom the messages would be delivered to the priority audience.

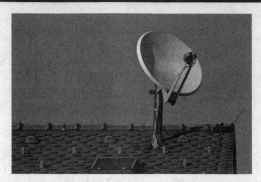

© foto.fritz/Shutterstock.

Through the formative research process, Olivia and her staff found the need to reach both parents and their young children. Many parents reported they would like to hear about the campaign on various radio stations that were classified as reaching young adults or those reaching Spanish-speaking or other ethnic-focused media channels. Parents felt that waiting rooms at prenatal or WIC clinics would be appropriate ways to promote the campaign. Additional channels determined to be important included infographic and print-based content material, specifically through web- and social media-based sources. These channels were believed to be important because campaign materials were readily available and were attractively designed to appeal to both parents and their young children. Finally, from the 2Min2X campaign implementation guidelines, Olivia and her team recognized that children could receive material and be shown video segments in their Head Start, preschool, or K-6 environments during snack time. These materials could be brought home by the children and promoted to a parent or caregiver.

Process evaluation is used to keep track of and assess campaign activities to identify areas for fine-tuning campaign communication efforts. Because priority audiences reside within and are interdependent with the larger society, campaign planners must attempt to involve these larger social systems (such as business organizations and government agencies) in supporting and participating in campaign activities. Furthermore, to make sure the campaign's health promotion goals and activities are fully implemented and established into the life of the priority audience, the campaign planner should design strategies for the audience's long-term involvement and the institutionalization of these activities as a regular part of the consumer's daily life. An excellent strategy for such institutionalization is to empower priority audience members to get personally involved with implementing and managing campaign programs. In doing so, they have a greater stake in achieving campaign goals, and the campaign activities become part of the audience's normative cultural activities.

Olivia discovered that the 2Min2X campaign was readily accessed using geographically focused analytics set up by the 2min2X website. Olivia also learned that messages on radio stations, in particular, prompted spikes in the campaign website for the county's geographical area. Staff at the WIC and prenatal clinics indicated to Olivia that when the website was emphasized on the print material and social media forums, these resources were well received. With this information, Olivia and her staff found sufficient evidence that their planned approach to use health communication methods had promising indications that children's brushing behaviors would be changed. This confidence was particularly strengthened as evidence from other communities and published works were found.

evaluations reorients campaign planners to the unmet health needs of the priority audience, inevitably leading campaign planners back to the first stage of the model (planning), where they identify new health promotion goals for future communication campaigns.

▶ Practical Application of the Health Communication Process

This section provides practical, real-life examples of health communication in community health promotion, including primary and supportive strategies. In particular, the application of two successful primary strategies and two supporting health communication campaigns are used to demonstrate the health communication process.

Health Communication as a Primary Strategy

Health communication as a primary strategy is most appropriate when the goal is to increase awareness or knowledge about a particular health issue among members of a certain population. Many primary strategy examples have been applied in public health settings, with two well-known ones being the *One and Only One* and *Great American Smokeout* campaigns.

One and Only One

The *One and Only One* campaign is an example of health communication as a primary strategy.[30] This campaign started because healthcare providers were using syringes more than once, which meant patients were being exposed to infections such as hepatitis and HIV. The campaign aims to increase awareness of safe injection practices among both healthcare providers and patients. The main idea of the campaign is that by following safe injection practices, unnecessary infections can be prevented. The goal of the *One and Only One* campaign is to "ensure patients are protected each and every time they receive a medical injection."

This campaign uses a variety of multimedia materials to convey its message including print posters, flyers, pocket cards, infographics, videos, electronic images, and so forth. In addition, the campaign also utilizes a variety of social media platforms, including Facebook, Twitter, Pinterest, YouTube, and others. On the campaign website, toolkits are available for healthcare providers and state and local health departments. These toolkits allow local areas to customize the campaign and use the resources as part of their websites, in healthcare facility waiting rooms, at health fairs, and in other public gatherings. In addition, educational materials for healthcare providers and patients are available on the *One and Only One* website (see Additional Resources).

The *One and Only One* campaign began with 20 founding coalition members. It has now evolved to include over 100 diverse partner organizations that are committed to improving patient safety and health care. This is an example of how communities can collaboratively work and use health communication to raise awareness and improve health.

Great American Smokeout

Another example of health communication as a primary strategy is the *Great American Smokeout* (GAS) sponsored by the American Cancer Society.[31] The GAS began in the 1970s and is now an annual event held on the third Thursday of November, with the purpose of encouraging smokers to quit tobacco use for just one day in anticipation that they will become permanently smoke free.

Health education specialists in local communities and in health systems can sponsor events to support the GAS. The GAS website provides toolkits with ideas and resources for individualizing the experience. For example, a display in a main gathering area of a worksite such as a lobby or cafeteria can include a display of educational pamphlets or brochures that highlight the risks of smoking and tips for quitting tobacco use. Worksite events may include employees signing quit cards and promising to be smoke free for the day or longer. Employees also could be provided with the opportunity to register for smoking cessation classes either onsite or at a nearby location. For people who are creative, videos can be made highlighting successful quitters and recognizing their accomplishments. Another health communication method could be classes or presentations such as a lunchtime seminar on smoking cessation or a related topic. The GAS website provides many social media tools and technologies to communicate the no smoking message. These include a Quit for Life mobile app, cover images for Facebook and Twitter accounts, options for telephone counseling when trying to quit smoking, Instagram images, print ads and much more. In one community, a partnership was created between the schools and local supermarket to promote the no smoking message. Students drew pictures relating to smoking and health on paper grocery sacks. On the day of the GAS, store patrons' groceries were placed in these bags.

Mass media channels can also be used in an event such as the GAS. The health communication method could include a press conference held at a local elementary school with a press release being the supporting material. The news story could highlight students who have pledged to be smoke free and not use tobacco during the GAS. It could also emphasize the health risks of smoking and the reasons to quit.

⑦ DID YOU KNOW?

The Centers for Disease Control and Prevention, National Institutes of Health, and National Cancer Institute each have an office of communications that directly reports to the agency director.

Health Communication Supporting Other Strategies

As previously mentioned, health communication is rarely used as an independent strategy to address a public health need. In a multicomponent approach, however, a health communication strategy is an integral part of all other health promotion strategies, whether policy, engineering, health services, or community mobilization. The successful implementation of these strategies relies, in part, on effective health communication. The following scenarios are illustrations of cases in which strategies other than health communication were the primary focus, but in which health communication was relied on to fully and effectively implement the strategies.

The Bully Project

The Bully Project (TBP) was formed to implement a school and community-centered campaign around the film *Bully*.[32] The documentary showcases five youth who endure persecution from their peers, and discusses the bullying of children and teens in U.S. schools. The TBP website points out that more than 13 million young people experience some form of bullying (physical, verbal, or online) each year.[32] The negative outcomes of bullying includes depression, anxiety, interpersonal violence, substance abuse, poor social functioning, poor school performance and attendance, and suicide.[33]

When TBP started its campaign in 2011, the primary goal was to educate children by sharing materials for teachers to implement lessons from the film. The project, however, also emerged as a way to impact adults in the school community. Currently, TBP promotes mobilization and policy advocacy through localized teams in 40 states to address bullying laws in their communities. As such, TBP is an example of a secondary communication campaign. It uses communication to advance local mobilization and policy advocacy rather than simply using information to affect awareness.

The TBP website has many resources and tools available for educators, students, parents, and advocates in the school's environment. A popular resource known as *10 Million Kids* urges schools to become involved using many organizing and message materials.[34] To launch the campaign, school staff view *Bully* and begin to prepare for conversations with students. The goal is to create strong, caring school communities involving many stakeholders—students, staff, parents, and elected officials (mayors, legislators). Materials are available not only for school screenings, but also through hosted community events such as home screenings/parties and community screenings.

TBP has produced positive impacts. For example, according to TBP's website, schools in over 3,000 cities and 7 countries have reached approximately four million students. In essence, though bullying occurs within a larger social context, TBP uses communication to affect relationships developed in the school in order to set the stage for communities to help reduce bullying.

Prescription Drug Disposal

With the increase in deaths due to opioid abuse, law enforcement agencies, health officials, and community members have come together to find solutions. One approach has been to reduce access to unused prescription medications. Recent federal regulations have made it easier for people to dispose of medications they no longer need by designating sites in communities as permanent drop-off locations. Other key activities in this ongoing effort are one-day "take back" events held in the spring and fall of each year in communities across the United States.

These take back events are an opportunity for people to stop by public sites such as grocery stores or pharmacies that have been designated as drop-off places for unused prescription medications. In 2016, there were over 4,000 community partners and just over 5,000 sites that participated. Since the start of the take back events, over seven million pounds of unused prescriptions have been collected.[35] Promotion of these biannual events include use of communication tools such as news releases, Twitter posts, billboards, and fliers, among others. To publicize the permanent drop-off locations in Washington State, for example, the local poison control center hosts a website where people can search for the location nearest them.[36]

In addition to reducing the supply of prescription medications, the Drug Enforcement Agency works with community partners to provide community outreach with information and awareness about drug abuse prevention. Their website provides a wealth of information that teachers, parents, and others may use.

---

⑦ DID YOU KNOW?

Many public service announcement campaigns include a mascot—Smokey the Bear, Woodsey the Owl, Vince and Larry the Crash Test Dummies, McGruff the Crime Dog, Daren the Lion for D.A.R.E., and more. Only Smokey the Bear, however, has his own zip code. That is because he was receiving a lot of fan mail from kids around the United States.

▶ Overcoming Challenges to Effective Health Communication

Perhaps, the most common barriers encountered in implementing the health communication process include limited or no audience input and the subsequent lack of audience feedback and pretesting. Why are these components often overlooked? The simple and most common cause is a lack of time or resources. It is true that seeking such consumer input and feedback takes time and costs money. To improve the odds of an effective program and maximize long-term impact, these barriers should be hurdled in whatever way possible. Audience members can provide valuable input into message design and implementation strategies through a process of "user-centered design," as they have in-depth personal knowledge and experience with the ways priority audiences communicate.[31,32]

Certain legitimate circumstances may warrant not seeking an audience's perspectives. One example is risk communication, which involves the immediate need to notify key officials and audiences that may be affected by a health danger. In cases such as these—when the urgency of the message is more important than how the message will be received and accepted by the audience—there are justifiable reasons to avoid audience perspectives. Fortunately, most messages are not designed for these kinds of conditions.

Barring a nonsupportive administrator, having few resources, or having nonresponsive priority audiences, many of these barriers can be overcome. Perhaps, the most effective way to jump the hurdle of lack of audience input and feedback may be to plan for it when budgets are created, discuss its importance to key stakeholders and administrators, and learn as much as possible about it as a barrier. From the authors' perspectives, some of the most enjoyable community health projects engaged in were due to the direct involvement with audiences.

⑦ DID YOU KNOW?

The first phone call from a mobile phone (or what we now call cell phone) was made in New York City in 1973.

▶ Conclusion

Health behaviors and health status are influenced by a variety of factors; therefore, the use of strategic communication intervention to address these health problems must also be multifaceted. Knowledge and awareness about health, disease, wellness, or risk factors within a focus population are not enough to significantly improve the health of a community. A system or environment that facilitates, encourages, and supports healthy lifestyles must exist. Consequently, health communication is rarely used as an independent strategy in community health. Rather, health education specialists use several strategies to address a particular health issue within the community.

The process presented in this chapter is useful in planning effective messages that link a combination of strategies. This process also is important in helping the reader obtain essential audience perspectives to select appropriate methods for the health problem faced by a priority population. By considering the unique health problems of a community, the most important health information needs of an audience can be identified and campaign goals can be established. Campaign messages needed to reach and influence priority audiences must be developed from the audience perspective. These strategies include strategic message design, selecting the settings where the audience can best be reached, and determining the best channels for reaching the intended audience. Relevant theory and research are used to guide strategic health communication interventions as well as to evaluate their effectiveness and future directions for intervention.

⑦ DID YOU KNOW?

Public health posters became more prominent during World War I to warn soldiers about potential risks of sexually transmitted diseases and alcohol. Famous French artists, including Lucien Levy-Dhurmer and Jules-Abel Faivre, helped create some of the posters in Europe.

Key Terms

Audience analysis Formative evaluation research conducted to learn about the experiences, orientations, and communication competencies of priority campaign audiences.

Audience segmentation The process of breaking down large, culturally heterogeneous populations into smaller, more manageable and more homogenous priority audiences for health promotion campaigns.

Channel The route through which communication or message delivery occurs (e.g., interpersonal, small group, organizational, mass media, community, technology).

Channel analysis A process that helps determine which communication settings, channels, and methods will most likely appeal to the priority audience.

Consumer orientation Designing the campaign from the unique cultural perspective of the priority audience and where members of the audience are involved.

Formative evaluation Gathering relevant data about the health issues and audience factors relevant to designing a health communication campaign.

Formative research Gathering inputs from a priority audience and performing assessments to better understand that audience. Formative research involves audience, market, and channel analyses.

Health communication interventions The crafting and delivery of messages and strategies, based on consumer research, to inform and influence individual and community decisions that enhance health.

Market analysis Examines the fit between the focus of interest and important market variables within the priority audience.

Marketing mix The combination of product, price, place, and promotion strategies created to support consumers performing a behavior.

Needs analysis Formative evaluation research conducted to learn about the specific health issues being addressed by health communication campaigns.

Pretesting Evaluating the impact of communication strategies on priority audiences before implementing these strategies within health promotion campaigns.

Priority audience Distinct groups that are like each other in key ways and have a high likelihood of responding to a given message, service, or product in similar or predictable ways.

Process evaluation Gathering relevant data about the ways that representative audience members are responding to campaign messages to guide refinement of the messages.

Segmentation The process of dividing a population into distinct segments based on characteristics that influence their responsiveness to interventions such as products, services, or messages.

Setting The place where the priority audience can be reached most effectively.

Social marketing The systematic application of marketing principles to create the conditions for social and behavior changes that improve the quality life for individuals and for the community.

Strategy A general plan of action that may encompass several activities and that considers the characteristics of the priority population.

Summative evaluation Gathering data about the influences of the campaign on achieving desired cognitive, behavioral, physiological, and economic outcomes.

Supportive material Tangible items needed to support the communication methods or messages by enhancing the message, improving its acceptance, strengthening its appeal, summarizing its main points, and complementing the message.

References

1. Department of Health and Human Services. (1998). *Healthy People 2010 objectives: Draft for public comment.* Washington, DC: Office of Public Health and Science.
2. Kreps, G. L., Query, J. L., & Bonaguro, E. W. (2010). The interdisciplinary study of health communication and its relationship to communication science. In L. Lederman (Ed). *Beyond these walls: Readings in health communication* (pp. 2–13). London, UK: Oxford University Press.
3. Maibach, E. W., Kreps, G. L., & Bonaguro, E. W. (1993). Developing strategic communication campaigns for HIV/AIDS prevention. In S. Ratzan (Ed.), *AIDS: Effective health communication for the 90s* (pp. 15–35). Washington, DC: Taylor and Francis.

4. Department of Health and Human Services. (2004). *Making health communication programs work: A planner's guide* (2nd ed.) (NIH Publication No. T-068). Washington, DC: Office of Cancer Communications, National Cancer Institute, National Institutes of Health. Retrieved May 1, 2017, from http://www.cancer.gov/publications/health-communication/pink-book.pdf

5. Kreps, G. L., & Maibach, E. W. (2008). Transdisciplinary science: The nexus between communication and public health. *Journal of Communication*, *58*(4), 732–748.

6. Rogers, E. M. (1996). The field of health communication today: An up-to-date report. *Journal of Health Communication*, *1*, 15–23.

7. Kreps, G. L. (2014). Health communication, history of. In T. L. Thompson (Ed.), *Encyclopedia of health communication* Vol. 2 (pp. 567–571). Los Angeles, CA: Sage Publications.

8. Kreps, G. L., & Neuhauser, L. (2015). Designing health information programs to promote the health and well-being of vulnerable populations: The benefits of evidence-based strategic health communication. In C. A. Smith & A. Keselman (Eds.), *Meeting health information needs outside of healthcare: Opportunities and challenges* (pp. 3–17). Waltham, MA: Chandos Publishing.

9. Kreps, G. L. (2006, June 7). One size does not fit all: Adapting communication to the needs and literacy levels of individuals. *Annals of Family Medicine* (online, invited commentary). Retrieved May 1, 2017, from http://www.annfammed.org/cgi/eletters/4/3/205

10. U.S. Department of Health and Human Services, Healthy People 2020. *Health communication and information technology.* Retrieved May 1, 2017, from http://www.healthypeople.gov/2020/topics-objectives/topic/health-communication-and-health-information-technology

11. National Prevention Information Network, Centers for Disease Control and Prevention. *Health communication strategies.* Retrieved May 1, 2017, from http://npin.cdc.gov/pages/health-communication-strategies

12. Kreps, G. L. (2012). Health communication. In J. M. Rippe (Ed.), *Encyclopedia of Lifestyle Medicine and Health* (pp. 542–546). Thousand Oaks, CA: Sage Publications.

13. Kreps, G. L. & Neuhauser, L. (2015). Designing health information programs to promote the health and well-being of vulnerable populations: The benefits of evidence-based strategic health communication. In C.A. Smith & A. Keselman (Eds.), *Meeting health information needs outside of healthcare: Opportunities and challenges* (pp. 3–17). Waltham, MA: Chandos Publishing.

14. Centers for Disease Control and Prevention. (2004). CDCynergy Social marketing Edition: Your guide to audience-based program planning: The study and use of communication strategies to inform and influence individual and community decisions that enhance health.

15. Centers for Disease Control. (2003). *CDCynergy 3.0: Your guide to effective health communication.* Public Health Foundation.

16. Roper, W. L. (1993). Health communication takes on new dimensions at CDC. *Public Health Reports*, *108*, 179–183.

17. Center for Communication Programs. (1998). *Strategic communication: Making a difference.* Baltimore, MD: School of Hygiene and Public Health, Johns Hopkins University.

18. Kreps, G. L. (2014). Health campaigns. In W. C. Cockerham, R. Dingwall & S. Quah (Eds.), *The Wiley-Blackwell encyclopedia of health, illness, behavior and society* (pp. 769–772). New York, NY: Wiley-Blackwell.

19. Kreps, G. L. (2014*).* Evaluating health communication programs to enhance health care and health promotion. *Journal of Health Communication*, *19*(12), 1449–1459.

20. Lefebvre, C. & Flora, J. (1988). Social marketing and public health intervention. *Health Education Quarterly*, *15*, 299–315.

21. Bandura, A. (1986). *Social foundations of thought and action: A social cognitive approach.* Englewood Cliffs, NJ: Prentice Hall.

22. Rogers, E. M. (1983). *Diffusion of innovations.* New York, NY: Free Press.

23. Prochaska, J. & DiClemente, C. (1984). *The transtheoretical approach: Crossing traditional boundaries of therapy.* Homewood, IL: Dow Jones Irwin.

24. Forthofer, M. S. & Bryant, C. A. (2000). Using audience-segmentation techniques to tailor health behavior change strategies. *American Journal of Health Behavior, 24,* 36–43.

25. Slater, M. D. (1996). Theory and method in health audience segmentation. *Journal of Health Communication, 1,* 267–284.

26. Slater, M. D., Kelly, K. J., & Thackeray, R. (2006). Segmentation on a shoestring: Health audience segmentation in limited-budget and local social marketing interventions. *Health Promotion Practice, 7,* 170–173.

27. Kotler, P. & Roberto, E. (1989). *Social marketing: Strategies for changing public behavior.* New York, NY: Free Press.

28. Bryant, C. (1998, June). *Social marketing: A tool for excellence.* Paper presented at the Eighth Annual Conference on Social Marketing in Public Health, Clearwater Beach, FL.

29. Neiger, B. L., Thackeray, R., Merrill, R. M., Miner, K. M., Larsen, L., & Chalkley, C. M. (2001). The impact of social marketing on fruit and vegetable consumption and physical activity among public health employees at the Utah Department of Health. *Social Marketing Quarterly, 7,* 9–28.

30. Centers for Disease Control and Prevention and the Safe Injection Practices Coalition. *One and only one campaign.* Retrieved June 20, 2017, from http://www.oneandonlycampaign.org/

31. American Cancer Society. *Great American Smokeout.* Retrieved June 20, 2017, from http://www.cancer.org/healthy/stay-away-from-tobacco/great-american-smokeout.html

32. The Bully Project. Retrieved June 20, 2017, from http://www.thebullyproject.com/

33. Centers for Disease Control and Promotion. (2014). *The relationship between bullying and suicide: What we know and what it means for schools.* Retrieved May 1, 2017, from http://www.cdc.gov/violenceprevention/pdf/bullying-suicide-translation-final-a.pdf

34. The Bully Project. *10 million kids.* Retrieved June 20, 2017, from http://www.thebullyproject.com/10m_kids.

35. U.S. Department of Justice, Drug Enforcement Administration. *National take-back initiative.* Retrieved June 20, 2017, from http://www.deadiversion.usdoj.gov/drug_disposal/takeback/

36. Washington Poison Center. *Take back your meds.* Retrieved June 20, 2017, from http://www.takebackyourmeds.org

Additional Resources

Print

National Commission for Health Education Credentialing, Inc. (NCHEC), & Society for Public Health Education (SOPHE). (2015). *A Competency-Based Framework for Health Education Specialists-2015.* Whitehall, PA: National Commission for Health Education Credentialing, Inc. (NCHEC) and Society for Public Health Education (SOPHE).

Acquiring the Tools for Applying Community and Public Health Education Methods and Strategies

Herschel de Vercha/Dreamstime.com.

CHAPTER 6

Developing Effective Presentation and Training Skills

Heather M. Wagenschutz, MBA, MA

Keely S. Rees, PhD, MCHES

▶ Author Comments

Very few can cram the night before a final exam and achieve an "A." Even fewer can quickly assemble and present a polished health education session or training. There is an "art" to the construction and facilitation of presentations that requires patience and practice. Do not allow the growing pains of becoming a savvy presenter and trainer discourage you. Over time, you will learn how to give great presentations in a variety of settings and embrace the importance of planning, organizing, and preparing methods that are impactful and rewarding. This chapter has been designed to help in the presentation process, from researching the topic and priority population to evaluating the presentation's effectiveness—and all that goes on in between.

🔍 CHES COMPETENCIES

1.5.1   Identify and analyze factors that foster or hinder the learning process.
1.5.2   Identify and analyze factors that foster or hinder knowledge acquisition.
2.4.3   Organize health education/promotion into a logical sequence.
3.1.1   Create an environment conducive to learning.
3.2.1   Develop training objectives.*
3.2.3   Identify training needs of individuals involved in implementation.*
3.2.4   Develop training using best practices.*
3.2.7   Evaluate training.*
3.2.8   Use evaluation findings to plan/modify future training.
7.1.3   Tailor messages for intended audience.
7.1.7   Deliver messages using media and communication strategies.

*Advanced level competency

Reprinted by permission of the National Commission for Health Education Credentialing, Inc. (NCHEC) and Society for Public Health Education (SOPHE).

▶ Introduction

Health education specialists teach, train, and advocate health promotion and disease prevention, which beckons a polished presentation skill set. Public speaking provides an opportunity to impress, educate, persuade, and sell others on concepts and ideas that directly affect individual and community health status. Presenting is challenging, but it can be enjoyable and provide tremendous intrinsic and extrinsic rewards when properly planned. The **method** is a particular procedure specifically carried out to disseminate information, objectives, and resource materials.[1] In essence, it is how presenters go about presenting information for audience adoption. A method can also refer to a specific part of the intervention, lesson, or presentation.[2] It is the methods of the presentation that dictate how well information is received and retained. Planning for presentations, including its methods, will increase the likelihood the audience will receive and connect with the intended messages and help inspire them to implement positive behavior changes.

▶ Steps for Conducting Effective Presentations and Trainings

Health education specialists create and use presentations for imparting information in almost every setting in which they work. These can include: (1) planning, developing, and designing health education and training programs; (2) presenting lectures and training groups or individuals; and (3) instructing and counseling clients or the public on specific health issues. Effective presentations help to educate the public, and therefore, serve as a critical part of public health and healthcare systems. This chapter will focus on seven key areas for conducting effective presentations and trainings, including (1) knowing the audience, (2) identifying goals and objectives, (3) gathering and organizing materials and resources, (4) identifying and selecting appropriate methods, (5) implementing the presentation, (6) preparing for questions and answers, and (7) gathering feedback.

Know the Audience

Knowing the general audience, topic, and expectations are the first steps to planning a presentation. An audience could consist of, for example, young people in schools, individuals attending a personal behavior change seminar, professionals attending a workshop or training, members of a community coalition committee, or community volunteers working as an advocacy group. Each group has unique needs and expectations. Information about the listeners such as ages, occupations, religions, politics, attitudes, beliefs, moods, and feelings is needed to be effective in the presentation.[3]

Presentation expectations are influenced by the setting in which the program takes place such as a boardroom, auditorium, classroom, or community center. Prior to the presentation, the health education specialist should find out who will be attending, what needs to be covered, and the time frame allotted for the presentation. Effective speakers must be able to adapt their presentation to the surroundings. For example, the approach a health education specialist uses in presenting blood-borne pathogens in a manufacturing setting may be quite different from that used for presenting the same information to public health nurses at a health department. Health education specialists are able to better adapt when they consider audience composition, knowledge levels, and attitudes. Those who prepare by gathering information prior to a presentation make better connections and impressions with their audiences and are more likely to adapt to meet the needs of the audience than those who do not.

Identify Goals and Objectives

Once the health education specialist has a clearer picture of the audience, the overall rationale of the presentation (main goal) can be better developed. A goal may cover a single session, a series of sessions, or an entire training or workshop. **Goals** tend to be broad and more abstract, but serve as the overarching principle that guides presentation direction. The health education specialist should envision the presentation and decide what will be provided to participants. In other words, what should a participant be able to understand, examine, or apply? Once determined, objectives can then be developed. **Objectives** contain specific, measurable, observable changes. They also serve as a road map for learners to better understand expected outcomes. Objectives are the foundation in an instructional exchange so that health education specialists and their audiences can understand the presentation's purpose. An organized set of objectives will help in planning and delivering information and help to designing assessments.

One historic resource for developing objectives is Bloom's Taxonomy.[4] Bloom's Taxonomy is often represented as a pyramid and is hierarchical; meaning, the learning at the higher levels cannot happen until prerequisite knowledge and skills are attained at lower levels. Put another way, participants have to "know" something before they can "comprehend," "comprehend" before they can "apply," and so on (**TABLE 6.1**).

TABLE 6.1 Associated Action or Performance Verbs Using Bloom's Taxonomy Revised	
Learning Level	**Other Ways to Express this Learning Level**
Remember	Recognize, recall
Understand	Interpret, exemplify, classify, summarize, infer, compare, explain
Apply	Execute, implement
Analyze	Differentiate, organize, attribute
Evaluate	Check, critique
Create	Generate, plan, produce

Data from Armstrong, P. *Bloom's Taxonomy*. Retrieved July 7, 2017 from www.cft.vanderbilt.edu/guides-sub-pages/blooms-taxonomy/

COMMUNITY CONNECTIONS 6.1

Monique, a health education specialist at the Brazos County Public Health Division, was asked by the local superintendent of prisons to give a two-hour program on human trafficking to 20 women at a local correctional facility. As Monique prepared for the meeting, she gathered handouts and the PowerPoint presentation she had used effectively many times with college students, knowing that she would need to assess her current audience to revise the information. She also called the superintendent back to ensure her materials were appropriate. Upon arriving at the facility, she discovered two of the women could not read beyond a fourth grade level and several of the women only spoke Spanish as a primary language. Thank goodness, her handouts included pictures and she had brought materials in Spanish. The information she had previously used with college students would have been too complex, and her original handout materials prepared for a young university audience would not have been appropriate for the incarcerated audience. Monique was pleased she had taken time to inquire about and consider the characteristics of her audience.

Assembling objectives involves complexity because of variables, including (1) ownership of the objective (participants or presenter), (2) length of the program (one time versus ongoing), (3) complexity of the objective, (4) abilities and experience of individual participants, (5) structure of the program (e.g., individual, group, makeup of group), (6) attitude of the participants (e.g., forced participation versus free selection, self-efficacy), and (7) learning styles of participants (e.g., multiple intelligences, cultural influences). For instance, consider an analogy of baking a cake. The objective is to teach someone to successfully follow directions and bake a six-layer cake. For some people, following baking directions is simple. Others have problems when attempting to bake. The instructor needs to decide what method or methods should be used to teach cake baking. Reexamination of the variables previously listed can help the instructor determine how these might affect the methods chosen. So, if the participants really wanted to bake a cake, would any of these variables affect their effort? If, for example, the instructor only had 30 minutes to teach baking to the group, would it have an impact on the end result? Does the fact that there are six layers to this cake influence the task? If the participant never so much as cooked an egg, would it influence the methods chosen? If there were 30 people in the group, should the instructor conduct the baking activity differently? If the individual was required to participate in the activity, what might the instructor do differently?

⊙ DID YOU KNOW?

When considering which presentation methods to incorporate in the classroom or community settings, the participants' learning styles can help guide what to choose:

Auditory Learners
Like to be read to
Like to read out loud
Like to use mnemonics to help learn material
Like to talk with others about their ideas

Visual Learners
Like to learn from reading, taking notes, and using worksheets
Like to use highlighters to outline important facts
Like to see a visual representation of the information
Like to use multimedia materials such as computers and transparencies

Kinesthetic Learners
Like to move around to learn new information
Like to take frequent breaks
Like to use rhythms or music to learn
Like to learn in different settings

Gather and Organize Materials and Resources

Creating effective presentations requires finding and assembling credible resources. This is becoming more and more difficult, especially in today's world of nonstop news and data. In addition to being reliable and accurate, sources must be trustworthy. Health education specialists must be able to judge the credibility of information that appears on the Internet and through social media. Keeping a lookout for opinion platforms and political agendas are less obvious today, thanks to savvy marketing. In fact, a 2016 study found that even the most tech-savvy younger generation was, "… duped by sponsored content and did not always recognize the political bias of social messages."[5] For all sources utilized, it must be determined if the author is presenting neutrality or advocating a specific viewpoint.

The authors of a source for information should be well known and respected in the field of study. Some sites like *Wikipedia* are crowdsourced by users (general public), not experts, which means anyone can edit the content. Checking the date of published information is also important. Although some sources may be decades old and still contain accurate information, other content areas experience rapid advancements and changes and will require sources to be more current. Additionally, presenters can use health sites associated with reputable institutions such as a respected university or government program.

Many resources are available at the local, regional, state, and national levels. Materials obtained from journals should be peer reviewed with cited references. Health education textbooks often provide appendices that list additional resources. Valid and reliable resources can provide inspiration for future ideas, act as supplements to the method (e.g., handouts, data), or aid in ensuring content delivered is accurate and up to date.

Organizing a presentation means thinking from the learner's viewpoint. Focus should be on what topic concerns the audience the most and in what order should it be delivered. There are many ways to organize information that can address the audience's needs (**TABLE 6.2**).

Identify and Select Appropriate Methods

Sometimes, a presenter is popular simply because of the way he or she presents; yet, limited

---

TABLE 6.2 Content Delivery Organization Techniques

- *Chronological order.* Presents the facts in the order they happened.
- *Problem and solution.* Begins with defining the problem and ends with how it was remedied.
- *Inverted pyramid.* The initial opener of a presentation summarizes the who, what, when, where, why, and how, and then presents facts in decreasing importance.
- *Deductive organization.* Starts with the opposite—a generalization that usually includes a theme or point supported by many facts and observations (scientific papers and sales publications often organize things this way).
- *Inductive organization.* Begins with specific examples and instances, and then leads learners to the general idea that data or research support.

---

learning occurs. Selecting fun or popular methods, however, is not always in the best interest of the priority population. Selecting appropriate presentation methods is first and foremost about utilizing processes that will help achieve desired program goals and objectives. This is not to say that methods cannot be fun, but rather their selection should be part of a planning process that reflects both theoretical and ethical elements. Health education specialists must select presentation methods that can enhance program goals, achieve targeted objectives, and ensure ethical codes of conduct are followed.

Methods become the critical strategies for delivering the content and subsequently helping participants achieve the objectives. There are many ways to address the targeted content and achieve objectives (**TABLE 6.3**). A presentation outline or plan encapsulates methods for delivering content and provides direction for the presentation. **FIGURE 6.1** provides a sample presentation outline for the initial session of a sample 10-week stress management program.

TABLE 6.3 Presentation Methods

Method	Focus	Characteristics and Comments
Appraisals or inventories	Assessment of needs, attitudes, behavior, interests, skills	Provides quick overview and on-the-spot assessment; be wary of reliability and validity issues
Audiovisuals	Cassettes, slides, overheads, posters, displays, books	Works for multiple intelligences (MI)
Brainstorming	Group participation; quick generation of ideas	Avoid discussion; seek total involvement
Case studies	Review and critique true event	Aids analytical thinking
Computer-based	CD-ROM, software programs, Internet- based assignments, chat rooms	Hits MI; can be dynamic; need to validate accuracy; may require training
Critical incidents	Similar to case study but without ending; can be made up	Provides critical thinking and problem-solving skills
Debates	Explore both sides of an issue (e.g., drug laws, abortion, teen rights, health care, advertising)	Works best with structure
Demonstrations	Provide visual performance of a skill (e.g., first aid, self-care, computer skills, cooking)	Helps visual learners; aids skill development
Dramatizations or skits	Can be scripted or improved	Works best with active participants and practice
Experiments	Can be done in session or on own	Ethical concerns; ranges from simple to complex
Fishbowls	Small inner circle discusses topic; outer circle can critique or partner up	Variation of debate
Games	Model TV games or be creative	Helpful review of material; fun
Large group discussion	Follow-up or part of lecture; can be structured or unstructured	Allows for questions; opportunity to check for learning

(Continues)

TABLE 6.3 (*Continued*)

Method	Focus	Characteristics and Comments
Lecture	Knowledge; attitudes	One-dimensional; verbal learners
Problem solving	Focus on dilemmas such as peer pressure, conflicts, stress	Helps to use problem-solving methods
Role playing	Participants act out scenarios; can be totally, partially, or not structured	Remind them it is a role; voluntary; needs processing
Sentence completion	Participants complete sentences with health implications	Follow-up discussion needed to process
Skill practice	Follow-up to demonstrations; pairing of learners helpful	Provide feedback; sequence properly
Small group discussion	Participants address issue prior to or as a follow-up to lecture or large group discussion	Have clear directions; move around groups to assist; keep focused
Values clarification	Participants choose sides or rank priorities	Helps clarify priorities for different dilemmas; often situational

Methods should match the content being delivered. This comes from having a clear idea of what information should be delivered, how in-depth the presentation will be, and the developmental stage of the audience. Health content greatly varies (from impersonal to very personal), so health education specialists need to be aware of what methods will best blend with the audience and materials. For example, sexuality educators teach material that touches on values, beliefs, and attitudes regarding personal information. The methods used in these programs need to gradually progress from less threatening to more in-depth activities. The educator needs to do this without running the risk of offending the audience by using methods deemed as inappropriate.

Certain methods may be acceptable to one culture or group while being completely unacceptable to others. Health information is closely tied to one's values, beliefs, cultural nuances, geographical issues, and other personal attributes. Thus, it is the educator's responsibility before using a method to ensure it is respectful and in accordance with the majority of the participants. Cultural issues include an individual's racial or ethnic background, religious beliefs, gender, age, familial background, disability, sexual orientation, language skills, geographical location, and political beliefs. The more a health education specialist can find out about the audience, the less likely the presentation will falter.

Health education specialists should also use methods that work for their particular personality and expertise as well as the role they are serving in the educational setting. Is the role as facilitator, trainer, teacher, workshop leader, or a combination of these? Based on the role served, they can then modify a lesson or presentation to suit the types of information being disseminated.

Target Audience: In-Service Teachers

Topic: Stress Management

Objectives
1. Participants will identify four common stress problems experienced by teachers and students (knowledge).
2. Participants will discuss how stress has affected their roles as teachers and affirm their motivation for the program by discussing two reasons they want to participate in this program (attitude).
3. Participants will develop a stress management plan (skill).

Key Content

1. Definitions of stress
    Types of stressors
    Effects of stress
    Coping strategies
    Preventing stress

2. Possible motivations
    Have more energy
    Improve body image
    Improve self-esteem
    Reduce health risks
    Improve life expectancy
    Ease pain

3. Elements of coping skills
    Different types of techniques
    Massage therapy
    Music and relaxation exercises
    Exercise
    Diaphragmatic breathing
    Meditation skills
    Journaling

Methods

Method	Content Focus	Instructional Aids	Time
Lecture/Discussion	Defining Stress Effects of stress	Handout	30
Brainstorm/Lecture	How stress affects teacher and student performance Motivation for reducing stress	Marker Board	15
PowerPoint/Music	Overload stress	Computer/Projector	10
Break			10
Small group work	Stress management strategies Stress management planning	Butcher paper	25
Group discussion	Strategies Potential obstacles to implementing		15
Closure	Key concepts learned		15

FIGURE 6.1 Presentation Outline.

The sequencing or order of the methods also needs to be considered. Methods that focus on skills should occur after the participants have adequate tools (e.g., knowledge, observations) to address skill-based activities. Although there are logical sequencing guidelines, it is beneficial for the health education specialist to be prepared with a variety of presentation methods, to adjust to the dynamics of the group, and to not be afraid to experiment with sequencing of the methods. In addition, methods should be selected that add variety to programs rather than overusing a single method.

Whether a session is delivered at a school, the community at large, or in a small group, the health education specialists must create an experience that is engrossing. Traditional "sit and listen" lecture style is an easy go-to method, but tends to lack engagement. It can be overused because presenters feel like they have more control, but these rarely produce long-term information retention, knowledge application, or behavior change. There is a range of adequate, good, and great teaching methods to consider for audience engagement (**TABLE 6.4**).

Many presentation methods exist other than those listed in Table 6.3. The types of methods used are restricted only by a lack of presenter creativity. Being creative as a presenter is less about innate talent and more about hard work. The presenter must think of different ways to present the material and get the audience involved, trying different methods to see what works best. It is not always the method that is "good" or "bad," but the dynamic makeup of an audience and how a presenter relates to the members.

TABLE 6.4 Presentation Methods for Participant Engagement

Adequate
More facilitator centered, participants are passive, lower retention rates with information for learners

- Lecture

Good
More participant centered, interactive, moderate retention rates with information for learners

- Discussion
- Group work
- Collaborative learning
- Puzzle/Jigsaw
- Pre- and Post-quiz

Great
Most participant centered, highly interactive, highest retention rates with information for learners

- Role play
- Simulation
- Debate
- Fishbowl
- Brainstorming, Mind mapping
- Experiments
- Skill practice

Data from Paul, A. M. (2013, January 9). *Highlighting is a waste of time: the best and worst learning techniques.* Retrieved July 7, 2017 from www .ideas.time.com/2013/01/09/highlighting-is-a-waste-of-time-the-best -and-worst-learning-techniques/; Weimer, M. (2012, July 26). *10 ways to promote student engagement.* Retrieved July 7, 2017 from www .facultyfocus.com/articles/effective-teaching-strategies/10-ways-to -promote-student-engagement/

⑦ DID YOU KNOW?

There is a great deal of variation with how learners remember (and forget). Retention depends on:

- The learners' prior and existing knowledge.
- The learners' motivation to learn.
- The types of the learning methods used.
- The contextual cues in the learning and remembering situations.
- The time allocated for learning to be retained.

Source: Data from Work–Learning Research, http://www.work-learning.com/catalog.html

Implement the Presentation or Training

After determining the audience needs, developing presentation or training objectives, gathering resources, and identifying methods that will help meet the predetermined objectives, the presentation or training is ready to be delivered. An organized presentation will lay out the objectives to be met, start with an opener, review any background material needed for the current presentation, and then get to the heart of the material. Sometimes, a presenter will take questions during a presentation (especially if it is part of a longer training with several components), while at other times these are left to the end.

Effective presentations involve employing speaker characteristics that may be practiced and learned (**TABLE 6.5**). Effective speakers understand these skills and use them to their advantage.

Effective presenters are aware of the messages that the body (nonverbal) and voice (verbal) convey to the target audience. For example, part of understanding the words "Be careful!" comes from a person's movement, tone, and facial expressions. While saying "Be careful!" and trying to create the impression of a warning, the body moves with a quick jerk, the tone is high and shrieking, and the eyes are wide open. The picture is complete for the audience. These components of communication offer more than just uttering sounds. The presenter connects feeling to the sounds, and the feelings help make a presentation dynamic. How a message is communicated may be just as important as what is said.

Use of both verbal and nonverbal skills can help a speaker connect with the audience and ensure the content is conveyed.

TABLE 6.5 Characteristics of Effective Speakers

- *Considerate.* Listening to and validating the concerns, opinions, and reactions of participants shows that the speaker values the audience's input as much as his or her own.
- *Genuine.* Making up information, giving false compliments, or using overdramatic wording can lead the audience to believe that the speaker is only there to be liked.
- *Trustworthy.* Good speakers create trust by being honest and sincere and using credible sources of information. If the data seem out of date or debatable, the audience may ignore what is being said.
- *Enthusiastic.* The excitement that surrounds a speaker who genuinely appears excited about the information being presented is catchy. Enthusiastic presenters maintain audience attention because they convince the audience that the information they are presenting is exciting, interesting, and important.
- *Humorous.* Appropriate humor personalizes the topic and allows the speaker to make light of subjects that can be complex or intense.
- *Proficient in subject.* Being prepared and well versed in the topic being presented shows dedication and commitment. Having a degree of proficiency in the topic increases credibility and trustworthiness from the audience's perspective.

Verbal Cues

The manner in which the presenter speaks has a direct impact on the conclusions an audience makes about the presentation, and subsequently the message being delivered in whole. What a presenter says and *how* it is said has a great deal to do with the entire success of the presentation. It is important, therefore, to consider how accurate and clear the message sounds to others. Principal **verbal cues** a presenter should use to help the audience connect with the presentation include word accentuation, pitch, tone, pace, volume, word choice, and proper grammar (**TABLE 6.6**).

Nonverbal Cues

Nonverbal cues are those impressions given to a person, group, or audience through facial expressions, body movements, and other gestures. Nonverbal cues aid the presenter in a smooth presentation delivery by reconfirming the meaning behind a spoken word. Usually, the first impression audiences pick up from presenters is the way they *appear*, such as standing tall, staring at the ground, or fidgeting with objects (**TABLE 6.7**).

Practice heightens awareness of verbal and nonverbal cues, thus ensuring a positive impression in a real presentation. Using a presentation evaluation form may be helpful when practicing presentation skills.

TABLE 6.6 Verbal Cues

- *Word accentuation.* The process of emphasizing certain words to let the listener know that a word or phrase is particularly important. Effective speakers are able to slow their pace in midstream to highlight important words or phrases without the audience being consciously aware of this tactic. A short pause following an accentuation generally helps drive the importance of the point.
- *Pitch.* This is associated with voice octave and can fluctuate from low to high. Like word accentuation, variation in pitch can be used to emphasize points. For instance, raising and lowering the pitch can create doubtfulness or uncertainty (e.g., "I think so"). Placing a higher pitch at the end of a phrase demonstrates uncertainty or questioning (e.g., "They are?"). A lower pitch usually represents endorsement (e.g., "It can be done"). Variation in pitch is a useful technique in situations where the speaker wants to elicit emotional reaction or support.
- *Tone.* Consists of the patterns in which a pitch is placed. Using a chant-like tone or a monotone can have a numbing effect on an audience. Listening to someone who speaks in a monotone detracts from maintaining interest levels, however fascinating the topic may be. When practicing speeches, it may be helpful for presenters to record their voice and listen to it for tone fluctuations.
- *Pace.* This is acceleration or deceleration of the presentation. Sometimes, a speaker will slow the pace of a speech to create a sense of intrigue or suspense. Speeding up momentarily could represent an increasing level of excitement. Too much speed, however, may confuse an audience because of lost words and pronunciations. Speakers should make sure the tempo is comfortable for the audience. If members of the audience appear confused or irritated, ask if the presenter could repeat what was said, or when they begin talking among themselves in order to find out what was missed, then the pace may be too fast. The presenter should ask the audience if the pace is adequate if individuals appear confused or frustrated.
- *Volume.* This should be raised and lowered according to where the presentation is taking place (e.g., a large or small room, outdoors or indoors). The speaker should always ask the audience if the volume is adequate. If not, the speaker should make adjustments rather than asking the audience to "just move closer." It is not the responsibility of the audience to make sure a speaker's volume is satisfactory. It is the speaker's role to monitor whether the audience can hear and to change volume to accommodate the listeners. Knowing the makeup of the audience beforehand may aid in planning appropriate voice volume. Older populations may have diminished hearing of high-pitched and soft-spoken sounds. Appropriate voice volume also is dependent on the room setup and structure. For longer rooms, speakers should aim their voice toward the back of the room, so those sitting near the back have a better chance of hearing. A room that is short in length yet wide requires less volume from the speaker, but more turning while speaking to ensure individuals sitting at both sides of the room can hear.
- *Use of words.* Includes word choice and use of proper grammar. Poor grammar or inappropriate choice of words can leave a negative impression of the speaker from the audience. Many times grammatical errors sprinkled through a speech can distract listeners and draw attention away from the content of the presentation. Likewise, use of regional colloquialisms or local jargon by a presenter may lead to misunderstandings by the audience.

Prepare for Questions and Answers

Following a presentation with a question and answer segment can be an effective means to convey concern for the audience and to gauge their understanding of what was presented. Staying relaxed and in control, while adequately and accurately responding to audience questions is important. In addition, the presenter should make direct eye contact with the individual asking the question and repeat the question aloud for other participants to hear.

Although question and answer sessions are easier to implement in smaller groups, they also need to be included in larger settings. The

TABLE 6.7 Nonverbal Cues

- *Posture.* Good posture conveys confidence and expertise. Proper posture necessitates standing tall, with the chest slightly out and the head back. Presenters who stand with feet shoulder-width apart, hands at the waist, and weight concentrated on the balls of the feet appear attentive. Speakers who sit in a chair or hide behind tables may appear awkward if they do start to move around the platform. Standing center stage without any of the previously described crutches makes for a strong first impression. Equally important is the ability to adapt posture to the type of presentation. The erect, stoic posture associated with a formal presentation may be intimidating or awkward for an informal setting. Similarly, resting on a table, which may be appropriate in an informal situation (e.g., facilitating a support group), would be inappropriate in a formal setting.
- *Eye contact.* Lack of eye contact may show distrust, apprehension, nervousness, lack of confidence, trepidation, or boredom. In contrast, appropriate eye contact portrays confidence and connects the speaker with the audience at a personal level. Effective use of eye contact includes connecting briefly (one to two seconds) with different listeners throughout the presentation. The speaker should take care not to focus on a single individual for an extended period of time, but rather scan the audience and focus periodically on individuals randomly. Each person in the audience wants to feel a part of the presentation. Effective use of eye contact can allow this connection to occur.
- *Body movement.* Body movement can create different degrees of intimacy, warmth, and friendliness. Speakers who move freely demonstrate a greater level of comfort with themselves and the topic and tend to maintain a higher level of audience interest. Arm and hand gestures are appropriate ways to express feelings. Waving arms and hands about during a comment like "What can we do?" has a greater impact than if arms were resting on the podium or at one's side. Gestures like pointing or giving the "okay" sign help to clarify or define a point. Body movement is not effective, however, unless the speaker has a purpose behind the movement. Highly scripted presenters who carefully choreograph each movement can appear unnatural. Too much movement, however, can become distracting rather than enhancing. Overuse of arm movement can convey hyperactivity or nervousness. Similarly, pacing may become irritating to listeners trying to hear a trailing voice. Effective speaking involves being able to remain in one spot until a natural break occurs in a thought process (e.g., the end of a concept), allowing the speaker to move without disrupting the flow of information. In general, a speaker should avoid changing positions until a thought has been finished. Similarly, a speaker should not start a new thought until all movement has stopped and the speaker is firmly positioned.
- *Facial expressions.* These can be used can be used to pull the audience toward unspoken insinuations. For example, lifting the eyebrows at the end of a question may show a desire for a response. Grimacing while reading the latest immunization rates for infants could be used to show the need for improvement. The sincerity of a presenter can be conveyed to the audience through facial expressions.

COMMUNITY CONNECTIONS 6.2

Monique recently attended a statewide conference sponsored by the state department of health and human services. As she listened to the keynote speaker, she noticed he made little eye contact with the audience and often stared at a point in space. He often stood in one place and slumped over his notes, went over his allotted time, and failed to entertain questions from the audience.

Monique was distracted by the negative nonverbal cues. Was the speaker nervous, uninterested in the topic, or simply unconscious of the real messages being sent? Lack of attention to nonverbal cues ruined what could have been a valuable presentation. Monique knew from experience that posture, eye contact, body movement, and facial expressions were all important nonverbal cues that helped make for a more effective presentation.

presenter should anticipate questions and prepare answers ahead of time, when possible. Sometimes, it can be intimidating for members of an audience to question a presenter, so it may be helpful to write some questions ahead of time and ask "friendly" members of the audience to ask them, if needed. This may open the way for more reluctant audience members to join. In addition, the way in which a presenter responds to questions from the audience will influence whether others will feel free to ask questions. If an answer to a question is not known, the presenter should acknowledge it and tell the group an answer will be disseminated to all participants in a reasonable time frame.

Gather Feedback

Participant feedback is valuable in gathering information about how to improve presentations and other training efforts. Information related to the appropriateness of objectives, content, and methods should be collected. When collecting data, it is desirable to avoid yes or no responses and helpful to allow for subjective comments about the methods used in the presentation. This **process evaluation** typically occurs in the form of objective and subjective responses (**FIGURE 6.2**).

Evaluation results that reveal any component of the presentation or training was ineffective, confusing, or uninteresting should be investigated as to why, where, and how to improve. Evaluations can measure different parts of the session: reaction, learning, impact, and results. Each slice uncovers the level of impact on the participant. Evaluations provide progress or evidence that a component is "working" or "worthwhile" in a presentation or training.

It is equally important for presenters to critique themselves and make use of peer evaluation. This can easily be done when there are copresenters or trainers. Being open to such honest reviews will likely help the health education specialist find ways to enhance presentation efforts.

▶ Tips and Techniques for Effective Presentations and Trainings

Know the Purpose and Material

The presenter should be mindful of the central purposes of the presentation, which are to persuade, instruct, or inspire. One way to ensure

---

Session Title or Topic _____   Presenter's Name _____

1. What (if anything) did you like best about this session/seminar/course?

2. What (if anything) would you change about the session/seminar/course?

3. What constructive feedback do you have about how the presenter could improve?

4. Overall, this session was (check one)
   ☐ poor   ☐ fair   ☐ good   ☐ great   ☐ outstanding

5. I would recommend this session to another person (check one)
   ☐ Yes   ☐ No   ☐ Unsure

General Comments:

FIGURE 6.2 Process Evaluation Questions.

this happens is by asking the question "So what?" while developing the presentation. For example, a speaker may say, "The number of Americans suffering from type 2 diabetes will increase rapidly over the next ten years." So what? What does this mean to a group of high school students or to employees within a worksite? An effective health education specialist will show how this connects to the audience in order to create direction. An example of the same opening statement but with first considering the question "So what?" is: "In the next decade, type 2 diabetes will increase at a rapid pace. What this means for healthcare workers is that we need to work more closely with county and city wellness groups to try to alleviate the soaring costs associated with mismanaged patients."

Focus on Presentation Design

It is quite difficult to offer a prescription for great presentation design when there are so many factors involved that affect design decisions, such as type of audience and content being delivered. It is enough to cause almost all health education specialists to squirm in their seats as they madly plug away at creating their presentations. As for the software available to create the presentation, many professionals approach it one of two ways. They either become overwhelmed with all the design and format options available to them and avoid having to figure it out by sticking with the less than exciting default settings, or they get so excited at all the design possibilities and everything they can do with the software that they suddenly become the Picasso of presentations, adding outrageous sound effects, wild slide transitions, and odd, out of place graphics that require a certain level of interpretation to follow along.

The unfortunate trend is a lot of presentations have reached a point at which everyone in the audience knows what to expect, and the visuals that were intended to complement the presenter's spoken word more often than not just get in the way. But armed with a few basic design rules, health education specialists have the power to avoid creating the mundane and predictable presentations that haunt audience members long after they exit the room. The design process should be viewed as

an opportunity to separate oneself, organization, or cause from all the others out there. It is a time to show the audience passion for the topic being presented, so they also might experience it as well. A presenter has a captive audience that is often hoping for the best, but in reality expecting far less. By following a few basic rules, the presenter can exceed the audience's expectations and leave them wanting more.

Rule 1: Less Is More

Numerous PowerPoint-type presentations typically involve a whirlwind of bulleted, small text crammed onto each slide and a presenter who reads each slide line by line. As the audience members catch on and realize the presenter is reading to them, they will often read ahead, creating a situation in which the presenter and audience are out of sync. This disconnect can lead to audience members only listening to a portion of what is being said and drawing their own conclusions.

Slides that contain a lot of small text usually mean the presenter is either an ineffective presenter or does not know the information well enough and is using the text-filled slides as a support mechanism. Large amounts of small text are also used because many believe more text is more convincing, though the opposite is true. By using a larger font size (e.g., 30 point), the presenter is forced to list only those points carrying the most weight and must have a good understanding of the material being presented. With fewer bulleted prompts to lean on, it becomes the presenter's task to elaborate each point rather than read to the audience, making for a presentation that keeps the attention of those in attendance. In the end, it comes down to a single question: If the audience can understand the presentation simply by reading a copy of the slides, why is the presenter even there? The slides are not meant to do the presenter's job, which is to convey the overall message. They are merely there to emphasize crucial points and visually complement the presenter's comments Without some kind of explanation from the presenter, what is written on the slides should mean very little to the audience.

Rule 2: Image Is Everything

Cheap-looking images are avoided in well-planned presentations. This includes the majority of images and clipart bundled with whatever presentation software is being used. Good presentation design stands out from the crowd, something extremely difficult to achieve with pictures that practically everyone in the audience has already seen or used at one time or another. Images used should be unique, high quality, and support a point in the presentation.

Images selected for inclusion on the presentation slides should be kept consistent. Illustrations should have a similar look and feel. Inconsistent imagery translates into design chaos. Also, style and fonts used matter within the presentation. Curly, flamboyant, carnival-type fonts have their place in design, but that place is not within the realm of PowerPoint-type presentations. Fonts used should be distinct and easy to read for audience members in both the front and the back of the room. The key is to have the audience focusing on the presenter, not the pretty words on the screen. Additionally, colors used within the presentation should be considered. Too much or too little contrast between the text and background colors can result in audience irritation and, eventually, disinterest.

The audience is not looking for a circus act. Words that tumble, dance, or swing into view only serve as a distraction. Although it may seem boring, it is usually best to stick with the default text animation. The same holds true for slide transitions. A presentation is not the time to demonstrate crafty video transition skills. It is better to stick with the default transition or another variety that is quite simple.

Rule 3: Be Original

When thinking about the layout of design elements (e.g., header, subheaders, body text, images) within a presentation, there is often the mind-set that one must follow the templates that come with the software. Those templates force the presenter to follow a rigid layout. Keep in mind the presenter's task is to make a statement,

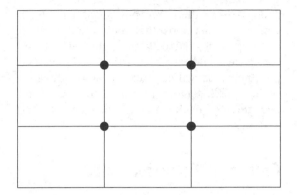

FIGURE 6.3 Rule of Thirds.

and doing so involves taking the time to create a unique visual complement to the verbal presentation. A decent level of originality can be achieved simply by following what photographers and artists refer to as the "rule of thirds." When applied to presentation slides, the rule works as follows: Imagine dividing the slide into thirds both vertically and horizontally (**FIGURE 6.3**). All important design elements within the slide are placed where the lines intersect, called *power points*. The logic behind this rule is placing design elements near these power points rather than directly in the center or scattered elsewhere that creates more interesting and powerful visuals. Within PowerPoint, the guides can be set to create an outline for the rule of thirds. The example in **FIGURE 6.4**

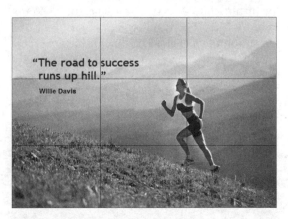

FIGURE 6.4 Rule of Thirds Applied.
© Sportstock/iStock/Getty.

shows a slide with the text positioned horizontally along the upper horizontal line while the woman running is aligned with the right vertical line. Audience members will first notice the woman, and their eyes will naturally follow the direction of her implied movement until they reach the text, thereby making a connection between text and image.

Prepare a Discussion Guide

A discussion guide can be a helpful tool to enhance a presentation. The guide may consist of a brief outline and talking points or discussion questions related to the presentation. The guide can highlight major themes and messages, provide background content, suggest related activities, and list resources for more information. It provides the audience with an outline for the presentation, copies of presentation slides, a convenient tool for note taking, and a way to take home the information from the presentation. A discussion guide also may include information about how to reach the speaker (e.g., address, phone, email), should members of the audience have further questions after the presentation.

Rehearse the Presentation

It is important to become familiar with the material and content that will be presented. Rehearsing for a presentation is not about memorizing or turning into a robot. When presenters do not rehearse, it is like handing in a rough draft of a paper for the final grade. Although there are some individuals who have the unique ability to give polished presentations even when preparing at the last minute, the vast majority of people cannot rely on finesse and innate ability. Rehearsing helps the brain run like a well-oiled machine with less malfunctions. Distractions during rehearsal should be minimized so the presenter can actively work through the flow of a presentation or training session until it feels connected and complete. Success is as much about the quantity of practice as it is the quality.

Some health education specialists may prefer to rehearse in the privacy of their home, while others do it at work, perhaps even asking a colleague to serve as a participant during the test run. Presenters also can set up a phone or tablet, record the presentation, and review the video (or have someone else review). Whatever the practice choice, rehearsal will help manage "butterflies" and nerves and take the presentation from a well-thought-out plan to reality. Practicing also increases confidence and checks for pacing and timing of different segments within a presentation.

The approach of "I'll figure it out when I get in front of them" is simply not advisable. Is there a formula for how much to rehearse? It depends on how comfortable the presenter is with the subject and the complexity of the session. A timer should be used during a presentation run-through to determine its length. Time should be added for buffers, questions, and participation. If rehearsals are running over, both the content and methods should be assessed. Decisions should be made during rehearsals on what can stay (if there is extra time) and go (if running over time). It helps to use imagination and envision the training session playing out with the audience from start to finish.

Develop Engaging Openers

Presentations will go most smoothly if they capture participants' attention from the beginning. By sharing a story, the health education specialist can often get on the same page with participants, helping to establish early rapport and relatedness about the subject matter.

In the field of health communication, for example, **storytelling** has been an effective tool for motivating health behavior change.[6] It involves what most people desire—feeling human connection. Personal experience **narratives** from real people experiencing authentic health behavior challenges can promote observational learning and may help to increase a participant's self-efficacy.[7] For example, "witness role models" talk about or witness their cancer experiences to an audience. Narratives coming from someone of the same gender, age group, and socioeconomic background can help position health behaviors as important or normative. More studies are revealing how narratives "…can produce knowledge gains, attitude change and behavior change."[8]

These narratives can be easier (and more pleasant) for audiences to understand and create an environment with a feeling of engagement. Relevant stories, anecdotes, or other narrative formats can resonate with the listener. Online presentation forums such as *TED Talks* and the *3 Minute Thesis* exemplify the art of storytelling using personal narratives.

Narratives are shown to be effective because they put a spotlight on real people who model what is possible (e.g., healthy behaviors) as well as, perhaps, demonstrating the consequences of what happens when not implementing a behavior change. Narratives also give listeners a chance to become immersed, even involved and invested, into a storyline. As a result, barriers are curbed and the participant feels as if he or she can accomplish the behavior change. Last, narratives may prompt emotions such as sadness, happiness, fear, or anger, which can motivate better choices and health outcomes (**TABLE 6.8**).

Narratives, just like an overall good presentation, should ultimately tell a story. There is a beginning (something happens), a middle (something unfolds; a turning point), and an end (something is realized or resolved). Presenters or their speakers and guests at the session who appropriately display genuine emotion along with teachable moment stories can add a powerful layer to learning. Having someone tell their narrative will require a process of organizing and rehearsing, similar to how the health education specialist prepares for a presentation.

Use Distilling to Keep on Point

Sometime in their lives, learners likely have been in a class or presentation and felt frustrated when the presenter gets lost on tangents or provides too much information. A good presenter

TABLE 6.8 Narrative and Nonnarrative Openers
Example of a nonnarrative health education session opener "The Human papillomavirus (HPV) is a common STD, with an estimated 60 percent of sexually active people contracting it at some point in their lives. HPV can infect anyone who has ever had a sexual encounter. HPV is spread through skin-to-skin contact, not through an exchange of bodily fluid."
Example of narrative health education session opener "In college I learned I had contracted HPV after a 9 month, monogamous, sexual relationship. An abnormal pap smear discovered it two years after I graduated. The type of HPV I had ended up needing multiple rounds of cryo (freezing the cervix) surgery. It was confusing, scary, and upsetting."

can help participants stay engaged by learning how to refine the focus and trajectory of the presentation. Presenters can increase the odds of attention and connection during a presentation

COMMUNITY CONNECTIONS 6.3

Recently, Monique was invited to attend a United Way banquet at which the guest speaker was the director of a local teenage pregnancy prevention center. The speaker began by telling a real-life story of a 14-year-old pregnant girl who was surrounded by violence and poverty. After this very effective attention-getting story, the body of the presentation focused on a new approach to working with at-risk teens in lower income areas. At the end of the presentation, the speaker referred back to the story that was used to open the presentation. Monique left the presentation with a sense of hope and motivation to help prevent teen pregnancy. She also knew she would try adding a story to the beginning of a future presentation to increase audience attention.

if they also know how to distill. **Distilling** tends to use more universal/plain language, so the core message for the audience can be explained without participants getting lost in the information or jargon. A well-distilled presentation is clear *and* memorable.

An effective way of distilling is for presenters to stay focused on relevant information and watch for "too much information" pitfalls. This occurs when presenters find it hard to focus on a primary goal and start to make all information important. Another pitfall includes presentations that contain complicated medical or scientific information. This can be overcome by explaining to participants up front, "Today's session is complicated. We do not want to get stuck in the weeds and get away from what is most important. If you would like more details, please talk with me after the session or follow up with an email." This acknowledges there is a magnitude of information for the session, but for the sake of time and brain bandwidth, material will stay focused. If hearing the smaller, more complex details is desired and if there is time, the presenter can certainly adjust and accordingly adapt.

To help make information stick, presenters must find a universal language to more efficiently and effectively communicate with their participants. Information must be presented in terms the entire audience can understand; the goal is to meet the presentation's objectives, not to show one's expansive vocabulary.

⊘ DID YOU KNOW?

A good rule of thumb would seem to be that if you ask a member of the audience a week later about your presentation, they should be able to remember three points. If these are the key points you were trying to get across, you have done a good job. If they can remember any three points, but not the key points, then your emphasis was wrong.

Data from Bourne, P. E. (2007, April 27). Ten simple rules for making good oral presentations. Retrieved July 7, 2017 from http://www.ncbi.nlm.nih.gov/pmc/articles/PMC1857815/

⊘ DID YOU KNOW?

Language is important in a presentation. Participants may relate better to concrete versus abstract words because there is clarity in their meaning. Words such as *spoon, table, green*, or *hot* are more easily understood than more abstract words such as *success, good*, or *love*.

Data from Friedlander, J. *Abstract, concrete, general and specific terms.* Retrieved July 4, 2017 from http://grammar.ccc.commnet.edu/grammar/composition/abstract.htm

---

▶ Overcoming Challenges to Effective Presentations and Trainings

Effectively presenting information to a group comes with plenty of challenges, all of which can be overcome with practice. More common challenges and strategies for overcoming them are presented below.

Build Trust

Trust is an important factor for individuals to buy into messages. Presenters need to ensure a lack of trust does not become an issue associated with a presentation. Building ground rules, especially for longer presentations and trainings, is one of the first ways a health education specialist can develop a trusting relationship with participants. Ground rules lay the foundation for a psychologically safe environment. In addition, there are numerous icebreakers that can be included in a presentation to help build a trusting environment between the participants and the presenter, and among the participants themselves.

Be Flexible

An issue that can cause stress is an overestimate or underestimate of the amount of time a method or activity will actually take. Many times a presenter will allot 15–20 minutes for an activity on paper, but discover in real time it only took 10 minutes or lasted as long as 30–40 minutes. Being flexible is probably the best way to overcome time issues. Having extra activities ready to implement if time runs under, and having a backup outline if an activity runs over, can help keep the presentation running smoothly. Knowing when to move on or let an activity continue is an important skill that will develop with time and practice. Newly practicing health education specialists should rely on a watch or timer to aid in timing. In addition, using a timeline or a matrix to help outline the presentation from start to finish can greatly reduce these kinds of problems.

Reduce Presentation Anxiety

Public speaking is a common fear, and many presenters will experience anxiety before and during a presentation. Sweaty palms, trembling, and a dry mouth commonly manifest stage fright. A presenter can use various techniques to decrease the anxiety caused by public speaking (**TABLE 6.9**).[9]

Reduce Distracting Mannerisms

In addition to effective verbal and nonverbal cues, a speaker needs to be aware of distracting verbal and nonverbal **mannerisms (TABLE 6.10)**. For example, most speakers have a favorite nuisance word or phrase that tends to be inserted between thoughts and during lulls in the presentation. Words such as *um, okay, like, you know*, and *ah* may be irritating and distracting to the audience. With overuse of these words, the audience begins to anticipate the next utterance of the nuisance word drawing attention away from the information being presented. With practice, speakers can train themselves to connect thoughts without using nuisance words or phrases.

Nonverbal distracting mannerisms such as fidgeting with one's jewelry or other item, twisting a finger in a necklace, or constantly pushing hair

TABLE 6.9 Strategies for Reducing Presentation Anxiety

- *Organize.* Organization will provide confidence in the material and allow focus during the presentation.
- *Visualize.* Seeing oneself visualize delivering the presentation with enthusiasm, mentally rehearsing the sequencing of the presentation can help build confidence.
- *Practice.* Nothing can take the place of practicing the presentation. Sometimes, it is helpful to have colleagues critique the practice sessions.
- *Breathe.* Deep breaths can help alleviate tension and resulting muscle tightness.
- *Focus on relaxing.* Calmness comes from focusing on being relaxed rather than thinking about the tension of presenting. Consciously altering thoughts to a more relaxing theme can help clear the mind of tension-filled thoughts and insecurities about the presentation.
- *Release tension.* Tightening muscles throughout the body and then releasing them while breathing deep releases tension prior to the presentation.
- *Move.* Gesturing or moving about may be a way to release some of the built-up tension. Speakers who find themselves clenching the podium or standing stiff and erect due to tension may find movement a welcome relief.
- *Maintain eye contact.* Eye contact helps reduce the feeling of being removed from the audience. It also helps speakers feel as if they were talking to a person one-on-one and lessens their focus on the vastness of the audience. Connecting with an individual in the audience builds confidence that the presentation is being understood.

behind an ear can distract from a presentation. While presenters may not be aware of the distracting mannerisms, the audience becomes keenly aware and irritated with these actions. Practicing in front of a mirror or peers or videotaping and

TABLE 6.10 Strategies for Overcoming Distracting Mannerisms

Mannerism	Strategy for Overcoming
Nuisance word	When ending a thought or sentence, be sure to close your mouth and avoid uttering sounds. Practice speaking short unrelated points while focusing on the transition between thoughts or sentences.
Fidgeting with personal item	Use arms and hands during explanations. If hands are part of the presentation, they are less likely to roam and distract the audience. Make a point of being able to see your hands out of the corner of your eyes throughout the presentation. Keep pockets empty to avoid the temptation of playing with keys and loose change. When finished writing with marking pens or chalk, place them on the table so that hands remain free to communicate. Style hair so it stays out of your face and eyes.
Fixating on a point in the back of the room or on the ground; no eye contact	Maintain eye contact with audience members, especially at the start of every new idea.
Pacing	Walk to a predesignated spot in the room and stay there until the point being made is complete. Be aware of the audience having difficulty in following your movement.

critiquing the presentation can aid in identifying these mannerisms and other distracting practices. Peers could use a checklist to identify unwanted presenter mannerisms (**FIGURE 6.5**).

Do Not Fret Over Technology Malfunctions

The use of technology is a way to make presentations come alive. Presentation software (e.g., PowerPoint), sound bites, videos, and music add dimension. There are occasions, however, when audiovisual elements can malfunction: the graphics did not correctly display, the music did not play on cue, the microphone cut out, or the computer locked up. In these instances, it is best to adapt, adjust, and move on. Computers sometimes seem as if they have an agenda of their own, so handouts of the main ideas and key points should be brought as backups to the slides. It is important

not to dwell on the problem or over-apologize, because this only magnifies the mistake and takes away from the presentation.

Anticipate Difficult Audience Members

Some audiences may include a select few whom consciously or unconsciously seek to negatively influence the presentation. This is especially true with controversial presentations such as sex education or environmental issues. These participants demand extra attention for a variety of reasons. The initial response may be to give up authority for fear of confrontation. This may affect the audience's perception of the speaker's competence. It is always best as a presenter to listen and respond without defensiveness. Often, these individuals just want to be heard and will retreat if they feel validated.

Distracting Mannerism		*Number of Times Observed*	
Nuisance word	_____	Word: _____	
Fidgeting with personal item (e.g., hair, tie)	_____	Item: _____	
Fidgeting with writing implement	_____	Item: _____	
Adjusting clothing, jewelry	_____		
Fixating on ground/back of room	_____		
Pacing	_____		
Hands in pockets	_____		
Arms crossed	_____		
Poor posture	_____		
Low voice volume	_____		
Speed (too fast or slow)	_____		

FIGURE 6.5 Distracting Mannerisms Checklist.

COMMUNITY CONNECTIONS 6.4

During a program, when Monique shared with parents at the local high school on the benefits of comprehensive sexuality education, an audience member disagreed with the benefits of risk reduction activities in the curriculum. Monique intently listened to the woman speak, even though she knew her information was not based on evidence or best practices. Once she finished, Monique simply thanked her for her opinion and reminded the group that as parents they were the ultimate sexuality educators for their children; the woman quietly listened to what Monique had to say. Monique was reminded that listening skills were extremely important for a presenter. By acknowledging the woman's points, without necessarily agreeing with them, she ensured control as the presenter while demonstrating comfort with opposing opinions.

▶ Expected Outcomes

The primary mission of presentations and trainings should be to accomplish goals and objectives. Objectives should be realistic, with short-term impact objectives focused on knowledge gains, affective changes, or skill development. One of the more difficult tasks for beginning professionals is to decide the degree of change necessary for participants. For example, what percentage of the audience needs to successfully grasp the knowledge for a presentation to be considered successful? A presenter needs to be cautious of setting objectives that are unrealistic such as lowering sexually transmitted infection rates after a three-day knowledge-based program.

One of the outcomes of a presentation that is extremely important to health education specialists is the opportunity to grow as professionals. There are very few substitutes for real-world practice. As a result, new professionals will find growth opportunities from early career presentations. Focusing on what went well and what can be improved should lead to an expectation of self-confidence that can come out of every presentation. As with most areas in life, the more practice and effort that go into the presentation, the more satisfaction likely will result. Students often dislike participating in and delivering in-class presentations in their preprofessional preparation; however, many health education specialists report back to the faculty months or years later on how beneficial the practice and feedback was for them. Additionally, through proper planning and meaningful evaluation, presenters can gain confidence in their ability to both accomplish objectives and deliver effective presentations utilizing appropriate methods.

▶ Conclusion

Learning the art of exceptional presentation preparation and public speaking is essential for health education specialists. Public speaking does not always mean a crowd of people and a podium; it involves a variety of opportunities for sharing health education messages. Regardless of setting, the more proficient the speaker, the more likely it is the audience will absorb information that will assist them in taking action.

Developing effective presentation and training skills thrive under a solid planning process. Health education specialists start with learning about the audience, gathering and organizing valid and reliable materials, ensuring up to date and applicable content, and selecting methods that will allow for greater learner engagement and retention. Putting it all together with rehearsals allow the body and brain to coordinate a polished product. Finally, gathering and reviewing feedback in the form of evaluations supply a continuous quality improvement loop so that future iterations can be the best possible in meeting participant needs.

Key Terms

Distilling Extracting the essential meaning or most important aspects of a presentation.

Goal An outcome a session will achieve by a specific point and time.

Mannerism A habitual gesture or way of speaking.

Method A particular procedure specifically carried out to disseminate information, objectives, and resource materials.

Narrative A spoken or written account of connected events that tell a story.

Nonverbal cues How the message is delivered through facial expressions, body movements, and other gestures.

Objective What students will be able to do after they have completed a session or course.

Process evaluation Assessment of what was implemented or presented; measures the process of the presentation and if participants liked it versus if they learned from it.

Storytelling Sharing a story in a presentation either by the presenter or another individual to connect with the audience; part of a narrative.

Verbal cues How the message is delivered through voice techniques.

References

1. Oxford dictionaries. Retrieved July 6, 2017, from http://en.oxforddictionaries.com
2. Gilbert, G. G., Sawyer, R. G., & McNeill, E. B. (2014). *Health education: Creating strategies for school and community health* (4th ed.). Sudbury, MA: Jones and Bartlett.
3. Jackson, M. *How to communicate with a diverse audience*. Retrieved July 7, 2017, from http://mitchjackson.com/diverse-audience/
4. Bloom, B. S. (Ed.). (1956). *Taxonomy of educational objectives, handbook I: The*

cognitive domain. New York, NY: David McKay Company, Inc.

5. Stanford History Education Group. *Evaluating information: The cornerstone of civic online reasoning*. Retrieved July 6, 2017, from http:// sheg.stanford.edu/upload/V3LessonPlans /Executive%20Summary%2011.21.16.pdf

6. Haigh, C. & Hardy, P. (2011). Tell me a story— a conceptual exploration of storytelling in healthcare education. *Nurse Education Today*, *31*(4), 406–411.

7. Institute for Healthcare Improvement. *Storytelling—it's news*. Retrieved July 6, 2017, from http://www.storynet-advocacy.org/news /IHI%20April-30-2015.shtml

8. Thompson, T. & Krueter, M. W. (2014). Using written narratives in public health practice: A creative writing perspective. *Preventing Chronic Disease*, *11*, 130402.

9. Mandel, S. (1987). *Effective presentation skills*. Los Altos, CA: Crisp Publications.

Additional Resources

Print

National Commission for Health Education Credentialing, Inc. (NCHEC), & Society for Public Health Education (SOPHE). (2015). *A Competency-Based Framework for Health Education Specialists-2015*. Whitehall, PA: National Commission for Health Education Credentialing, Inc. (NCHEC) and Society for Public Health Education (SOPHE).

Internet

HealthIT.gov. *Find quality resources*. Retrieved from HealthIT.gov http://www.healthit.gov /patients-families/find-quality-resources

Medline Plus. *Guide to healthy web surfing*. Retrieved from http://medlineplus.gov /healthywebsurfing.html

National Center for Complementary and Integrative Health. *Finding and evaluating online resources*. Retrieved from the http://nccih .nih.gov/health/webresources

Scanlan, C. (2003, June 20). *Writing from the top down: Pros and cons of the inverted pyramid*. Retrieved from http://www.poynter .org/2003/writing-from-the-top-down-pros -and-cons-of-the-inverted-pyramid/12754/

TED Talks. Retrieved from http://www.ted.com /talks

The Institute for Healthcare Improvement Open School Team. *Collecting patient experience stories*. Retrieved from http://www.ihi.org /education/ihiopenschool/resources /Documents/CollectingPatientExperience Stories.pdf

The University of Queensland. *3 Minute Thesis*. Retrieved from http://threeminutethesis .uq.edu.au/

Verner, S. (2017.). *Six smart ways to organize writing content*. Retrieved from http://busy teacher.org/4838-6-smart-ways-organize -writing-content.html

CHAPTER 7

Developing and Selecting Resource Materials

Katherine Delavan Plomer, MPH

Robert J. Bensley, PhD, MCHES

▶ Author Comments

Katherine: I have been a health educator for the last 25 years, working across a broad spectrum of topics, including HIV/AIDS, school health, cancer prevention, tobacco prevention and control, health literacy, and professional development. Throughout my career, I have been involved in selecting and developing health education materials for a wide variety of audiences. Health information can be confusing and overwhelming for many people. In the current information age, health education specialists have the difficult job of clarifying and communicating vast amount of available health information to wide and varied audiences. Health education specialists can provide an important service by creating easy to understand and audience-centered materials that allow everyone, regardless of reading ability, language status, or other barriers, to receive the health information they need to take care of themselves and improve their lives.

Robert: Over the past 15 years, I've spent a lot of time building and implementing theoretically driven public health technology solutions focused on changing behaviors associated with WIC parent-child feeding, child care center feeding practices, food preparation and cooking skills, weight management, blood pressure management, breastfeeding support, CPR skill acquisition, and college student sexual health practices. The systems we've built have relied heavily on developing, selecting, and delivering thousands of bilingual web-based links, videos, infographics, and internally developed PDF resources directed at assisting users' progress toward active behavior change. Narrowing the plethora of potential resources for a personalized plan of action can be a daunting task, and the skills shared within this chapter will help in providing a framework for tackling a project such as this.

🔍 CHES COMPETENCIES

2.3.4	Apply principles of cultural competence in selecting and/or designing strategies/interventions.
2.3.7	Tailor strategies/interventions for priority populations.
2.3.8	Adapt existing strategies/interventions as needed.
2.3.9	Conduct pilot test of strategies/interventions.*
2.3.10	Refine strategies/interventions based on pilot feedback.*
2.4.6	Select methods and/or channels for reaching priority populations.
5.2.4	Evaluate emerging technologies for applicability to health education/promotion.
6.1.2	Identify valid information resources.
6.1.3	Evaluate resource materials for accuracy, relevance, and timeliness.
6.1.4	Adapt information for consumer.
6.1.5	Convey health-related information to consumer.
7.1.2	Identify level of literacy of intended audience.
7.1.3	Tailor messages for intended audience.
7.1.4	Pilot test messages and delivery methods.*
7.1.6	Assess and select methods and technologies used to deliver messages.
7.1.7	Deliver messages using media and communication strategies.

*Advanced level competency

Reprinted by permission of the National Commission for Health Education Credentialing, Inc. (NCHEC) and Society for Public Health Education (SOPHE).

▶ Introduction

In the age of technology, health information is available almost immediately—anywhere, anytime. Information is available through a quick keyword search on the Internet or comes without invitation through traditional and social media channels. For instance, anyone can write a blog espousing their health philosophies or recommendations, medical advice websites make people feel like they are able to diagnose their own illnesses, and sales of prescription drugs and "miracle cures" are directly marketed regularly to the public through websites, television, and glossy magazine ads. People are bombarded everyday with advice, warnings, and even inaccurate health information. With all of these stimuli, how can health education specialists develop or select materials that engage those who need to be reached? How can materials be designed so they are effective, functional, and motivating? How can health professionals make sure accurate, science-based information is as appealing as what exists in health advertisements? Health education specialists are continually challenged to cut through the noise and misinformation to get accurate and scientifically based health education resources disseminated, read, believed, and acted upon by the public.

Throughout this chapter, several themes vital to making health education resources relevant and useful to populations recur. The cardinal rule is to select or develop resources that present messages simply and clearly so key messages and action steps standout. A second essential rule is to pretest materials with the **intended audience**. They are the only ones who can accurately say what works and what does not. Involving the intended audience in the production of materials can mean the difference between materials being used or ignored.

The list of different types of resources available to the health education specialist is too vast to describe each in detail here. This is because resource materials basically include any type of print or web material designed to convey a message. This includes brochures, flyers, advertisements, webpages, online videos, online web tools, newsletters (both printed and online), infographics, PDFs, games, apps, posters, billboards, bookmarks, placemats, bumper stickers, grocery bags, refrigerator magnets, car magnets, comic books—the list is staggering. Being able to effectively evaluate the use for existing resources and develop new materials to fill in the gap is an essential skill health education specialists need to master. It should be no surprise then that one of the seven major responsibilities for a health education specialist, as defined by the National Commission on Health Education Credentialing, is to "serve as a health education/promotion resource person."[1]

▶ Steps for Selecting or Developing Materials

Before Selection or Development Begins

The amount of health education resources available is immense, and knowing how to evaluate them and what to use is a key skill for all health education specialists. Plenty of discussion and planning needs to take place before the first word is written or materials are selected or designed, because developing an educational piece or assessing existing material for adoption is an investment of personnel time and project resources. Basic fact sheets and information for most major health problems already exist online. New materials for this type of content should not be created, unless they are important for reaching a specific priority population that needs something unique for the information to resonate. The effort health education specialists will most likely focus on is choosing the mode of communication, and then finding the materials that best fit education and program goals. Is the audience millennials? Search for available resources online (e.g., websites, blogs, videos). Hoping to reach seniors? Do not count out web-based materials, but think about more traditional print forms of outreach. Knowing where to look and what criteria to use in selecting materials is key. Verifying new materials are needed and time, staff, and resources can be committed to the task before development begins

will increase the likelihood that the end product serves its purpose.

Questions a health education specialist should ponder prior to creating materials include the following:

- *Why is this material needed?* The need for developing the product may arise from any number of causes such as requests for unavailable materials, the results of a needs assessment, available materials being out of date or inappropriate for a particular audience, available materials being too expensive to purchase, a health emergency (e.g., Ebola outbreak), or the emergence of a new public health issue (e.g., Zika virus).
- *What is the best way to reach the priority population?* The decision on mode of communication should be based on the intended audience and how they prefer to access information.
- *How will this material fit with the program's existing goals and services?* Will the material be used to promote the program's services, supplement presented information, or distributed as an educational tool in and of itself? For example, a nutrition program may use a poster to advertise its services and at the same time provide basic tips on healthy eating.
- *Are there existing materials that could fill the need or do new materials need to be developed?* This question can be answered by looking at existing materials both within and outside an organization, as a plethora of web-based materials that are likely to fit the need and can be used free of charge exist.
- *What materials are available?* Government sites such as the Centers for Disease Control and Prevention (CDC), national and state departments of health, or other government agencies have many materials that have been already developed and are available for download. These materials are open for use by the public and do not have copyright restrictions. Additionally, finding materials can consist of conducting an Internet search to find other major companies, nonprofit organizations,

universities, and experts working in a topic area and checking out materials they have already developed. But remember, nongovernment resources will need permission for use due to copyright and other ownership issues.

Develop or Select the Material

People generally access health information to fulfill a need—whether it is knowledge on how to manage an illness, information on where to go for services, concern over a health issue, or personal interest in a topic. Materials are effective if they take into account the intended audience and their information needs, are attractive and current so the consumer is motivated to engage with the material, and are clearly designed so key messages stand out.

The following seven steps will help to organize and plan material development and selection.[2] These steps can be applied to any form of materials or resources.

Step 1: Define the Intended Audience

Before material development or selection begins, it is important to have a clear understanding of the needs, interests, and culture of the intended audience. Many factors will determine the intended audience; for example, a program may have a defined audience to serve or an individual or group of individuals may request information be developed (e.g., breast cancer survivors may request information on diet and exercise strategies to maintain their health). Other factors to consider are who is most at risk for a given health problem (e.g., injection drug users are a high-risk group for HIV/AIDS) and who might have missed previously developed messages (e.g., Vietnamese women may not be informed about cervical cancer screening due to a lack of culturally and linguistically appropriate materials).

Step 2: Gather Information about the Intended Audience

It is important to gather as much detailed information as possible about the intended audience.

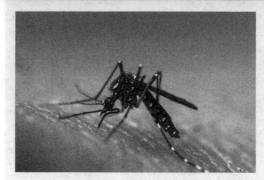

© Joao Paulo Burini/Moment/Getty.

Bekah works at a county health department in an area where the Zika virus and other mosquito-borne diseases are potential health threats. She has been given the task of developing materials to distribute at physicians' offices, at community health and WIC clinics, and through the health department website. Bekah began her work by conducting an Internet search for materials already available on the Zika virus. She discovered CDC had an extensive communications page with materials already developed, several local health departments had developed their own materials, the American Medical Association had materials and a webinar on Zika, and the U.S. Department of Health and Human Services maintained a blog on the subject. Bekah's audience will be the community at large, but the populations most at risk for complications include women who are pregnant or may become pregnant.

Finding out about demographics, needs, interests, concerns, knowledge, values, attitudes, beliefs, barriers to behavior change, motivators, cultural habits, and language preferences allows for the development of audience-centered messages and appealing materials. This information is critical in helping to determine the goals and objectives for the material as well as how the information and messages will be presented.

Finding data on a selected audience can be accomplished in a number of ways. Population level data can be found relatively easily by searching databases at the federal, state and local level.

COMMUNITY CONNECTIONS 7.2

To learn more about the knowledge, behaviors, and concerns of pregnant women in her area, Bekah spoke to several doctors and conducted two focus groups with pregnant women at community health clinics. She learned many pregnant women did not think the risk of contracting Zika was very high, and when the use of repellents was discussed, they were reluctant to use them due to perceived safety concerns. They felt the risks associated with the health repellent outweighed the risk of contracting the virus. None of the materials Bekah reviewed addressed this concern, so she knew she needed to develop an informational piece about the safety of using insect repellents during pregnancy.

For example, community data profiles for all counties in the United States are collected and reported by the CDC on the Community Health Status Indicators page of their website.[3] Healthdata.gov is another example of a site with access portals to many datasets.[4] Community health data can also be found by reviewing results of large surveys such as the Youth Risk Behavior Survey or other population-based surveys.[5]

Local data can further be acquired through focus groups, in-depth interviews with community members, or surveys. Gathering these data is important to truly understand the specific needs and characteristics of the intended community audience. Local data collection will help to tailor materials so they are relevant and responsive to local population needs.

Step 3: Develop Goals and Objectives for the Product

Setting goals and objectives focuses the direction of the material and helps separate what the audience "needs to know" from what is "nice to know." The process for setting goals and objectives should be driven by what is learned from researching the intended audience: What are effective motivators for the intended audience? Do knowledge gaps

exist? What are their barriers to change? Failing to set goals and objectives can result in creating material that is unfocused and too broad to meet the population's needs. Knowing these needs will also help determine the key messages most likely to resonate with the intended audience. Objectives should be limited in number and should focus on the change desired from the reader rather than on facts or principles (**TABLE 7.1**). The tendency is to want to provide a lot of information in case people "want" to know it or it "may be useful." Focusing on the "need to know" information makes key messages clearer and materials better focused on behavior change messages. For example, a message on how and why to reduce cholesterol may be lost in an infographic that puts too much emphasis on the differences between HDL and LDL cholesterol. Including members of the intended audience in this phase will help ensure that goals and objectives are appropriate and achievable.

Step 4: Develop or Select Content and Visuals

Content can be developed or selected once goals and objectives have been determined. Again, participation by the intended audience in this phase is key and can greatly enhance the product and save time later in making revisions. This stage involves deciding how best to present the intended message. For example, what motivates

TABLE 7.1 Sample Goals and Objectives for a Zika Virus Fact Sheet

Goal: Pregnant women will learn about the safety of insect repellent and how to use repellents and other methods to reduce their risk of infection.
Knowledge objective 1: Women can identify two mosquito repellents that are safe for pregnant and breastfeeding women.
Knowledge objective 2: Women can identify at least one non-repellent strategy to reduce their risk of mosquito bites.
Behavioral objective: Women will commit to applying mosquito repellent when engaging in outdoor evening activities.

COMMUNITY CONNECTIONS 7.3

Bekah, in consultation with her community advisors, began to develop content and visuals for her Zika protection material. The intended audience was pregnant women and with her population being racially and ethnically diverse, she wanted to make sure she included pictures that represented the community. To develop the key messages about using insect repellent, Bekah used her knowledge of the Health Belief Model to make sure her intended audience knew it does not matter whether there is 1 mosquito or 1,000, everyone is at risk for contracting Zika if even one infected mosquito is present (perceived susceptibility); Zika can cause severe consequences for the fetus (perceived severity), and applying insect repellent is an effective and safe way to prevent a serious infection (perceived benefits).

COMMUNITY CONNECTIONS 7.4

Bekah showed the insect repellent fact sheet to her colleagues at the health department and gave them a checklist for providing feedback on layout, writing style, and content. She changed some technical information on frequency of applying repellent based on review from an outside content expert. Because she could not provide all the information she wished in the fact sheet, she reviewed several websites and added the web addresses to her resource so those seeking more information would know where to find it.

---

the intended audience to engage in the behavior and what barriers exist? It is essential at this stage to incorporate behavior change theory and models and to decide how to formulate messages based on theoretical principles. This development phase also requires decisions regarding layout and presentation of the material.

Step 5: Internally Review and Evaluate Material

Material should be extensively reviewed internally before it is submitted for pretesting with the intended audience. Proofreading will help identify spelling, punctuation, and other errors. Coworkers, other health education specialists, and graphic designers should review material for accuracy, spelling, grammar, and design. A video, game, or app should be watched or tested internally to discover any glitches or content that needs to be corrected. A content expert should review the information for currency and accuracy, if needed. For example, it would be appropriate for an oncologist or representative from the American Cancer Society to review a web video that focuses on treatment options for breast cancer.

Step 6: Pretest and Revise as Necessary

Developing or selecting health education materials is time consuming, and one step frequently omitted due to time constraints is **pretesting** the material with the intended audience. However, this is one of the most important aspects of resource development that should *not* be overlooked, as it helps ensure materials are well understood, responsive to audience needs, and culturally sensitive.[1] The pretest needs to take into account a variety of important factors, including how the material looks, whether the recipient of the information understands the key messages and feels capable of following recommendations, and whether the material is offensive in any way. The creator of the material cannot accurately assess if the material is acceptable—only the intended audience can provide this input.

The following elements should be assessed when pretesting materials[2,6,7]:

- *Visual appeal.* Is this something someone would want to pick up or watch? Are the colors, images, format, and layout appealing? If the material does not attract attention and invite further attention, it will not be utilized.
- *Comprehension.* Is the content understandable? If key messages are not clear or are misunderstood, the material will not be useful. Make sure to use common language and

define any words or phrases that may be misunderstood.

- *Self-efficacy*. Do people feel they can do what is being asked? Many health messages are ineffective because they are seen as unrealistic. For example, someone overweight who has tried to lose and maintain weight may feel ashamed by not being able to manage weight by materials that focus only on guidelines for healthy eating. Materials that do not address the true barriers associated with weight management may not be effective.

- *Cultural acceptability*. Is the message in any way offensive? Does it seem relevant? Images or messages acceptable to one culture may have an entirely different connotation in another. Similarly, recommendations that make sense to one group may not seem relevant to another. For example, a vegetarian healthy eating campaign would not be best suited for populations who live in "food deserts" and experience food insecurity where residents only have limited ability to purchase fresh fruits and vegetables. Messages that are stereotypical about populations may also be offensive. The best way to ensure a resource is not offensive is to have it reviewed by members of the intended audience.

- *Persuasion*. Do people feel compelled to act? Do they feel the message is relevant to them? Was the message in the material convincing enough that the intended audience would know, for example, regulations surrounding newly implemented tobacco-free policies?

Individual interviews, focus groups, and written feedback forms can be used to pretest materials. In addition, the ease of using available online surveying services (e.g., SurveyMonkey) provides the capability to easily email materials or a link to a resource and have pretesters respond to any number of questions about it. The written feedback form or online survey should be pretested prior to use to ensure questions are clear and will provide the needed feedback. It should be made clear to pretesters that the questions are not intended to be a quiz, but rather to elicit feedback on the material. All questions should be worded in a neutral

language to avoid biasing the pretester. Ideally, 25–50 members of the intended audience should review materials. If this is not realistic, pretesting with at least 5–10 people is better than not pretesting the material at all.[2] If major changes are suggested as a result of the pretesting, the material should be reviewed again by members of the intended audience before the revised version is distributed.

Step 7: Disseminate the Material

Development plans should include how best to distribute materials so they are accessible and seen by the intended audience. How will they be disseminated? By email? Handed out during a presentation or program? Distributed in mass quantities at a health fair or cultural event? As a link in a Facebook post or a web link in a tweet? Available to download from an organization's website? If the intent is for the intended audience to download, it is important to make sure it is easy to do so and there are options that allow those without updated software and slower Internet connections to easily print. This may be as simple as making sure the final product is saved as a PDF, because PDF viewers (e.g., Adobe Acrobat) are free rather than in a specific document format (e.g., Microsoft Word), which all users may not have.

If part of a social media campaign, what are the best apps to use? Instagram? Facebook? Twitter? A combination? If it is an on-demand webinar or video, will a link be sent to the intended audience so they can access it directly or will a promotional campaign be conducted to entice people to a website to find the material there? In designing the most effective dissemination plan, remember to think about the intended audience and how and where they get their information.

COMMUNITY CONNECTIONS 7.6

Bekah had the fact sheet printed for community distribution. She created a colorful version to post on the health department website, but due to budget constraints, the fact sheet for in-person distribution was printed in crisp black type on light-colored paper. Fact sheets and a link to the health department's website were sent to OB/GYN offices, distributed at community health and WIC clinics, and passed out at community health fairs. Links to the online version were distributed as messages in the health department's Twitter campaign and posted on the Department's Facebook page.

▸ Tips and Techniques for Developing and Selecting Resource Materials

Most public health materials are developed for broad constituencies. There are many ways to get health messages out to the community and printed materials—whether actually printed or accessed as a link via the Internet that could essentially be printed—that still play a huge role in how health education specialists educate and motivate the public. Each project is unique, but there are some general principles that can be followed to make a resource attractive, clear, and appropriate for the intended audience.

Determine Appropriate Content

Deciding on and prioritizing the information to include in a resource is the cornerstone to disseminating the health message. More information exists on a topic than there is room for sharing it, and often—especially if a team creates written material—there are different views on what content is important. The following guidelines help to ensure the ending product does not try to cover too much material, and what is covered is reinforced for the reader:

- *Limit goals and objectives.* Prioritize goal and objectives to one or two main points. Trying to fit too much information in any one resource will make it difficult for the reader to retain *any* of the information.
- *Present important information first.* Mention main points up front, reinforce throughout, and organize logically in the order in which the reader will use the information.
- *Summarize important points.* Summarize key points at the end, particularly if a lot of information has been communicated, to reinforce action steps and refocus the reader on the key points of the material.

Adjust for Health Literacy and Reading Level

Most public health materials should be developed for readers with limited literacy. The National Assessment of Adult Literacy, released in 2003, revealed that 30 million adults struggle with basic reading skills and only about 12% of adults have proficient health literacy skills.[8] **Health literacy** is defined as "the degree to which individuals have the capacity to obtain, process and understand basic health information and services needed to make appropriate health decisions."[9] Health literacy is comprised of many factors including cultural and conceptual knowledge and listening, speaking, mathematics, writing, and reading skills.[9]

Much of the work in the health literacy field has focused on assessing the **readability** of health materials in relation to the education level of the reader. Education level is the measure most often used to estimate reading ability, but people generally read at a level below their last completed grade. It is estimated that 50% of the U.S. population cannot read a book written at the eighth grade level and 45 million Americans are functionally illiterate and read below a fifth grade level.[10] As such, when developing materials for the general public, it is best to aim for a fourth to sixth grade reading level, with seventh to eighth grade being the highest level. A higher level can be used if writing for a specific audience, but even an "educated" reader can appreciate a simple, direct, and well-written message. A common misconception is that writing materials at sixth grade reading level is the same as writing materials suitable for a sixth grader, which can imply a tone of writing designed for a child. Writing at a reduced reading level really means simplifying materials by reducing sentence length, explaining unfamiliar terms, and adjusting word selection to use simpler and more familiar words.

⑦ DID YOU KNOW?

More than 300 studies have found health-related materials far exceed the average reading ability of U.S. adults.

Data from Committee on Health Literacy Board on Neuroscience and Behavioral Health. (2004). *Health literacy: A prescription to end confusion.* Washington D. C.: The National Academies Press.

A number of readability tests are available for determining reading level. Many word processing programs have built-in readability tests and online formulas to test the readability of a document and are easy to access. Most **readability formulas** (e.g., SMOG, FOG, and FRY) are based on a system that compares the number of sentences to the number of polysyllabic words within a passage. Materials that contain several short sentences consisting of short words will score at a lower reading level.

Readability formulas provide a gauge of how easy or difficult a resource is to read. Formulas do not, however, provide a complete picture. Readability formulas should be one measure, but not the only way an educational piece is evaluated. These formulas do not take into account context, accuracy of language used, clarity of style, design, or the reader's experience or culture. Combining a readability formula with other evaluation methods, including pretesting and tools such as the Suitability Assessment of Materials (SAM), will provide the most accurate picture of how easy or difficult a document is to read. SAM provides a systematic way to review and rate print material in six categories: content, literacy demand, graphics, layout and typography, learning stimulation and motivation, and cultural appropriateness.[6] The tool provides specific criteria for rating material as superior, adequate, or not suitable in each of the six categories.

Readability and understandability is key for online materials too, so first review Internet sites that will be cited to make sure the information is easy to understand and navigate. In addition, numerous webpage readability sites exist, where readability scores are calculated on an inputted webpage address. Materials should also be compliant with W2C accessibility guidelines (www.w3.org/wai), which ensures access to the web by everyone regardless of disability and, for government publications, adherence to Section 508 guidelines (www.usability.gov/accessibility).

⑦ DID YOU KNOW?

Improving readability or "writing in plain language" is more than just good practice—it is a requirement for the federal government. In 2010, President Obama signed the Plain Writing Act of 2010, which requires federal agencies use clear communication that the public can understand and use. In 2011, he issued a new executive order aimed at "Improving Regulation and Regulatory Review." This order states that regulatory systems must ensure regulations are accessible, consistent, written in plain language, and easy to understand.

In addition to making sure information is written at an appropriate reading level, the following writing style guidelines will make a resource easier to read[2,11]:

- *Use common words*. Substituting words e.g., using *shot* for *injection* or using the word *flu* rather than *influenza*) makes materials much more understandable to people. Stick to common words whenever possible to create the easiest materials to read (**TABLE 7.2**). As a general rule, use words with fewer syllables whenever possible.

TABLE 7.2 Substituting Common Words to Increase Ease of Reading

Word	Substitute
carcinogens	cause cancer
hypertension	high blood pressure
contraception	birth control
injection	shot
physician	doctor

TABLE 7.3 Active versus Passive Voice

Active:	Eat five servings of fruits and vegetables a day.
Passive:	Five servings of fruits and vegetables should be eaten every day.
Active:	Exercise three times a week for good health.
Passive:	Get regular exercise in order to have good health.

- *Use concrete language.* The more exact and concrete the language, the clearer the message. Spell out the exact recommendation whenever possible. For example, "Don't ever text when you're driving."
- *Use a conversational tone.* Writing in the third person is often the norm in writing. Using the second person *you*, however, can be effective in personalizing information and focusing the message directly on the reader. For example, "Stop exercising if you feel short of breath."
- *Explain technical terms.* Technical words, especially medical terms, are often unfamiliar to people and can be difficult to understand. Technical terms do not necessarily need to be avoided but should always be defined or explained. For instance, *mammogram* is an important term to understand in relation to breast cancer screening. A mammogram might be described as an "X-ray of the breast."
- *Write in an active voice.* Using active rather than passive phrases is more direct, action oriented, and how people tend to talk with each other (**TABLE 7.3**). Vivid and active phrases make it clear to readers exactly what is expected of them and what action to take.
- *Use short sentences.* Sentences should be kept short when possible. Sentences that are too long and cover too many points can be confusing.

- *Use slang words with caution.* Slang should be used with caution because it is not always appropriate and may offend some people. On the other hand, it is useful to use terms with which the priority audience is familiar and to which they can relate. Also, take caution in using common social media acronyms (e.g., IMHO, YOLO), as not all populations may be accustomed to their meanings.
- *Add interaction.* The more readers interact with the material, the more likely they are to remember and incorporate the information. Interaction can be added to materials by making PDFs fillable forms by adding checkboxes and text boxes, posing questions for readers to answer, or adding links to other sites, videos, or resources that provide ability to delve deeper into specific aspects of the content (**FIGURE 7.1**).

⑦ DID YOU KNOW?

The English language itself can get in the way of writing clearly. Consider the following examples:
- The bandage was wound around the wound.
- After a number of injections my jaw got number.
- I had to subject the subject to a number of tests.
- The way the bully responded was pretty ugly.

Am I at Risk for Breast Cancer?

You may be at risk for developing breast cancer if you can answer "yes" to any of the following*:

- I have a family history (mother, grandmother, sister) of breast cancer.
- I have a personal history of breast or ovarian cancer.
- I began my period before age 12.
- I began menopause after age 55.
- I have been exposed to great amounts of radiation (x-rays, treatments).
- I have the "breast cancer" gene.

*Even without one or more of these risk factors, you could still be at risk for breast cancer.

FIGURE 7.1 Adding Interaction.

Focus on Layout and Design

Layout is the combination of text and graphics on a page, and a balance between the two is important. A well-designed layout is one that works for the audience, organizes information in a way the reader will use it, and attracts attention. The following design guidelines aid in the development of an effective layout for health education materials[2,11]:

- *Create a cover or opening statement that grabs the reader's attention.* Many people will take only a few seconds to determine whether they want to read a resource. If the cover or opening statement does not appeal to the reader or provide enough basic information on the content, people may not peruse any further.
- *Leave ample white space.* Crowded materials make it difficult for readers to sort through relevant information. Text should be balanced with graphics, graphical elements (boxes, lines, tables), and white space. White space may increase the length of the material, and a common mistake is to cut out white space to preserve content. Before doing this, the content should be reviewed to determine if unnecessary information can be eliminated or any language tightened. Hyperlinking to additional content for a web-based resource is another way to preserve space.

- *Use headings to separate text.* It is best to organize related information under an appropriate heading, as this guides readers through the text. It also helps in directing readers back to sections of information that may be more relevant to their needs.
- *Use bullets and numbering to highlight key points.* Using bulleted or numbered lists makes it easy for readers to identify main ideas without sorting through unnecessary information. Each list should have a simple, instructional heading. Lists should be limited to five or six items and if more room is needed, subheadings can be used. Lists also aid in the presentation of sequential information.
- *Use a jagged right edge.* Readers have an easier time reading text with a jagged right edge (left justified). Right or full justification makes it difficult for a reader's eyes to follow text down the page.
- *Use generous line spacing.* As a rule of thumb, multiple spacing should be used to separate paragraphs.
- *Use horizontal print rather than vertical.* People are accustomed to reading from left to right across a page. Vertical print can challenge even strong readers.
- *Avoid orphan lines.* Orphan lines are those that do not fit on the same page or in the same column as the rest of the text. The layout should be rearranged so that a minimum

of two lines is set off by themselves. It is better to move a whole paragraph or section to the next page than to leave a line stranded.

- *Plan materials so important ideas follow appropriate reading pattern.* Most readers of print materials are right-eye dominant, meaning they first look at the upper left corner and then crisscross diagonally across the page (in a "Z" pattern) toward the bottom right corner. Therefore, the most important idea should be in the upper left with a final key message flowing to the bottom right corner. On a webpage, readers tend to view the screen using an "F" pattern, where the reader scans the top line horizontally from left to right, moves quickly to a second line and scans left to right, then scans vertically the remaining elements, occasionally following a left-to-right horizontal scan of anything else of interest.[12]

- *Design with mobile in mind.* Mobile access to the Internet continues to expand, and globally is the primary method for accessing the Internet.[13] Mobile access to online health education represents a major shift in how users interact with information, resulting in differences in usage patterns and levels of engagement.[14] This is because many websites were initially designed with fixed device (e.g., laptop, desktop computer) as the mode for access, but are now being primarily accessed through a mobile platform.[15] Mobile screens are smaller in size as compared to a fixed device, making it more difficult for users to engage in material developed with a bigger screen in mind.[15] If the primary audience is likely to be mobile users, then the material needs to be designed as such. This means a responsive design needs to be considered, where the webpage adjusts dependent on device accessing it rather than just the shrinking in size to fit a smaller screen. If that is not a possibility, then the material being developed needs to have less content and simplified messaging to account for the smaller viewing space. It is always better to err on the side of "less is more," and create materials with less content and imagery so it is likely able to be read regardless of device accessing it.

Follow Typestyle Guidelines

Poorly chosen fonts, typestyles, or type size can greatly impair readability. An abundance of literature is available that describes the intricacies of print and font choices, and common typestyle guidelines for printed educational materials include the following[2,11]:

- *Use appropriate type size.* With print material, it is best to use either a 12–14-point type size. Larger sizes may be used to highlight main ideas, themes, headings, or titles. Anything smaller is difficult to read. Web material tends to scale down a font size (10-point), as the limited space on a webpage necessitates a reduced font size. Plus, it is easy for web users to adjust their screen or webpage viewing size or expand the webpage itself in order to adjust the font for readability purposes.

- *Choose fonts carefully.* Although it may seem creative or fun to use more than two fonts, it can make the material appear cluttered and be more difficult to read. When using two fonts together, it works best to combine a serif font with a sans serif font (**FIGURE 7.2**). With print material, serif type (letters have extensions or "feet" on the ends) is easier to read than sans serif type (letters do not have extensions on the ends). Sans serif is appropriate when trying to convey a sense of formality or professionalism. In contrast, serif is less formal and conveys a "softer" feeling. However, this differs with web-based content, where sans serif is easier to read on the screen.

SERIF (with feet)   **SANS SERIF (without feet)**

FIGURE 7.2 Serif and Sans Serif Type.

Script fonts are appropriate when trying to convey softness, sensitivity, or elegance, but can be difficult for readers and should be used sparingly. As such, it is important to use a large enough type size when using script. This is true for both print and PDF web materials that are designed to be printed. With webpage content, it is best to use the fonts (e.g., Arial, Calibri) most likely to be part of any web browser, as those are what people are familiar with and will appear regardless of browser or device.

Specific fonts can be used to elicit a specific feel or emotion. For instance, use of courier can captivate a retro feeling associated with a typewriter. In contrast, overuse of a specific font can detract from the message. An example is the overuse and misuse of comic sans when trying to convey a childlike or informal writing style.[16]

- *Consider color.* There are many options for print color. Black is by far the clearest. So, sticking with dark colors like navy blue, dark green, or burgundy if choosing a color other than black is best. The print chosen should contrast with the background color, so a white or light background works best with dark type. In the event the background is a dark color, then 100% white should be used for the text, as black text on a dark background is difficult to read. Ability to read certain colors due to visual impairment also needs to be considered.
- *Emphasize a word or main idea.* Capitalization, boldface, and italics are meant to enhance a point. If they are used for more than a few words at a time, it becomes difficult to read the text and to distinguish important ideas. Full capitalization is hard to read and conveys a message of "shouting" (**FIGURE 7.3**).

Also, underlining should be used sparingly or not at all. Underlying was a cue for the printer to change the typeset to italics before computer word processing was available.

- *Use visual cues such as arrows, circles, or boxes to call attention to important points.* Setting important information aside in a text box or circling an important word or phrase provides emphasis. Arrows can be helpful in pointing the reader to a specific spot on an illustration.

Select Appropriate Graphics and Images

Appropriate graphics and images can greatly enhance the effectiveness of health education materials. Clear graphics can make a complex idea or procedure more easily understood, improve recall of information, and increase readers' interest in a written piece. The use of graphics, graphic organizers, and pictures has been shown to increase memory retention, recall, comprehension, and adherence.[17,18]

Graphics and images relieve the monotony of large volumes of text and can reduce text by illustrating important points. They can, however, confuse the reader if they are not linked to the educational purpose. Applying the following guidelines to the use of graphics and images will ensure they help the reader and do not detract from the educational message[2,11]:

- *Use graphics and images that aid in communicating the message.* Graphics and images should help the reader comprehend and follow the message. Individuals who have a difficult time comprehending text tend to

THIS IS AN EXAMPLE OF USING ALL UPPERCASE LETTERS. WHICH DO YOU THINK IS EASIER TO READ, THIS PARAGRAPH OR THE ONE IMMEDIATELY FOLLOWING?

This is an example of using a mixture of upper- and lowercase letters. Which do you think is easier to read, this paragraph or the one immediately preceding it?

FIGURE 7.3 Inappropriate Use of Capitalization.

use graphics and images as a guide. Therefore, a graphic should be placed near the text that illustrates the idea. Do not include a graphic or image just for the sake of having one. It will distract the reader and could be confusing if it does not help communicate the message.

- *Use simple drawings as opposed to complex graphics.* Simple drawings do not contain large amounts of detail and are easily recognizable. Complex graphics generally contain shading and intricate detail. As such, complex graphics may not be understood by the viewer or may lose their clarity.
- *Use captions to explain graphics.* A caption below a graphic explains what is depicted.
- *Use graphics and images that are appropriate for the intended audience.* If the material is intended for the general public, graphics should depict positive health behaviors. Ideally, a person should be shown acting out the positive health behavior being described.
- *Use culturally appropriate graphics and images.* Graphics and images should depict a culture in a realistic and positive way. It is important, however, to avoid stereotyping or making assumptions about people or behaviors (e.g., not every family is made up of two parents, a boy, a girl, and a family dog). Graphics and images should be pretested with the intended audience to be sure they are not perceived as stereotypical, offensive, or irrelevant.
- *Use recognizable graphics and images.* Anything displayed should be recognizable to the intended audience. For example, some may not recognize a picture of the lungs unless it is put in the context of where the lungs are in the body.
- *Leave ample white space around graphics and images.* As with type, sufficient white space reduces clutter. This will help the graphic or image draw the eye into the type rather than vice versa. Also, wrapping text around the graphic or image should be avoided, as it is often hard to read.
- *Use varying sizes of graphical elements.* Graphics that are all the same size are not very interesting. Instead, varying element sizes adds interest and shows what is most important. Size should depict the relative importance of each image.
- *Anchor graphics and images to the edge of the page.* Graphics and images should not be floating in the middle of the page but rather anchored to the edge of the page to help balance with the text.
- *Consider image size when creating web material.* Even in today's world not everyone has high-speed access to the web. As recent as 2016, 10% of all Americans lacked access to a high-speed Internet connection, especially in rural and tribal land populations.[19] A multi-megabyte image can dramatically impact load time on a slow connection, resulting in users becoming impatient; the likelihood for abandoning a site increases dramatically when load time is more than a second or two. Mobile users expect the load time to be even faster.[20,21]

Visualize Data and Information

Much of what public health professionals communicate to the public is data—how many people are impacted by a particular health issues, for example, what percentage of a given population is at risk, what trends are in a disease progression, and what do evaluation results mean. Deciding the story the data is supposed to tell and then finding ways to visually relay key messages of that story through data presentation is an art and a skill. Data can be displayed in many more ways than just through a bar graph or pie chart, which may provide greater impact. New techniques are evolving for data visualization in presentations and materials (see Additional Resources).

Infographics have become a popular way of presenting complex data in a visual way. Pictures can make data more accessible by taking it out of charts and putting it into a pictorial form (**FIGURE 7.4**). Originally designed as maps using data to represent geography,[22] infographics have become part of a larger data visualization tendency for communicating statistics, trends, and connections in a way that resonates with people.

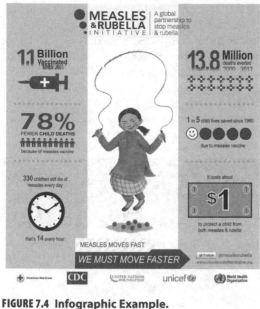

FIGURE 7.4 Infographic Example.
Courtesy of Centers for Disease Control and Prevention.

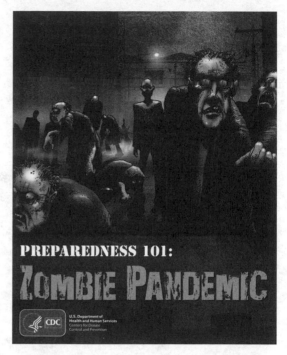

FIGURE 7.5 CDC Emergency Prepardness Campaign.
Courtesy of Centers for Disease Control and Prevention.

Creating infographics involves the same steps as creating other materials. Determining goals and objectives for the infographic, researching the priority audience, and designing the infographic with users' needs in mind are important. There are many companies and websites that provide free infographics creation (e.g., Piktochart, infogr.am, Canva). Generally, the "free" level has the most limitations in options of how to represent information and further flexibility and options become available with a subscription or fee. Other tools like PowerPoint are providing upgrades that allow charts and graphs created more easily for use in infographics.

Comics and **photonovels** are also visually interesting and effective ways to provide health information. Photonovels can make health information accessible to low literacy and other audiences by providing technical information with visuals, minimal wording, and a compelling story line.[23] CDC created one of their most popular emergency preparedness information campaigns using this format to capitalize on the mainstream entertainment popularity of a "zombie apocalypse" (**FIGURE 7.5**).[24] Fotonovelas for Latino audiences have been widely utilized and popular for

many years and shown impact with various health issues.[25,26]

The medium of photonovels has been brought to life using motion comics. For example, the CDC created an effective HIV/STD prevention motion comic in 2011 and reported encouraging results for the 15- to 25-year-old age group for which it was designed.[27] Traditional comics can be brought to life and others can be created using whiteboard animation through websites like Videoscribe, RawShorts, and others.

Use a Variety of Internet Resources

The proliferation of the web over the past two decades has resulted in the availability of numerous resources, in many different formats, available for use by health education specialists. Static and interactive webpages, downloadable PDFs, video streaming, blogs, webinars, gaming, and social media channels are commonly available resources that can be used for health education and promotion interventions. However, even though extensive health information exists online, the lack of any required process for approving online content means much of it is of questionable content and quality. For example, the proliferation of marketing and advertising on websites and social media that masquerades as education means it is important to assist audiences in understanding the difference as they look for information online. Criteria in **TABLE 7.4** can be used to help evaluate credibility of web-based materials or sites to use for educational purposes.

Webpages

Webpages come in numerous forms and can be singular pages with content or multiple pages

TABLE 7.4 Web Materials Checklist

Criteria	Positive Signs	Caution/Red Flag
Who sponsors the site/created the material?	■ The site is sponsored by a reputable, known organization or person. ■ The site's purpose is education and not sales. ■ There is clear information about the site's sponsor in the "about" section.	■ The site sponsor is unknown. ■ The site sponsor is a vendor or merchant. ■ No information is provided about who sponsors the site.
What is the site's/material's purpose?	■ Educate. ■ Inform.	■ Sales. ■ Promotion of product or service.
Original source of information.	■ Peer-reviewed research. ■ Evidence-based information.	■ Own studies. ■ Anecdotal information. ■ Unknown.
Who reviews the site/material? Is the information current?	■ Curated by reputable organization. ■ Commitment to objectivity. ■ Reviewed and updated on a regular basis.	■ Site not reviewed. ■ Information is out of date. ■ Cannot tell when information has last been updated. ■ Bias is clear.
Does the site ask for personal information?	■ No—that's good! ■ Could be okay if the purpose is to further inform you.	■ Collecting personal information to sell something. ■ Provides or sells personal information to other organizations.

Data from U.S. Food & Drug Administration. Quick tips for buying medicines over the Internet. Retrieved from http://www.fda.gov/drugs/resourcesforyou /consumers/buyingusingmedicinesafely/buyingmedicinesovertheinternet/ucm202863.htm; National Center for Complementary and Integrative Health. (2014). Finding and evaluating online resources. NCCIH Pub. No. D337. Retrieved from http://www.nccih.nih.gov/health/webresources

across a site. Some may be interactive in nature, where input (rather than a simple click) by the user drives the next series of content or pages displayed. The concept and varying functions served by websites and webpages are numerous, and include anything from a simple list of content associated with a health issue to a theoretically driven and interactive behavior change system. However, both the development and a thorough discussion of different types and formats of webpages is far beyond the scope of this chapter. Many websites and checklists exist for determining factors that influence credibility of websites, which usually include examining the author of the content, domain extension (e.g., .org, .gov., .com, .edu), date last updated, cited sources of content, existence of advertising, hyperlinks within the content, writing style and site design, and other factors. Website and individual webpages can be a great resource to share with a priority population, as they can easily be linked to from various social media apps, the health agency's website, within news articles or other print articles, as resources within web-based interventions[28] and other dissemination avenues.

PDFs

Many infographics and other graphically designed materials are accessible as PDFs that can be easily downloaded, printed, emailed, or linked to from other social media and webpages. Previously shared guidelines associated with developing print materials mostly hold true for PDF materials as well, due to the nature of the PDF actually being a document rather than a webpage.

Video Streaming

Numerous videos are available on web-based multimedia sites (e.g., YouTube, Vimeo) focusing on a variety of health education topics, public service announcements, "how to" skills such as a cooking demonstration, and other content. Some are posted by reputable organizations while others are self-made. Videos can be a great tool for sharing information or demonstrating skills, and can appeal to different populations by being able to further explain complex concepts, keep the audience engaged, and elicit a wide variety of emotions. Videos can be helpful for limited literacy and older audiences, as they do not rely on the written word, or they can be coupled with content such as a recipe to show necessary cooking skills associated with preparing the meal.[29] Accessibility, however, is important. Slow connections cause videos to stop frequently for buffering, which can be a frustrating experience.

Blogs

Blogs can be an effective way for accessing new information and trends. Subscribing to blogs from universities, trusted sites, or reputable scholars and researchers can help health education specialists and priority populations stay current on latest trends and information. Many major organizations and researchers active in a specific field have a blog that can be followed. Before using content from or recommending a blog for educational purposes, it is important to first determine if any bias exists, the credibility of the institution or the author, and if information is kept current. Some bloggers begin their blog by providing information, and then switch to marketing to get followers to sign up for a skill-building course, subscription, or other products. Blogs sending readers to sites that want to sell them goods or services should be suspect, even when the information may be interesting and accurate. Information and education should be free, as is the case with CDC's blog covering a variety of topics in public health (see Additional Resources).

Webinars, Podcasts, and Learning Modules

Like blogs, a plethora of online learning modules, podcasts, and webinars are available that can be used to provide consistent information on a topic. They provide an easy, on demand way for people to get information at their convenience. Some points to consider when recommending a webinar, podcast, or learning module to others include (1) knowing goals and objectives for having someone access the site (What do you want them to do with the information they receive?) and (2) always review the online resource before referring someone to it (Can you sit through it? Is it interactive? Is it informative? Is it the right level of complexity? Is it correct and up to date?).

Gaming

Another rising method of health education is using games, even though they have been used in therapeutic health since the 1980s, when commercial video games were used as a form of distraction, which showed therapeutic benefits for reducing nausea in child cancer patients, and anxiety reduction.[30] More recent focus is on development of games merging health education theory with a popular technology for an interactive learning experience, with some games having shown a positive impact in changing behavior and increasing knowledge.[31] As with all other media, it is important to know the purpose for directing the intended audience to a given game and to check out the game first to make sure it is research based, relevant, and up to date.

Consider Special Populations

Older Audiences

Older adults may have greater difficulty with vision, memory, and chronic illnesses, all of which can impede comprehending material. Font size is particularly important when writing for older audiences. A general rule of thumb is to start with 12-point type and add a point for every decade after age 40. For instance, if a printed piece were to be directed toward postretirement individuals, the appropriate type size would be 14–16 points (ages 60–79). As an individual's eyesight diminishes, it is easier to read larger type.

Colors should be carefully chosen. Older populations tend to have a harder time reading light type on a dark background. Choosing colors with a strong contrast between the text and background, preferably dark type on a light background, can help minimize reading issues. Abbreviations, clichés, slang, and figurative language are to be avoided, as they may be unknown or confusing. Cues such as arrows, underlines, circles, and colors are useful in helping the eye focus on the most relevant information. A variety of graphics and images should be used to reflect the diversity of age, culture, and health status represented in the broad category of older adults.

---

⑦ DID YOU KNOW?

mHealth, short for Mobile Health, is "the use of mobile technologies to support the achievement of health objectives." According to a 2009 survey by the World Health Organization, 83% of the 114 member states utilize some sort of mHealth initiative. The most frequent mHealth initiatives are health call centers, emergency toll-free telephone services, managing emergencies and disasters, and mobile telemedicine (WHO).

Data from World Health Organization. (2011). *mHealth: New Horizons for Health through Mobile Technology.* Switzerland: WHO.

Culturally Diverse Audiences

Making materials culturally appropriate is essential for reaching members of different racial and ethnic groups. Recognizing distinctions between subpopulations is critical. For example, the categorization of Asian/Pacific Islander has a multitude of nationalities and cultures within it, so health education specialists should be careful not to broadly generalize about the population as a whole. Learning about the local population is important to developing relevant, appropriate materials. Many health messages are lost on members of minority populations because of poor translations, lack of attention to culturally specific motivators, and lack of involvement of the intended audience in the development and review of materials.[32] Reviewing materials designed for wide distribution assures multiple populations are considered and represented.

Translation of materials into other languages is another challenge. Messages should be developed, whenever possible, in the language of the intended audience versus being developed in English and then translated, as literal word-for-word translations from English often result in the loss of meaning of the material. When translation is required, a bilingual team representing the different ethnic groups or dialects of the intended audience should review the material. Three strategies health education specialists can use to create accurate educational materials, no matter what the language, include (1) back translation—translate the materials in one language and then independently translate them back into the first language, (2) decentering—simultaneously translate materials into both languages, adjusting both until they have equivalent meaning, and (3) extensive pretesting.[32]

---

⑦ DID YOU KNOW?

At least 350 languages are spoken in U.S. homes with one in five residents speaking a non-English language at home (USCB, CIS).

Data from U.S. Census Bureau. (2015). Census Bureau reports at least 350 languages spoken in U.S. homes. Retrieved from http://www.census.gov/newsroom/press-releases/2015/cb15-185.html; Center for Immigration Studies. (2014). One in five U.S. residents speaks foreign language at home, record 61.8 million. Retrieved from http://www.cis.org/record-one-in-five-us-residents-speaks-language-other-than-english-at-home

▸ Overcoming Challenges In Developing and Selecting Resource Materials

Manage Time

There is no such thing as developing a "quick infographic" or a "simple brochure." Often, the most clear and well-written materials—the ones that look like they must have been easy to develop—actually took the most time. It is better to be realistic up front and allow adequate time to develop and pretest written materials. The following factors should be considered when creating a development timeline for materials:

- *Number of people involved in development.* The more the priority population is included in the development process and the larger the team for developing materials, the longer it will take.
- *Material approval process.* Internal procedures and requirements and the proper approval channels can add significant time to development.

- *Pretesting process.* Developing pretest questions, finding people to help review materials, and incorporating feedback add time to the project, especially if results of pretesting reveal major changes need to be made to the material.
- *Software skills.* If new to material development software, additional time will be needed. A simple PDF can take time to conceptualize, research, develop, pretest, and upload to a site.

The development process almost always takes longer than anticipated. An important strategy for managing time is to have a clear action plan: What are the steps in creating the material and what is the timeline? Setting deadlines for the steps that need to be taken and sticking to them will help keep on track. Knowing who is doing what is also important in managing time: Who is developing the content? Who is doing the layout? Who is managing the upload to the website? Who is monitoring the social media channel? When multiple people are working on the material it is important to coordinate schedules and keep in constant communication. If key individuals in the organization need to approve the material, they need to keep abreast of the process and the timeline of the project. In addition, developing pretest questions and making contacts to find pretesters early in the project, instead of waiting until everything is finished, can positively impact the timeline.

Find Pretesters

Finding members of the intended audience to help pretest materials can be challenging. Depending on the nature of the material being developed, individuals with certain characteristics are needed for the most accurate review. For example, African Americans pretesters should review a fact sheet on diabetes written for African Americans. A local health clinic that serves primarily African American patients may have individuals willing to participate. Office staff can be enlisted to advertise in the clinic or utilize social media channels to recruit interested individuals.

Partnerships with community groups (e.g., senior centers, schools, adult education programs, health clinics) can assist in finding individuals who might be willing to help pretest materials. Online social networks may also be an avenue for getting feedback prior to sending out for pretesting to a larger audience. If possible, incentives for reviewing materials—whether it is money, grocery certificates, or a small gift of appreciation—let pretesters know their time and input is valuable.

Build Capacity in Graphics and Design

Finding graphics and images to use can be challenging, especially on a budget. Stock photo websites (e.g., Getty Images, Shutterstock) have photos, vectors, illustrations, icons, music, and videos for purchase. Subscriptions to these sites provide access to all or part of the content for a set period of time, and purchasing an individual photo or illustration or a package of images for a fee is also possible. Once images are purchased, they can be freely used in materials.

Using search engines like Bing or Google Images is another means for finding images. Thousands of images will come up on any given search but many are copyright restricted, so it is important to check copyright rules and properly cite illustrations as appropriate. It is possible in the tools section of major search engines to limit images only to those that are not restricted. Sites also exist that provide free, high quality images that are not copyright restricted or have limited restrictions (e.g., Morguefile, Creative Commons). Images can also be found through government sources such as free health education images in CDC's Public Health Image Library (see Additional Resources).

Being able to apply graphics and images to enhance the message is an art form that was previously left to graphic designers. Even though the availability of numerous publishing and illustration software packages has brought robust tools to the material developer, it does not necessarily mean the developer has graphic design skills. Many times it is the health education specialist who will be developing the materials. To overcome this challenge, bookmark folders can be set up and webpages added to it that have unique and interesting examples of the application of graphical elements, webinars or online learning modules exist that share graphic design skills, and online videos demonstrate certain aspects of how to apply graphic tools associated with specific design software.

▶ Expected Outcomes

Health materials, if properly developed, can be effective in providing information, motivating behavior change, and directing the priority population to needed services. The development process takes time and requires attention to many details such as content, typestyle, layout, readability, and cultural appropriateness. The step-by-step process and the tips and techniques provided in this chapter provide a solid framework to use in material development and selection, resulting in a number of intended positive outcomes.

Materials that Fit a Need

As was discussed early in the chapter, taking time to ask and answer key questions before beginning development is important. Answering preplanning questions will ensure all channels have been explored, the correct method is selected to reach the intended audience, the proposed material is clearly needed, and the material fits within a program's existing goals and services.

Clear and Understandable Materials

Each step in the development process provides important information to guide in the development of the material. Gathering information on the intended audience and developing goals and objectives for the product will ensure health education specialists understand the population they are trying to reach and materials developed or selected will have a clear purpose. Developing content and visuals in partnership with the intended audience and internally reviewing and externally pretesting materials will ensure they are accurate, clear, and motivating.

Audience-Centered and Culturally Appropriate Materials

Involving members of the intended audience in developing and pretesting materials is extremely beneficial. The most important outcome is creation of materials that are culturally appropriate and centered on audience needs, preferences, and motivators. Materials that are pretested with audience members are more credible and provide the community with a sense of ownership in the end product. Including audience members also helps health education specialists to better know the community, build relationships, and create partnership opportunities for future projects.

▶ Conclusion

Designing or choosing health education resources is an important job of health education specialists. Technology is increasing the access populations have to information and is providing new tools for health education specialists to disseminate materials. As such, the process of material development and review is continual, because health education materials can quickly become dated as new materials and content are created and disseminated—thanks to the Internet and other technologies—at an increasingly rapid pace.

Developing and selecting materials requires health education specialists to draw upon their knowledge and skills in many areas. Knowledge of behavior change theory and social marketing and health communication principles can aid in content and message selection. Skills in conducting focus groups and facilitating meetings are important in gathering input from the intended audience and working with a team to develop materials. Creating written materials also requires skills in writing, design, and readability assessment. Equally important is to constantly be aware of rapidly changing trends associated with the Internet, social media, and other technologies. Developing health education materials is one way health education specialists can utilize their many skills to communicate vital health information to the public, and can be a fun and rewarding part of the health education specialist's job.

Key Terms

Health literacy A person's ability to understand and process basic health information to make appropriate health decisions.

Infographic A resource consisting of visual images to represent information or data.

Intended audience The audience designated as the population to reach. Also referred to as the priority audience.

Layout The arrangement of text and graphics on a page.

Photonovel A resource consisting of sequential storytelling that uses photos instead of illustrations as the images.

Pretesting The process of testing materials with the intended audience through individual interviews, focus groups, or written forms to be sure materials are understandable, attractive, and culturally appropriate.

Readability How easy it is to read a document is based on such factors as approximate grade level, clarity of writing style, layout, design, and vocabulary.

Readability formula A mathematical formula generally used to calculate the approximate reading level of a piece of material. The formula takes into account the number of sentences in relation to the number of polysyllabic words within a passage.

References

1. National Commission for Health Education Credentialing. (2015). *Responsibilities and competencies.* Retrieved June 6, 2017, from http://www.nchec.org/responsibilities-and-competencies

2. National Institutes of Health. *Clear and simple.* Retrieved June 6, 2017, from http://www.nih.gov/institutes-nih/nih-office-director/office-communications-public-liaison/clear-communication/clear-simple

3. Centers for Disease Control and Prevention. (2016). *Community health status indicators.* Retrieved June 6, 2017, from http://wwwn.cdc.gov/communityhealth

4. U.S. Department of Health and Human Services. *Healthdata.gov.* Retrieved June 6, 2017, from https://www.healthdata.gov/

5. Centers for Disease Control and Prevention. (2016). *Youth risk behavior surveillance system.* Retrieved June 6, 2017, from http://www.cdc.gov/healthyyouth/data/yrbs/

6. Doak, C. C., Doak, L. G., & Root, J. H. (1996). *Teaching patients with low literacy skills.* Philadelphia, PA: J. B. Lippincott.

7. National Cancer Institute. (2004). *Making health communications work.* Bethesda, MD: National Institutes of Health. Retrieved June 6, 2017, from http://www.cancer.gov/publications/health-communication/pink-book.pdf

8. National Center for Education Studies. (2006). *The health literacy of America's adults: Results for the 2003 national assessment of adult literacy.* Retrieved June 6, 2017, from http://nces.ed.gov/pubs2006/2006483.pdf

9. Nielsen-Bohlman, L., Panzer, A., & Kindig, D. (2004). *Health literacy: A prescription to end confusion.* Washington, DC: National Academy Press.

10. Literacy Project Foundation. *Staggering illiteracy statistics.* Retrieved May 16, 2017, from http://literacyprojectfoundation.org/community/statistics/

11. Centers for Disease Control and Prevention. (2009). *Simply put: A guide for creating easy-to-understand materials* (3rd ed.). Atlanta, GA: Centers for Disease Control and Prevention. Retrieved May 16, 2017, from http://www.cdc.gov/healthliteracy/pdf/Simply_Put.pdf

12. Nielsen, J. (2006). *F-shaped pattern for reading web content.* Retrieved May 16, 2017, from http://www.nngroup.com/articles/f-shaped-pattern-reading-web-content/

13. Bold, W. & Davidson, W. (2012). Mobile broadband: Redefining Internet access and empowering individuals. In S. Dutta & B. Bilbao-Osorio (Eds.): *The global information technology report: Living in a hyperconnected world.* (pp. 57–66). New York, NY: World Economic Forum. Retrieved May 16, 2017, from http://www3.weforum.org/docs/Global_IT_Report_2012.pdf

14. Nicholas, D., Clark, D., Rowlands, I., & Jamali, H. (2013). Information on the go: A case study of Europeana mobile users. *Journal of the American Society for Information Science and Technology, 64*(7), 1311–1322.

15. Brusk, J. J. & Bensley, R. J. (2016). A comparison of mobile and fixed device access on user engagement associated with women, infants, and children (WIC) online nutrition education. *JMIR Research Protocols, 5*(4), e216.

16. Coles, S. (May 30, 2015). *What is bad about comic sans?* Retrieved from http://www.quora.com/What-is-bad-about-the-Comic-Sans-font

17. Kools, M., van de Wiel, M. W., Ruiter, R. A., Crüts, A., & Kok, G. (2006). The effect of graphic organizers on subjective and objective comprehension of a health education text. *Health Education & Health Behavior, 33*(6), 760–772.

18. Houts, P., Doak, C. C., Doak, L. G., & Loscaizo, M. J. (2006). The role of pictures in improving health communication: A review of research on attention, comprehension, recall and adherence. *Patient Education and Counseling, 61*, 173–190.

19. Federal Communications Commission. (2016). *2016 broadband progress report.* Retrieved June 6, 2017, from http://www.fcc.gov/reports-research/reports/broadband-progress-reports/2016-broadband-progress-report

20. Wahbe, A. (2015). *Page speed: Are slow loading times killing your growth?* Retrieved May 16, 2017, from http://www.shopify.com/enterprise/60726275-page-speed-are-slow-loading-pages-killing-your-growth

21. Work, S. (2011). How loading time affects your bottom line. [Web log post]. Retrieved April 29, 2017, from http://blog.kissmetrics.com/loading-time/

22. Thompson, C. (July 2016). The surprising history of the infographic: Early iterations saved soldiers' lives, debunked myths about slavery and helped Americans settle the frontier. *Smithsonian Magazine.* Retrieved May 16, 2017, from http://www.smithsonianmag.com/history/surprising-history-infographic-180959563/

23. Wahowiak, L. (2014). Health workers, artists partner to deliver messages via comics: Tools can influence health behavior. *The Nation's Health, 44*(7), 1–16.

24. Centers for Disease Control and Prevention. *Zombie novella.* Retrieved May 16, 2017, from http://www.cdc.gov/phpr/zombies_novella.htm

25. Unger, J. B., Cabassa, L. J., Molina, G. B., Contreras, S., & Baron, M. (2013). Evaluation of a fotonovela to increase depression knowledge and reduce stigma among Hispanic adults. *Journal of Immigrant and Minority Health, 15*(20), 398–406.

26. Chan, A., Brown, B., Sepulveda, E., & Teran-Clayton, L. (2015). Evaluation of fotonovela to increase human papillomavirus vaccine knowledge, attitudes, and intentions in a low-income Hispanic community. *BMC Research Notes, 8,* 615.

27. Centers for Disease Control and Prevention. (2011). *KABI Chronicles: The Edge Motion Comic Series.* Retrieved May 16, 2017, from http://npin.cdc.gov/KABIChronicles/index.html

28. Bensley, R. J., Brusk J. J., Anderson, J. V., Mercer, N., Rivas, J., & Broadbent, L. N. (2006). wichealth.org: Impact of a stages of change-based Internet nutrition education program. *Journal of Nutrition Education and Behavior, 38,* 222–229.

29. Bensley, R. J. & Rivas, J. (2017). *Health eKitchen.* Retrieved May 16, 2017, from http://wichealth.org

30. Kato, P. M. (2010). Video games in health care: Closing the gap. *Review of General Psychology, 14*(2), 113–121.

31. Giunti, G., Baum, A., Giunta, D., Plazzotta, F., Benitez, S., Gómez, A., … Bernaldo de Quiros, F. G. (2015). Serious games: A concise overview on what they are and their potential applications to healthcare. *Studies in Health and Technology Informatics, 216,* 386–390.

32. Sabogal, F., Otero-Sabogal, R., Pasick, R., Jenkins, C., & Perez-Stable, F. (1996). Printed health education materials for diverse communities: Suggestions learned from the field. *Health Education Quarterly, 23,* 123–141.

Additional Resources

Print

Evergreen, S. D. H. (2017). *Effective data visualization: The right chart for the right data.* Thousand Oaks, CA: Sage Publishing.

National Commission for Health Education Credentialing, Inc. (NCHEC), & Society for Public Health Education (SOPHE). (2015). *A Competency-Based Framework for Health Education Specialists-2015.* Whitehall, PA: National Commission for Health Education Credentialing, Inc. (NCHEC) and Society for Public Health Education (SOPHE)

Internet

Federal plain language guidelines. (2011). Retrieved from www.plainlanguage.gov

Centers for Disease Control and Prevention. (2015). *Everyday words for public health communication.* Retrieved from http://www.cdc.gov/ccindex

Centers for Disease Control and Prevention. (2016). *CDC Clear Communication Index.* Retrieved from http://www.cdc.gov/ccindex

Centers for Disease Control and Prevention. (2016). *CDC Clear Communication Index score sheet.* Retrieved from http://www.cdc.gov/ccindex/pdf/full-index-score-sheet.pdf

Center for Digital Games Research, University of California at Santa Barbara. *Health games database.* Retrieved from http://www.cdgr.ucsb.edu/database

Centers for Disease Control and Prevention. (2017). *Health Literacy.* Retrieved from http://www.cdc.gov/healthliteracy

Centers for Disease Control and Prevention. *Public health imagery library.* Retrieved from http://phil.cdc.gov/phil/links.asp

Centers for Disease Control and Prevention [Web log]. Retrieved from http://blogs.cdc.gov/publichealthmatters/

Emery, A. K. (2016). *The data visualization checklist.* Retrieved from http://annkemery.com/checklist/

Evergreen data: Intentional reporting & data visualization. [Web log]. Retrieved, from http://stephanieevergreen.com/category/blog/

Harvard. *Health literacy studies.* Retrieved from http://www.hsph.harvard.edu/healthliteracy/

Health Literacy Innovations. (2008). *The health literacy and plain language resource guide.* Retrieved from http://www.imiaweb.org/uploads/docs/hli_resources_guide.pdf

Infographics: A collection of health concept infographics created by NIH Institutes. Retrieved from http://www.flickr.com/photos/nihgov/sets/72157659983805859

McKinney, J., & Kurtz-Rossi, S. (2000). *Culture, health and literacy: A guide to health education materials for adults with limited English literacy skills.* Retrieved from http://healthliteracy.worlded.org/docs/culture/

University of Minnesota. *Creating patient education materials.* Retrieved from http://hsl.lib.umn.edu/biomed/help/creating-patient-education-materials

University of Wisconsin-Madison. *Games and simulation for healthcare.* Retrieved from http://healthcaregames.wisc.edu/index.php

U.S. National Library of Medicine. *U.S. Government medical stock image & footage.* Retrieved from http://www.nlm.nih.gov/services/stockshot.html

Weinstein, M. (2016). *25 places to find free images online that you will actually want to use.* Retrieved from http://www.searchenginejournal.com/25-places-find-free-photos-will-actually-want-use/153529/

Wright, T. (2016). Quick! Free! Updated! Graphics for your trainings & presentations. ETR. [Web log post]. Retrieved from http://www.etr.org/blog/pd-graphics2/

CHAPTER 8

Using Social Media

Robert J. Bensley, PhD, MCHES
Rosemary Thackeray, PhD, MPH
Michael Stellefson, PhD

▶ Author Comments

Robert: For me, it started with a computer science degree working as a Systems Engineer at IBM. At that time, none of *it* existed or was available to the public—laptops, cellphones, tablets, Internet, gaming, social media, apps. It was a world where big water-cooled mainframes ruled the scene, and data were only available to the ardent self-proclaimed computer geeks. When my community health education students start complaining about not being able to work their way through *Healthy People 2020* or some other public health database, I often times tease them with the reply, "Is that so? Try doing that with a stack of data punch cards." Fast forward 30+ years and the landscape has drastically changed. It seems new technologies and apps evolve on a daily basis, where just when you think you have the hang of one process a new method is staring you in the face. The rapid transference of information between and among people is amazing. Never before have we experienced such a vast spider web network of information sharing. This chapter is about using tools we call social media as a means for finagling our way into and through those networks—because it is the technology of the day. However, 30 years from now, the social media apps we have grown to know and love will likely be collecting dust on some shelf, right next to my stack of data punch cards.

Rosemary: I began my career working at a state health department where I felt I was finally a professional with my own desk in a cubicle. However, I did not have a computer and voicemail was nonexistent. The only computer on the second floor was a small Macintosh you had to reserve by writing your name on a paper calendar attached to a manila file folder. Fast-forward 15 years—I was mentoring university students in developing a marketing campaign for our public health major. The students were suggesting using social media, Facebook in particular, for the promotional strategy; I had no idea how Facebook worked or how we could use it. That marketing campaign sparked my research interest in how health agencies use social media to communicate with audiences. It was a natural fit with my research in social marketing and health communication that had started years before. I continue to be fascinated with how and for what reasons people use social media and enjoy discovering how health educators can use social media to promote health and prevent disease.

$\mathcal{P}$ CHES COMPETENCIES

1.1.3	Engage priority populations, partners, and stakeholders to participate in the assessment process.
2.2.1	Identify desired outcomes using the needs assessment results.
2.3.6	Identify delivery methods and settings to facilitate learning.
2.3.7	Tailor strategies/interventions for priority populations.
2.3.8	Adapt existing strategies/interventions as needed.
2.4.1	Use theories and/or models to guide the delivery plan.
2.4.6	Select methods and/or channels for reaching priority populations.
3.1.1	Create an environment conducive to learning.
3.3.7	Use a variety of strategies to deliver plan.
4.1.1	Determine the purpose and goals of evaluation.*
4.1.4	Adapt/modify a logic model to guide the evaluation process.*
4.4.4	Use available technology to collect, monitor, and manage data.
5.2.1	Assess technology needs to support health education/promotion.
5.2.4	Evaluate emerging technologies for applicability to health education/promotion.
6.1.4	Adapt information for consumer.
6.1.5	Convey health-related information to consumer.
7.1.3	Tailor messages for intended audience.
7.1.6	Assess and select methods and technologies used to deliver messages.
7.1.7	Deliver messages using media and communication strategies.
7.1.8	Evaluate the impact of the delivered messages.
7.2.5	Use strategies that advance advocacy goals.

*Advanced level competency

Reprinted by permission of the National Commission for Health Education Credentialing, Inc. (NCHEC) and Society for Public Health Education (SOPHE).

Michael: My academic career began as a graduate student in the mid-2000s when social media websites like Facebook were just beginning to become popular on college campuses. At the time, I thought social media was a cool way to keep in touch with friends from high school and family members, but I had no idea it could ever become useful for much else. Fast forward 10+ years, and social media has changed the world we live in. It allows us to share messages and content, recount stories and experiences with others, and build connections with people from all walks of life. However, in many respects, social media is now the "Wild West" for health information. Users can engage and interact with health-related content that may or may not be accurate or supported by empirical research. My passion lies in understanding how we, as health education specialists, can best leverage social media to help people prevent and manage behavioral risk factors associated with chronic disease. I've used community-engaged research methods to create *COPDFlix*, which is a low-computer literate social media resource center for Chronic Obstructive Pulmonary Disease (COPD) patients, informal caregivers (e.g., friends, family), and clinicians. *COPDFlix* allows users to collaborate and share self-management education videos on patient behavioral tasks critical for improving disease management and health outcomes such as smoking cessation, exercise, and medication use. This chapter lays the foundation for planning, implementing, and evaluating innovative social media strategies that can reach and engage priority populations such as those living with chronic disease. Moving forward, I see health education specialists playing a critical role in creating, managing, and monitoring health-related content available on social media.

▶ Introduction

There is no question that one of the most important innovations over the past 25 years has been the advent and expansion of the Internet. Those who were practitioners prior to the mid- to late-1990s can share stories about the many difficulties associated with critical health education activities such as accessing resources for populations, communicating information, advocating for health policy, and collecting population data. The numerous changes that took place with technology since the turn of the century, however, reduced these difficulties. Now well into the 21st century, the Internet has become an integral part of health education practice.

Looking back 15 years ago, no one had ever heard of Google, Facebook, Twitter, YouTube, Pinterest, Instagram, Snapchat, Pandora, iPhone, iPad, Android—because none of these existed. The Internet provided the platform that allowed these software applications ("**apps**") and devices to evolve and flourish. Now, jump ahead to the present and it is hard to believe a world without the multitude of advancements that evolved due to the rapid sharing of information associated with the Internet. With millions of websites and apps existing, it is obvious the Internet has grown to become an essential part of daily living both for health education specialists and the populations they serve.

This chapter focuses on one set of software apps and platforms that have evolved from the ability to rapidly share information combined with the human need for social interaction. Commonly referred to collectively as **social media**, these apps were born onto the Internet, have evolved over time, and will undoubtedly continue evolving as new desires, needs, and capabilities arise.

---

⑦ DID YOU KNOW?

The Federal Trade Commission has developed guidelines for people who develop mobile health apps. These guidelines ensure developers create apps that are in compliance with all the rules and regulations designed to protect consumers.

The Rise of Social Media

The advancements in technologies have opened the door for informal communication to thrive. As such, the communication framework is no longer one-way, top down, but rather multidimensional and directional. What began as primitive bulletin boards, chat, and online news portals in the late 1970s and early 1980s, evolved into advanced blogging with file and link sharing, multiuser messaging and gaming, and profile creation in the 1990s. Over the past few decades, the Internet has provided users with the ability to create networks of friends, microblogging, video, music streaming, and sharing, and live broadcasting. These software **platforms** continue to evolve as the devices on which they run (e.g., computer, laptop, tablet, smartphone, smartwatch) also continue evolving. Collectively, the term **technology** includes the collection of devices and software apps that run on them, which are powerful tools available for improving the health of populations. As such, health education specialists need to think strategically about how to use these tools for promoting health and preventing disease and illness.

At the onset of the Internet, "experts," who were the recognized content providers, shared information with the masses. By the late 1990s, the ability to create member communities through AOL and other apps started to change the Internet top-down approach thinking. In 2001, the online free encyclopedia, *Wikipedia*, was launched and became one of the first apps to break this mold of expert-generated information by providing the capability for a social network to determine what is considered relevant and necessary information. This, and other initiatives occurring around the same time, opened the door for the current communication approach of being more "bottom up." More bottom-up approaches consist of user-generated messages, and people seeking and finding information from a variety of sources and sharing it with others.

Social Media Framework

Social media can be defined as "activities, practices, and behaviors among communities of people who gather online to share information, knowledge, and opinions using conversational media. Conversational media are web-based apps that make it possible to create and easily transmit content in the form of words, pictures, videos and audio."[1] From this, it is evident that social media is not a single app but rather a broad collection of apps that are designed to be an avenue for a variety of information sharing opportunities. Literally, hundreds of social media apps currently exist on the web, each with its own unique purpose and presence in the social media world. These apps can be categorized in a number of different ways, most commonly in terms of function. Social media can be thought of in terms of both the platform in which it is delivered and how it is used. Six types of platforms that are commonly considered to make up the collective social media are described, with additional description of some of the more popular apps being used:

- *Social Networking.* These network sites allow users to connect and share with others who have similar backgrounds and interests. Facebook, Instagram, LinkedIn, and Snapchat are popular examples of social networks. Facebook is particularly good at hosting discussions, promoting causes, or sharing content. To customize content for each user, Facebook has over 100,000 indicators of relevance it considers when displaying posts. Many health interventions, resources, programs, and social support groups live on Facebook due to its popularity and large audience.[2] Instagram is an image- and video-based blogging platform where users can capture and share up to one minute of their life, environment, or community with others who subscribe to, or "follow," their account.[3] It is especially popular among millennials, where almost 6 out of 10 Internet users between 18 and 29 years have an Instagram account.[4] Users can personalize images and videos by choosing from a variety of filters to emphasize or de-emphasize colors, adjusting audio on videos, and "geo-tagging" images to identify the date and location of images or videos.[5]

- *Blog Comments and Forums.* These online forums provide the ability for individuals to engage in conversations by posting and responding to community messages. Comments are typically centered on the specific subject of the posted blog. Numerous blogging sites exist on the web, which are typically focused on specific or niche issues.

- *Microblogging.* This shortened version of blogging allows users to share short, written entries with their followers, which can include links to websites or other social media. Being "micro," these apps are typically one way rather than conversational and limit entry length. As of the edition of this text, Twitter was the most commonly used microblogging app. It is a social media website that allows sending out a stream of short messages called "tweets" which are limited to 140 characters. Twitter is a real-time application with approximately 6,000 tweets happening every second.[6] Content must be relevant and concise to capture the audience's attention.

- *Media Sharing.* These sites provide the ability to share multimedia such as photos, videos, and audio. Many of them provide the capability for maintaining a community profile and commenting on other members' uploads. For example, media sharing apps include YouTube, Vimeo, and Flickr. YouTube is a video distribution platform for content sharing. Users can view, upload, rate, and comment on uploaded videos. Over 800 million users watch over four billion hours of YouTube videos each month, and approximately 100 million people take a social action on YouTube every week by liking, sharing, or commenting on videos they watch.[7] Health-related topics on YouTube range from general health education to the latest medical treatments to homemade videos produced by individuals.[7]

- *Bookmarking.* Like it sounds, bookmarking sites allow users to save and organize online resources and websites. Tagging allows the bookmark owner to make links searchable and easier for their followers to find. Pinterest and StumbleUpon are popular bookmarking sites. Pinterest is a personalized platform for uploading, saving, and sorting images or "pins" through collections known as "pinboards." Visually appealing posts can be directed to an audience to catch their attention and stick out among the "noise." Once a health-related image is clicked on Pinterest, users are taken to an external site where they can find more information on a health topic.

- *Social News.* A means for bringing news articles to web followers, social news links are then designated by followers (e.g., by clicking "like"), which dictates where they appear in the list of recommended articles to read. For example, social news sites include Digg, Reddit, and WikiLeaks.

Looking at social media in terms of usage, social media is like an ecosystem, where the focus is on how the different platforms and apps are used rather than grouping by platform types. Different platforms and apps cross functionality, resulting in social media being viewed more as an interconnected ecosystem that consists of six main primary usages[8]:

- *Publishing with blog platforms.* These include wikis, hybrid publishing/sharing (e.g., Wordpress, Blogger, Wikipedia, Tumblr, Twitter).

- *Sharing with multimedia platforms.* Types include video, document, photo, music, links, and places sharing (e.g., YouTube, Instagram, Pinterest, Spotify, Delicious, Foursquare).
- *Messaging platforms.* Apps that provide the capability to send and receive short text, images, or videos (e.g., WhatsApp, Facebook Messenger, Google Hangouts, Skype, Snapchat).
- *Conversation platforms* (e.g., Github, Reddit).
- *Professional communication and collaboration tools.* These provide the ability for teams to communicate as a group through a social network (e.g., Slack, Yammer).
- *Professional, niche, and mainstream social networks.* These apps consist of connecting to multiple profile-based pages for the purpose of communicating and sharing content and "memes" through a virtual social network (e.g., LinkedIn, Facebook).

Social Media Prevalence

Internet penetration varies by country. While 88% of people living in North America use the Internet, only 77% of Europeans do, and 27% of those living in Africa.[9] In the United States, differences in Internet use differ by age, income, education, and geographic area, though the gaps between various groups are gradually getting smaller.[10]

COMMUNITY CONNECTIONS 8.1

Katilee is a health education specialist who works for a local county health department. Her position is funded in part from a CDC obesity prevention grant, awarded based on the higher than state and national childhood obesity and type II diabetes rates among elementary age children from lower income families within her community. The focus on the grant was to positively impact healthy food consumption behaviors prior to the child entering elementary school. Being highly proficient in a number of social media platforms, she began exploring using a social media approach for influencing key parent-child feeding skills among her community's population at greatest risk.

Likewise, cell phones are nearly ubiquitous in the United States. In 2016, 95% of American adults said they had some type of cell phone, with 77% reported having a smartphone.[11] Because many popular social media apps are delivered on a smartphone, it is important to understand who has access to these devices. For instance, smartphone ownership is lower among people who are older, who have less formal education, and have lower incomes,[11] while 65% of teens aged 13–18 have reported access to a smartphone.[12]

Who uses social media? An initial response is likely to be "It's a tool for millennials and Generation Z." True, these two generations were either born into or came of age in a world where the Internet has always been a dominant part of society. Millennials are those born between the early 1980s and early 2000s, while Generation Z (a.k.a. Gen Z) include those born from the end of the millennials to the present. As such, the millennials came to age at the onset of the social media evolution, whereas Gen Z have always lived in a world where these platforms have been plentiful. It is estimated that 92% of Gen Z has a digital footprint, meaning they have an online trail of where they exist.[13] As such, they are completely ingrained in the use of social media. But they are not the only ones accessing social media. It has been estimated that in 2016, approximately 75% of the U.S. population had a social media profile and two billion social media users existed worldwide, with Facebook alone accounting for 75% of those users.[11,14] Within the United States alone, this represents a 10-time increase in social media in the 10 years following 2005, which is the year when Facebook and YouTube both became available to mass audiences.[14]

But what about other age groups? Is social media confined just to those who grew up as the platforms evolved? Even though millennials and Gen Z have the highest percentage of generational member use in the United States, populations 30–49 years (80%), 50–64 years (64%), and 65+ years (34%) are also active users of social media, with Facebook over two times as popular as any other social media app.[4] For adults who go online, Facebook is the most common platform, with 79% of adults in the United States using it.[4] In contrast, the percentage of adults using other social media apps ranges from 24 to 32%, depending on the app. Younger populations are more likely to use apps that provide instant sharing (e.g., Twitter, Snapchat), whereas older population use is more related to profile-based social media (e.g., Facebook and LinkedIn).[4] In particular, almost 75% of Snapchat users are less than 34 years old; though overall, only 18% of social media users report using Snapchat.[15] Specific app use varies by a number of other demographics as well, with college-educated adults more likely to use social media than those with a high school or less education.[4] A higher percentage of women tend to use social media platforms (e.g., Pinterest use being two times higher in women than men), with the exception of Twitter and LinkedIn where usage rates for both men and women are more similar.[4,11] The most popular social media app, Facebook, is more likely to be used by women and younger age groups.[4] In contrast, some demographic groups have similar usage with certain apps, but differ with others. For instance, rural and lower income populations are less likely to use professional profile networking (e.g., LinkedIn) or microblogging (e.g., Twitter) than their counterparts, even though they have similar usage of broader social profile networking and bookmarking sites (e.g., Facebook, Instagram, Pinterest).[4]

ⓘ DID YOU KNOW?

The five-year period from 2002 to 2006 saw the birth of LinkedIn, MySpace, Facebook, Flickr, YouTube, and Twitter.

The multitude of the constantly evolving social media avenues has created a unique challenge for health education specialists. New apps continue to appear, as populations continue to expand their desire for both interacting and sharing information with others. As such, health education specialists need to rethink how to engage priority populations. Is social media a place to put health-enhancing messages, a means for inviting populations to become a partner in efforts to influence their health, and an avenue for monitoring patterns associated with attitudes, beliefs, and behaviors? What about the future and the new technologies, apps, and platforms that are bound to evolve? What role does the health education profession play in keeping abreast of or even influencing these future manifestations?

▶ Steps for Using Social Media in Health Education Interventions

There are a few key principles that health education specialists may want to consider when designing a strategic approach to social media.

The reason for the focus on principles, instead of the "how to" for specific platforms or tools, is that platforms constantly change. What is popular today may not be in five years. For example, among millennials, Snapchat is more common today than Facebook.[16]

⑦ DID YOU KNOW?

The first blogging sites began in 1999.

Before deciding how to use social media as part of an intervention, health education specialists must first identify the program goals and objectives. Knowing what the program is trying to accomplish should guide all intervention-related

COMMUNITY CONNECTIONS 8.2

Katilee's first step was to determine what and how the priority population uses social media. She formulated a number of questions to help guide her, including:

- What is their access to technology?
- What technologies and social media do they use?
- For what purpose do they use technology and social media?
- Where are they when they use technology?
- What is their comfort level with technology and social media platforms?

She started with a cursory search for web-based information informing population needs and usage associated with various social media platforms and

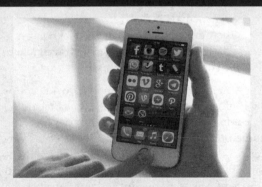
©Denys Prykhodov/Shutterstock.

apps. In addition to finding solid information regarding both general and population-specific social media usage rates, she came across a research study published in the *Journal for Nutrition Education and Behavior* that, in part, identified WIC client social media preference. She discovered the respondents involved in the study included WIC clients from agencies within her state. Findings reported 80% of clients who responded indicated they regularly use Facebook, with younger clients more likely to use it than their older counterparts. She also discovered that only 17% used Twitter and that 57% were interested in a virtual or online discussion group focused on WIC needs. Armed with these findings, she further searched for social media app engagement trends and found Pinterest to be primarily used by females (71%), with 57% of all pins focused on food-related content. Her results confirmed that only 37% of Twitter users are within her primary age group (i.e., millennials, ages 18–29), and even though a little more than half of Instagram users come from millennials, approximately half of them are males. Across the board, she discovered mobile access was a popular way for interacting with most of the available forms of social media primarily used by her priority population. Based on her findings, she decided to focus her efforts on millennial mothers who participate in the WIC program.

decisions. Once goals and objectives are established, health education specialists can follow these four simple steps to strategically decide if and how to use social media as part of the intervention: (1) understand how the priority population uses technology and social media, (2) identify intervention strategies, (3) select an appropriate social media strategy, and (4) determine what social media apps to use.

Step 1: Understand How the Priority Population Uses Technology and Social Media

Some questions to help guide determining the priority population's technology and social media usage include:

- What is their access to technology?
- What technologies and social media do they use?
- For what purpose do they use technology and social media?
- Where are they when they use technology?
- What is their comfort level with technology and social media platforms?

A number of sites and reports provide up-to-date information, patterns, and trends regarding access to technology, all of which varies based on numerous user characteristics. But as stated earlier, access is widespread and not likely to diminish in the near future, especially with the continual release of new technologies and ways of accessing and sharing information. For instance, in 2018, the annual smartphone shipments worldwide is expected to be 900% over what was shipped a decade earlier.[17] Smartphone growth, however, is projected to level off or even decline, while smartwatches, which were basically nonexistent prior to 2013 and only recently becoming popular as options for accessing the Internet and apps, are expected to grow 18% annually through 2021,[18] dependent on whether or not advances in apps and capabilities meet consumer needs.

The plethora of possible social media apps and how they are used is also constantly evolving. Social media users vary in the frequency in which

and the reasons behind why they visit sites (e.g., users are more likely to visit Facebook daily while Pinterest is weekly or less often).[4] The reasons people use social media varies by the individual, but in general people use it to solve problems. What most people are trying to solve with social media is how to stay connected. People want to stay connected with those who are important to them, causes they care about, and organizations or companies that provide products they use. As such, it is important for health education specialists to continually ask themselves: "Are we using this to solve a problem the priority population cares about?"

The frequency in which people use the Internet and social media for health-related purposes varies. Among youth, very few reported getting health information from social networking sites, but rather they were more likely to turn to Internet search engines to find information.[12] In contrast, 80% of adults reported going online to search for health information, but very few reported emailing a provider, tracking their health information online, or taking advantage of online support groups.[19] Similarly, consulting online rankings or reviews was not a common behavior, and posting reviews or comments, questions, or information was infrequent, with only 10–15% of respondents doing so.[20]

Social media users can be categorized into seven types based on their motivations for using social media: creators, critics, collectors, joiners, spectators, distributors, and inactives.[21] Those who are *creators* develop original content to publish or upload on various sites. People who are considered *critics* like to share their opinions by postings ratings or reviews or by contributing to online forums. *Collectors* represent the group of people who like to accumulate information through using RSS feeds, adding tags to pages or photos, or use platforms such as Pinterest to assemble ideas, photos, information, and more. People who maintain a social network site profile on a platform such as Facebook or LinkedIn are considered *joiners*. They may visit the site, but do not do much more than that. Similarly, *spectators* are those who read, watch, and listen

COMMUNITY CONNECTIONS 8.3

Being from the health department, Katilee sought out the WIC clinic, which was a program within her county health department. Katilee made an appointment with Kendra, a nutritionist in the WIC clinic, who informed her that their clinic does not have much of a social media presence outside of a Facebook page they maintain for posting clinic-related information such as hours of operation, eligibility guidelines, and occasionally a WIC food-approved recipe. She also shared they use wichealth.org, a national Internet-based parent-child feeding intervention, as the main source for their parent-child feeding behavior change intervention.

"Within wichealth clients have the option of sharing content and skills they receive with their own social networks via Facebook, Twitter, and Pinterest," Kendra told Katilee. "The metrics we have access confirm clients share through these apps some of the parent-child feeding skills we're providing them."

When further questioned about social media practices, Katilee discovered the clinic really did not have any plan in place for how best to reach clients through various social media apps but were definitely interested in working with her to do so.

to what is posted on various platforms, but they are not actively contributing to the discussion. In contrast, *distributors* are active users of social media, characterized by sharing, retweeting, or reposting information with others, but do not create it. Last, *inactives* are people who do none of these.

Step 2: Identify Intervention Strategies

Once the way the priority populations use social media is understood, the health education specialist makes informed decisions about what intervention strategies to include as part of the program. The majority of this book outlines several strategies or methods for influencing change (e.g., advocacy, coalitions, media, presentations,

health communication). Relevant chapters incorporate how social media can be used within the method. The role for social media within each of these interventions will depend on the program goals, objectives, and what is known about the priority population.

Step 3: Select an Appropriate Social Media Strategy

Once intervention strategies are selected, it is time to develop a specific social media strategy, which includes the purpose for using social media. Four primary purposes for social media exist: to communicate, to collaborate, to educate, and to connect. These strategies are not mutually exclusive, but the health education specialist will want to choose a primary purpose as it relates to the intervention.

Communication as a purpose means social media platforms are used for conversations with the priority population. This may be a one-way conversation for sharing information from the organization outward such as a local health department sharing changes to clinic hours, a community coalition asking for donations to the local refugee community, or the local American Heart Association advertising new weight management classes. One-way communication can be very valuable during disaster or outbreak situations. For example, during a 2015 mumps outbreak in Queens, New York, the New York Department of Health and Mental Hygiene ran a Facebook advertising campaign to alert residents about the outbreak and advised people with symptoms to stay home. The advertisement reached over 86,000 persons and the number who clicked on it was just over 4,000 people.[22]

Two-way conversations are when a response or answer is requested from the priority population. For example, a community coalition may ask for input on proposed new walking paths or for feedback on the new park that just opened in the neighborhood. Another example includes soliciting ongoing feedback about what is going well with the program and where opportunities for improvement exist. Truly, the advantage of social media is that it is social and can provide for interactions rather than static, top-down messages.

The second purpose for a social media strategy is to collaborate with the priority population. Health education specialists may want to create an environment where the priority population members are seen as co-collaborators in improving health and well-being. There may be interest in gathering from them user-generated content (UGC), which is content they author, create, or collect. For instance, a photo contest could be held to solicit photos that identifies where the neighborhood needs to be cleaned up in order to improve walkability. Another example could be local coalition members using social media to organize and join forces with community members to encourage the local health board passing of an ordinance.

Using social media for education is perhaps the most common approach in health education. Health education specialists may want to consider using social media for this purpose with caution. If a health organization has a presence on a social media site for a group of people who share common interests, such as a Facebook page for suicide prevention advocates, social media can help these individuals share information with each other or receive information from the organization. In contrast, as noted earlier, many people go online to look for information and use general search engines (e.g., Google) to perform that search. They may not think about going directly to a state or local health department, Facebook page or the Twitter account to find health information. In contrast, people may go to a social media site maintained by a specialized organization such as the American Cancer Society for expert information on cancer prevention. Using social media for dissemination of information to the public at large is not the best use of time or resources.

Utilizing social media for connections can be valuable when trying to establish communities of social support, and many apps provide the ability to create community groups.[23] Social media can unite people across time and space who share similar interests or concerns. For example, social

Katilee went back to the Internet to discover all she could about how millennial WIC clients interact with social media apps. A quick search for "WIC" and "Pinterest" identified a number of pinboards associated with various WIC clinics across the country and confirmed the plethora of pins associated with recipes and cooking. To her delight, she found a number of the food-related pins were focused on healthy foods and included a variety of WIC-approved foods. She also found a guide titled *Like Facebook, Love Your Community*, which is associated with using Facebook groups and pages as a means for building a community network. Finally, she started following a number of Facebook pages that had been created by women who represented her priority population and started paying attention to the types of posts being written or shared.

media can connect mothers who have children with special healthcare needs to share resources and ideas. To illustrate, the CMV Action UK is a charity in Great Britain that raises awareness of cytomegalovirus (CMV) and supports families of children born with CMV. Their Twitter account (@cmvactionuk) has over 3,000 followers.[24]

Step 4: Determine What Social Media Apps to Use

After determining the social media strategy, the next step is to determine the specifics about what social media apps to use. A variety of social media apps exist from which to select, and numerous sites exist that can help guide the direction of where social media is moving. Apps selection should match the technologies the priority population uses and for the reasons they use it. For example, if the priority population is not on Twitter, a Twitter account should not be created. If teens use Snapchat to share videos about their summer vacations and not about health, reconsider trying to reach them with humorous but relevant messages about how to protect their skin from the sun. It may be

Having found what she considered to be solid information about social media use, Katilee decided the next step should be to validate her findings by gathering input from clients participating in the county WIC clinic. She devised a data collection process that would involve WIC nutritionists presenting the social media concept to their clients and gathering feedback on what might be most useful for them and their interest in sharing relevant posts or pins with others within their own social networks. Kendra helped Katilee in sharing this with the other nutritionists in the clinic, and before too long Katilee had data from over 50 clients. The data confirmed what she suspected: clients primarily used their cellphones to connect with their social networks, were active users of Facebook, and followed a number of pinboards, especially those that provided recipes for preparing healthy foods, cooking video links, and links to recipe websites. Whether or not clients would like and follow a WIC-sponsored Facebook page or join a Facebook online discussion group sponsored by the WIC clinic was met with guarded responses. Many felt the current WIC clinic Facebook page really had little value that would necessitate their wanting to interact with it. In addition, they felt having the title of the page listed as the name of their WIC clinic stigmatized them in a way that they would not be willing to share anything from the page to their personal social networks. "Call it a 'eat fresh for life' page or something like that and I would be interested in following it," was a common type of reply.

beneficial to create shareable videos or images they will want to share with friends.

Part of the social media app decision must also be whether to join the conversation in which the priority population is engaged or whether it is best to try and encourage them to follow a new feed. Perhaps, starting a new weight loss class would mean creating a space where class members can connect and share. If the strategy is focused on collaboration for advocacy, it might be most effective for health education specialists

to join the topic of conversation in places where people are already talking about it.

▶ Tips and Techniques for Effectively Applying Social Media

Effective use of social media shows great potential to break down barriers in health education; however, there are few guidelines in place to assist health education specialists when using social media. These are particularly needed because health education specialists vary in their experience with social media. Previous social media experience is associated with greater self-efficacy for using social media in practice, and younger health education specialists with less work experience report higher social media self-efficacy compared to their older colleagues with more experience.[25] Moreover, health education specialists have high self-efficacy for developing objectives and identifying populations that would benefit from social media, yet they are less confident when providing technical support for implementing social media campaigns.[25] Regardless of previous experience or confidence using social media, there are some general tips and techniques health education specialists can use to more effectively apply social media.

Keep Abreast of New Social Media Avenues

A variety of social media tools exist for disseminating public health information on disease outbreaks, medical discoveries, and emerging health hazards. As a result, many health education specialists leverage various social media platforms to engage patients, clients, and consumers. Distinct populations access different types of social media based on their access to technology, which is often influenced by sociodemographic characteristics.[26] Factors such as these are important to consider when determining how social media should be integrated into a health education program.[27]

It is advisable to identify social media sites that are regularly accessed (daily or almost daily) by the priority population. Often, the best approach is to start with basic social media apps and sites that require fewer resources to administer early on, and then gradually operate additional accounts that require more expertise.[28] Some of the more popular apps include Facebook, Twitter, Instagram, YouTube, and Pinterest.

Social media channels should provide useful and actionable health information, resources, and support. For example, using images on social media captures users' attention and enhances message comprehension. Posts with images typically receive higher engagement than posts without images. Social media users seeking health information are more likely to click, share, comment, or like content of posts with photos, suggesting branded visual content may be more effective in facilitating health-related interaction on social media.[29,30]

Adopt a Social Media Policy

When progressing from dissemination to engagement, more resources are generally needed for social media development and maintenance. Therefore, carefully considering the resources and expertise necessary to operate different social media accounts is important.[28] Professional health organizations should have social media moderator policies and trainings in place.[25] For example, it is important to specify who to consult before posting content or responding to comments on social media pages. Basic social networking engagement activities such as hashtag use, creation of video tags, uploading video responses, and updating profile pictures should be covered.[31] Trainings should also include how to remove destructive posts that personally attack other users.[32]

A formal social media policy helps to establish structure and standards around social media use.[27,28] This policy should facilitate interactivity and respect the diversity of user demographics, cultural backgrounds, and opinions.[33] Social media policies in health education and promotion should address the following six guidelines[33]:

1. Communicate values and expectations.
2. Document best practices for posting and communicating on social media.
3. Protect individuals and the organization from pressures of expediency.
4. Consider Healthcare Insurance Portability and Accountability Act (HIPAA) protections to safeguard protected health information on social media.
5. Include a social media code of conduct for staff members and visitors.
6. Identify what content can be shared on social media and what content cannot be shared.

Health education specialists should also consider the following questions when creating a social media policy[27]:

- What are the penalties for creating an unauthorized account or otherwise breaking the social media policy?
- Who is authorized to represent the organization on social media?
- When is it appropriate to use an agency brand or logo?
- What processes are in place for staying current on privacy settings of each social media platform?

The Centers for Disease Control and Prevention has developed a comprehensive policy for posting to their social media pages that can serve as a starting point for policy development.[34]

Keep Social Media Activity Lively and Relevant

If left unattended, health-related social media conversations can become unpredictable, drift in directions that are frustrating to members, and sometimes even cause harm.[35] When little new content is added by moderators, social media sites devoted to health promotion tend to lack robust conversations around patient-centered health issues.[2] Three models are most commonly used to manage social media activities in public health and health education circles[31,36,37]:

- *Centralized model.* One group or individual has administrative authority with content created by or in collaboration with various staff members.
- *Decentralized model.* Content is created and managed by more than one individual, unit, or team, each of whom creates and maintains his or her own content.
- *Hub-and-spoke model.* A cross-functional core (hub) coordinates social media use centrally, but execution is left to individuals, units, or teams.

Some programs manage social media accounts with just a few staff members, while others have a dedicated full-time staff or teams. Others have found that employing a public information officer in a local health department is associated with adopting social media earlier, having more followers, and tweeting about specific public health topics.[38] Regardless of the size of or approach associated with the social media staff, collaboration between health communication leaders and health education content developers is important for establishing an effective social media management structure.[27]

Skilled social media moderators are essential for maintaining channels and maximizing engagement through scheduling messages, monitoring channels, and responding to posts. Moderators help to facilitate network engagement by infusing insight based on user interactions. Reviewing trends and discussions on social media can help moderators better understand user interests, knowledge, and existing misunderstandings or myths about a health topic.[28] Moderators can also provide valuable social support that clinicians are often unable to provide, such as providing tips for communicating with providers and sharing disease self-management education.[32] It is recommended that moderators not only share existing online health education resources, but also post UGC, which tends to increase the frequency of interactions and improve user engagement.[39]

To grow and manage a digital health presence on social media, one strategy suggests adopting a life-cycle approach to online community development.[40] This life cycle gradually evolves from moderating with less engagement to ensure participants have a safe space to communicate, to becoming more engaged by generating new materials, and UGC posts that spark extended peer-to-peer interactions. How much "hands-on" time moderators spend managing social media depends on time spent "listening," creating content, and directing friends, followers, and subscribers to the information they desire. Conversations around shorter term conditions that are easily treatable will require less moderator engagement, while longer term moderator support is often needed for health topics like chronic disease management. Long bursts of content flooding social media followed by little social activity makes for unproductive conversation and may cause people to tune out or stop following the page or feed.[27] Because of the potential for information overload, moderators should check into the social media frequently—for short periods of time—and involve multiple people in content development and distribution whenever possible.[27] A team-based approach to social media development can offer several advantages, ranging from a broader scope of times for message delivery to additional coverage and support for moderators. Delivering messages on social media in several formats from different voices can increase accessibility and reinforce important content.[27]

⑦ DID YOU KNOW?

"Podcast," believed to have been coined by Ben Hammersley in 2004, comes from combining "iPod" with "broadcast."

A common misconception about using social media is that it provides a podium for delivering a message. Instead, social media enables health education specialists to talk *with* their audience rather than simply talking *at* them. Talking with an audience on social media helps to build a sense of trust and adds a personal touch. To foster meaningful interaction on social media, health education specialists should consider developing a systematic social media awareness, outreach, and engagement "playbook" that includes the following:

- *Listen to social media conversations.* It is important to determine what health-related questions are being asked and what health-related topics are trending on social media. This "social listening" involves scanning social media interactions (e.g., discussions, posted comments, and sentiments) to understand what conversations are occurring. Visiting a variety of social media pages helps to generate a rich understanding of the intended audience and their culture.[28] Trend assessment can also include reviewing content of relevant websites or blogs[41] and analyzing consumer feedback posted to social media.[28]

- *Network with others who have similar health-related interests.* Health education specialists should strive to take social action on social media such as "liking" status updates and comments and cross promoting content from reputable partners, agencies, and influencers.[42] It is recommended to engage with federal government agencies (e.g., National Institutes of Health, CDC), professional organizations (e.g., American Public Health Association, Society for Public Health Education), nonprofit organizations (e.g., American Lung Association), and state and local health departments. Often, these groups will tag and mark their "favorite" posts, which enhances visibility. Other methods for enhancing social networking include answering questions on various health-related topics (e.g., how to register for health insurance plans, questions on common diseases and disorders), holding question and answer sessions with health experts in attendance, and writing accessible content in plain language.

- *Leverage social networks.* Effective social media managers leverage opportunities to expand the reach of their message. Repurposing evidence-based health content for social media communication is one efficient way to start a conversation with online community members. Another strategy is to identify and revive conversations that never concluded or answer questions left unanswered on social media. A general guideline is to devote at least 45 minutes per day to monitoring social media during business hours, with three hours per week devoted to message development and evaluation.[27] It is recommended to post to Facebook at least three times per week, with three to five hours per week spent engaging with users. On Twitter, it is usually sufficient to post at least once daily, with three to five hours a week spent listening to and managing feeds. Social media posts have a very brief shelf life due to the huge amount of posts being shared. On average, Facebook posts expire within three hours and a tweet's average lifetime is only about one hour. Therefore, it is important to promptly and professionally respond.

- *Edit social media content posting.* Social media content management involves administering digital content (e.g., text, images, video) in several stages, including: (1) creating, (2) modifying, (3) publishing/sharing, (4) monitoring, and (5) removal (if necessary). Content management should consider user accessibility and engagement and promote content on several social media websites to enhance visibility. Third-party social media management software (e.g., SproutSocial, Hootsuite) makes it easy to create an editorial calendar to schedule social media posts ahead of time. These software packages allow an administrator to program the time for when a message is to be sent out, holding it in virtual storage until the designated launch time, which could be any day or time of the week.[27] SproutSocial provides a "Social Inbox" tool that allows administrators to facilitate meaningful connections on social media through identifying users' specific questions and directly providing responses.

TABLE 8.1 can be used as a checklist of questions to consider when preparing media files and web links for posting to social media.

TABLE 8.1 Checklist for Posting to Social Media

- ☐ *Is it relevant?*
- ☐ *Is it original?*
- ☐ *Is it shareworthy?*
- ☐ *Is it easy to share?*
- ☐ *Does it relate to a bigger story?*
- ☐ *Is it likely to evoke an emotion that promotes a positive health behavior?*
- ☐ *Does it use clear, simple, active, plain language?*
- ☐ *Does it give your audience the chance to engage?*
- ☐ *Is it appropriate for your channel and audience?*
- ☐ *Is it accessible through different social media vehicles?*
- ☐ *Does the post request user feedback related to the media file or web link?*
- ☐ *Do you have a promotional plan to post the video on various social media pages?*

Data from Centers for Disease Control and Prevention. (2012). *CDC's guide to writing for social media*. Atlanta, GA.

Evaluate Social Media Campaign Implementation

Evaluation is a fundamental element that needs to be included in all social media activities.[42] Health education specialists should start thinking about evaluation early on when selecting an appropriate social media strategy (i.e., by at least Step 3 of the process described earlier). Data gathered during

COMMUNITY CONNECTIONS 8.6

Katilee formulated a social media plan consisting of creating a Facebook page titled "Eat Fresh for Life" that would contain relevant information about healthy recipes, links to shopping and cooking videos, and the ability to join different Facebook groups for small group discussions and chats. Her plan also proposed utilizing an "Eat Fresh for Life" pinboard, comprised of healthy cooking and eating recipes and video links. As part of her plan, she identified a schedule for moderating the social media approach, monitoring posts for relevance, ensuring new content appeared on a regular basis, and addressing questions or needs contained in threads. Katilee presented this plan to her supervisor and, upon approval, brought it to both her coworkers and Kendra, with the intent to finalize how best to market and promote the social media campaign within their community.

social media evaluations enable decision makers and staff members to: (1) learn from mistakes, (2) make program modifications, (3) monitor progress toward program goals, and (4) judge the success of programs in achieving short-term, intermediate, and long-term outcomes.[43] Health education specialists are trained to develop and evaluate programs guided by behavior change theory and Specific, Measureable, Achievable, Realistic, and Time-bound (SMART) objectives. It is especially important to consider what can be realistically achieved using the social media strategies selected.

Relevant questions to consider when developing the evaluation strategy include: (1) How can SMART program objectives be assessed?; (2) What are the expected short- and long-term outcomes of the social media activities?; and (3) How should social media implementation be monitored? Once evaluation objectives are specified, health education specialists should describe evaluation strategies using a logic model (**TABLE 8.2**).

Process evaluation is the most relevant type of evaluation used to assess social media use. It is defined as the measurement of factors that influence the success or failure of social media use, including tracking relevant metrics and performance indicators.[44] This type of evaluation provides health education specialists with data to assess the implementation of social media as part of an intervention or as a stand-alone tool.[44] Incorporating process evaluation into social media campaigns brings

TABLE 8.2 Social Media Logic Model

Inputs	Activities	Outputs	Outcomes	
			Short Term	**Long Term**
Example	*Example*	*Example*	*Example*	*Example*
Messages developed by communication specialists; personnel; internet access	Using Twitter to promote vaccination campaign to moms of young children	Tweets posted; tweets retweeted by others; followers of Twitter profile	Increased awareness of vaccination campaign; Increased visits to the immunization clinic	Increased likelihood of vaccinating children

Data from Centers for Disease Control and Prevention. (2011). The health communicator's social media toolkit. Atlanta, GA.

added value to the assessment of social media's usefulness in health communication, health promotion, and community health outreach efforts.[41] Relevant process evaluation questions include:

- What are the **inputs** or resources needed for the social media activities to happen? How can inputs be measured or counted (e.g., How many evidence-based videos have been developed for posting to YouTube?)?

- What are the **outputs** or resulting products of each social media activity? How can products of social media activities be measured (e.g., number of messages posted during a set period of time, number of friends/followers acquired over a specific time period, number of posted messages shared by others, insights or consumer feedback left on pages)?

⑦ DID YOU KNOW?

In 2005, the first video was uploaded to YouTube. The name? "Me at the Zoo."

Data from process evaluation enables key decision makers and other stakeholders to monitor and track both inputs and outputs on social media. Importantly, measures and performance indicators should adhere to **infodemiological** (i.e., study of determinants and distribution of health information on the Internet to improve public health) principles.[45] Within process evaluation, there are a variety of important performance indicators and metrics used to assess the reach, engagement, and implementation of social media programs and campaigns.

Reach is measured by the overall breadth and depth of network involvement, whereas evaluating the overall size of an online community and the extent to which network involvement grows over time assesses breadth. For example, on video sharing social media websites, a health education specialist might be interested in tracking the total number of subscribers according to specific user characteristics (e.g., what proportion of people living with COPD over the age of 40 subscribe to the *COPDFlix* YouTube channel?). Examining conversations and recording the frequency of page and post views over time often measure depth or exposure to social media. Monitoring the number of people who make contact with or view specific social media materials and applications is an important indicator of reach.

Engagement is measured by assessing the volume of interaction and responsiveness of network members. Performance indicators include **lower level engagement**, defined as the number of people who acknowledge agreement with or preference for content (e.g., marking a video as a "Favorite" on YouTube), and **higher level engagement**, such as the total number of people who participate in creating and sharing content to influence others in their social network (e.g., retweeting a post on Twitter). It is important to regularly review and record page-specific metrics (e.g., "likes," "shares," "comments") to monitor engagement with social media pages and/or feeds.

Evaluating the extent to which social media activities are delivered as originally intended assesses implementation. Fidelity measures track implementation of social media messages and campaigns to ensure that both content and applications are appropriately designed and delivered and match intended purposes.[40] Performance indicators include **user experience** as measured by sentiment and survey feedback. Advanced methods such as automatic textual analysis can seamlessly categorize user feedback by particular topics, and word clouds can capture word frequencies or important topics discussed on social media. **Loyalty** indicates the extent to which network members return to social media pages on a regular basis (e.g., hourly, daily, weekly). **Moderator responsiveness** or how reactive moderators are when interacting with members of their social network is also a key indicator of social media implementation. Metrics used to assess moderator responsiveness can range from the number of questions addressed by the moderator to the average amount of time needed to respond to network members' posts.

> ### ⑦ DID YOU KNOW?
>
> An algorithm called TensiStrength can detect the strength of psychological expressions for stress and relaxation among Twitter users based on the content of their tweets.

Data from TensiStrength, http://sentistrength.wlv.ac.uk/TensiStrength.html

▶ Overcoming Challenges with Social Media

As can be guessed, there are many challenges to effectively using social media for health education and promotion campaigns. Many of these are in direct response to the nature of social media itself, where health education specialists cannot control what, when, and how information is shared. This is dramatically different than many of the other methods shared in this book. For instance, health education specialists can control what is included on the print and Internet resources developed as well as how they are delivered to populations. This is also similar with traditional media, where health education specialists can control the messages and have some influence on how and when they are shared with the public. With social media channels, a whole new set of challenges arise.

Manage Misinformation

Social media serves as a robust platform for health information sharing. With these collaborative benefits, however, also comes potential for harm. Social media enables "nonexperts" to share their own health opinions very swiftly, without any real substantive checks in place to prohibit the spread of health-related misinformation. Evidence-based healthcare de-emphasizes anecdotal reports, such as individual patient stories or narratives, in favor of results from rigorously tested interventions and treatments.[46] The main limitation of health information shared on social media is overall lack of quality and reliability.[47] Unfortunately, health-related misinformation is often being shared on Pinterest, Instagram, and other visual social media websites.[48,49] Sharing misleading or fictional health information on social media has the potential to spread unverified health claims or "rumors" that can be very harmful, especially when consumed by vulnerable populations.[50]

While social media may indeed become the way of the future for adapting, conveying, and disseminating health information, it is important to remember that its use is largely unregulated, with limited oversight provided by trained health professionals. Many posts on social media are shared by users who do not even review what they are sharing.[51] As social media becomes more integrated into public health, health education specialists will likely play an important role in detecting and reporting potentially harmful health information that is being shared.[52] In this capacity, health education specialists should engage with the public to address health-related misconceptions or false information in a manner that is both nonconfrontational and enlightening. It is also important that health education specialists act as resource people on social media by sharing only high-quality educational materials and always directing the public to reliable sources of health information.

Reduce Agency Barriers to Using Social Media

The rate of social media adoption by health-related nonprofit organizations and government agencies is on the rise. For example, approximately 60% of state health departments use at least one type of social media to help meet their organizational objectives.[53] As this trend continues, there will be numerous opportunities for influencing and changing health behavior through social media.[47,54] As is often the case, however, bureaucracy surrounds organizations and government health departments, which limits employees from having access to social media while at work.[55] Integrating social media into the workflow of health-related organizations increases risks for negative outcomes such as breaches of patient confidentiality and unprofessional interactions caused by lack of etiquette.[52] Using social media for professional purposes requires users to formulate posts that reflect the official views and mission of their employer or organization. Current guidelines for social media use in the public health workforce emphasize several best practices[56-58]:

- Maintain patient confidentiality (e.g., HIPAA privacy rule states that clinical vignettes posted on social media concerning patients must have all personally identifying information and any revealing references removed).
- Monitor privacy settings on social media to limit the exposure of content to users outside of approved social networks.

- Declare personal and professional conflicts of interest.
- Maintain separate personal and professional profiles.

Minimal on-the-job social media training negatively affects health education specialists' self-efficacy to use social media to achieve work-related objectives.[25] Training health education specialists to become active communicators and disseminators on social media may help remedy the perception that health-related social media contains mostly inaccurate, corruptible, and biased information. As such, organizations and agencies should consider instituting policies and training programs that focus on how health education specialists can apply social media in the field.[25]

Measure Reach and Impact

In theory, social media technologies enable health education specialists to reach many people quickly with very little cost. Through use of analytics available with platform-specific data or other providers such as Hootsuite or Google Analytics, it is relatively easy to assess social media exposure such as likes or favorites, views, shares, and retweets. However, it is more challenging to accurately assess a broader reach and impact. For example, if Susan Jones retweets the health department's tweet, how many of her followers actually saw it? If a post is not favorited, does that mean nobody read it? What did people do because of seeing the message? Unless there is a click-through link, there is no way to know what action was taken. For example, is it known if the person who saw a post about breast cancer called her doctor to schedule a mammogram?

Attempting to quantify more than basic analytics is not impossible, but has some difficulties, particularly with identifying who should be part of the study population. A study aimed at reducing risky sexual behavior and sexually transmitted infections found that while about 800 people "friended" their Facebook page, researchers estimated that many more people viewed the page and content without friending it.[59] Because of this, the evaluators had a difficult time assessing the impact of their intervention.

Keep Up with Social Media Trends and Technologies

As has been shared throughout this chapter, one thing is for certain: social media is an evolving process that is still in its infancy in relation to how best to share health education and promotion messages to priority populations. What is popular today may be on the shelf tomorrow. A prime example of this is the social networking site MySpace. During the mid-2000s, MySpace was the most popular website and social networking app in the United States. That was short termed, however, as Facebook overtook that lead in 2009. It has been suggested that one reason for this change was due to the Facebook profile, where users established a profile based on their real information rather than a pseudonym common to MySpace. Users were ready to engage on a more personal basis and MySpace did not provide that capability. In the decade following MySpace's height of dominance, Facebook's monthly site visits were 3,000 times that of MySpace users.[60]

Trying to keep up with current social media trends can be exhausting. For instance, just when an agency feels they have a solid social networking presence on their Facebook site, the trends in social media use change. Although by 2017 Facebook led the world in monthly usage with over 1.8 billion active users, trends indicate a shift may be occurring due to **social media fatigue**, resulting in users engaging in more private messaging apps.[14,61] The top two messaging platform apps in 2017 (WhatsApp, Facebook Messenger) accounted for 2 billion active users worldwide.[14] Knowing when and how these trends might shift is critical for maintaining a social media presence. Even though it can seem daunting, health education specialists can keep up with trends by taking time to (1) follow social media experts (e.g., following their Twitter feeds), (2) subscribe to relevant social media blogs, (3) attend social media conferences or webinars, and (4) subscribe to social media YouTube channels and podcasting

sites. Regardless, it is critical health education specialists who are in tune with what is trending with social media options, as it is an ever-growing channel for delivering health education and promotion messages.

▶ Expected Outcomes

Rapid Dissemination of Messages

Skillful application of social media can surmount archaic dissemination boundaries of geography and time. The pervasive use of social media has created a vast global network that can quickly spread health information to mobilize action.[52] One example of the powerful effect social media can have on nonprofit organizations occurred after Facebook decided to allow users to post their organ donor status in their profile. The week after this feature was introduced, U.S. state organ donor registries experienced a 23-fold surge in donor pledges, presumably due to this social media effect.[62] Another example was the Amyotrophic Laterals Sclerosis (ALS) or Lou Gehrig's Disease Ice Bucket Challenge of 2014, which involved people pouring buckets of ice water over their heads and challenging others to do the same within 24 hours, or agree to make a monetary donation to support ALS research if they chose not to accept the challenge. Images of the Ice Bucket Challenge went **viral** on social media with people posting videos and/or pictures of themselves reluctantly embracing the "freezing cold" challenge. Between June and August of 2014, more than 1.2 million videos of people taking the Ice Bucket Challenge were shared on Facebook and it was mentioned on Twitter over 2.2 million times.[63] ALS awareness and donations ascended to unprecedented levels during this time frame due (in large part) to the virality of this social media campaign. These examples illustrate the power of social media to increase awareness of health-related news, discoveries, and initiatives to motivate the public to engage in healthy behaviors and support health-related causes. Caution should always be applied, however, before attempting to harness the power of social media to disseminate health messages.

Breadth of Exposure at a Low Cost

The initial investment to set up a social media account is free or low cost. If agencies seek UGC and utilize it as part of a social media strategy, the cost to the organization is none. However, the personnel required for ongoing content management associated with varying platforms can be time and resource intensive. Yet, overall, it costs little money for a potentially broad reach—hundreds, thousands, or millions of users may see the message.

For instance, one organization aimed to provide support groups for breast cancer survivors under the age of 45 years.[64] Traditional methods of recruitment to these support groups were not successful, resulting in only a handful of participants. After implementing a social media strategy using targeted advertising, however, they experienced nearly 5,000 daily unique visitors to their page. It was estimated this successful new social media advertising strategy only cost $1 per person.[64]

One issue to keep in mind about potential reach is the social media "half-life,"[65] which is the amount of time that passes when a post receives half of its engagements (likes, shares, favorites). **Half-life** for most social media platforms is estimated at less than an hour.[65] That means that after an hour or two has passed, the potential for any engagement has diminished, regardless of follower or fan base. As a result, regular posting of social media messages are critical for maintaining reach.

⊘ DID YOU KNOW?

Embedding an image within a social media post can increase the number of "likes" and comments the post receives.

Being "In Tune" with the Population

Incorporating a variety of social media tools into health education and promotion campaigns demonstrates the health agency is on top of current trends and understands the importance of meeting priority populations in the world in which they reside. The adage "build it and they will come" might sound impressive, but in reality health agencies in tune with the social media landscape understand it can be more effective to fit within that which is already built. Agencies with a social media plan are able to join the conversation already happening within the populations they are trying to serve and offer them a reason why they might want to follow the agency in return. By taking this approach, the adept at social media health education specialist is then able to contribute to the conversation rather than trying to convince the priority population to seek out and engage on their own. Social media minded health education specialists understand the importance of engaging with the story already unfolding instead of recreating a new means for delivering messages. For example, it is likely better to seek out the channels where a population is already talking about bullying-related suicides, and then trying to develop and entice the population to follow a new suicide prevention social media intervention. Health education specialists with a social media mindset also understand the wide range of platforms and apps available to them and, as such, are less likely to rely on what may be an ineffective approach for engaging with populations (e.g., health department Facebook page consisting of "information dump" rather than a forum for sharing).

▶ Conclusion

Of all the chapters within this book, it is likely this one will see the most change between now and the next edition. That is because of the specific nature of the topic, as social media continually evolves by the minute. In just the 11 seconds it took to read the first two sentences of this section, it is estimated 600 blog posts were written, 90 new users joined Facebook, 50 new users joined Pinterest, and 85,000 tweets were sent by users of Twitter.[6] There is no doubt social media has a presence in the lives of populations locally, nationally, and globally. That being the case, it is essential for health education specialists to pay attention to the technologies arising within this method of communication. Being social media proficient means being able to meet priority populations and impact change within the virtual environments in which they live, work, and play.

Key Terms

App Software applications that provide social media functions.

Engagement The volume of interaction and responsiveness of network members.

Half-life The amount of time that passes when a post receives half of its engagements.

Higher level engagement The number of people who participate in creating and sharing content to influence others in their social network.

Infodemiological The study of determinants and distribution of health information on the Internet to improve public health.

Inputs Resources needed for the social media activities to occur.

Lower level engagement The number of people who acknowledge agreement with or preference for content.

Loyalty Extent to which network members return to social media pages regularly.

Moderator responsiveness How reactive moderators are when interacting with members of their social network.

Outputs Resulting products of each social media activity.

Platform The format in which social media is delivered.

Reach The overall breadth and depth of network involvement.

Social media Websites and applications that enable users to create and share content or to participate in social networking.

Social media fatigue Result of societal overuse of social networking and media apps.

Technology The collection of devices and the software apps that run on them.

User experience The overall experience of a person using a website or app, especially in terms of how easy or pleasing it is to use.

Viral The rapid and wide circulation of an image, video, or other form of information from one Internet user to another.

References

1. Safko, L. & Brake, D. K. (2009). *The social media bible: Tactics, tools, & strategies for business success.* Hoboken, NJ: John Wiley & Sons.

2. Cole-Lewis, H., Perotte, A., Galica, K., Dreyer, L., Griffith, C., Schwarz, M., & Augustson, E. (2016). Social network behavior and engagement within a smoking cessation Facebook page. *Journal of Medical Internet Research*, 18(8), e205.

3. Gauthier, T. P. & Spence, E. (2015). Instagram and clinical infectious diseases. *Clinical and Infectious Diseases*, 61(1), 135–136.

4. Greenwood, S., Perrin, A., & Duggan, M. (2016). *Social media update 2016.* Retrieved June 6, 2017, from http://www.pewinternet.org/2016/11/11/social-media-update-2016/

5. Manikonda, L., Hu, Y., Kambhampati, S. (2014). *Analyzing user activities, demographics, social network structure and user-generated content on Instagram.* Retrieved June 6, 2017, from http://arxiv.org/pdf/1410.8099.pdf

6. Internet live stats. (2017). Retrieved June 6, 2017, from http://www.internetlivestats.com/

7. Pant, S., Deshmukh, A., Murugiah, K., Kumar, G., Sachdeva, R., & Mehta, J. L. (2012). Assessing the credibility of the "YouTube approach" to health information on acute myocardial infarction. *Clinical Cardiology*, 35(5), 281–285.

8. Cavazza, F. (2016). *Social media landscape, 2016.* Retrieved June 6, 2017, from http://fredcavazza.net/2016/04/23/social-media-landscape-2016/

9. Internet World Stats. (2017). *Internet usage statistics. The Internet big picture: World Internet users and 2017 population stats.* Retrieved June 6, 2017, from http://www.internetworldstats.com/stats.htm

10. Perrin, A. & Duggan, M. (2015). *Americans' Internet Access: 2000–2015.* Pew Research Center. Retrieved June 6, 2017, from http://www.pewinternet.org/2015/06/26/americans-internet-access-2000-2015/

11. Pew Research Center. (2017, January 12). *Mobile Fact Sheet.* Retrieved June 6, 2017, from http://www.pewinternet.org/fact-sheet/mobile/

12. Wartella, E., Rideout, V., Montague, H., Beaudoin-Ryan, L., & Lauricella, A. (2016). Teens, health and technology: A national survey. *Media and Communication, 4*(3), 13–23.

13. Beall, G. (2016, November 5). "8 key differences between gen z and millennials" [Web log post.]. Retrieved April 29, 2017, from http://www.huffingtonpost.com/george-beall/8-key-differences-between_b_12814200.html

14. Statista. (2016). *Share of adult Internet users in the United States who use social networking sites from 2005 to 2015.* Retrieved June 6, 2017, from http://www.statista.com/statistics/273035/share-of-us-adult-internet-users-who-use-social-networking-sites/

15. Aslam, S. (2017). *Snapchat by the numbers: Stats, demographics & fun facts.* Retrieved May 19, 2017, from http://www.omnicoreagency.com/snapchat-statistics/

16. Simpson, C. (2017, March 10). The dos and don'ts of reaching millennials via social media. *Adweek.* Retrieved May 16, 2017, from http://www.adweek.com/digital/courtney-simpson-startek-guest-post-the-dos-and-donts-of-reaching-millennials-via-social-media/

17. Bajpai, P. (2016, May 10). *The evolution of smartphone markets: Where growth is going.* Retrieved June 6, 2017, from http://www.nasdaq.com/article/the-evolution-of-smartphone-markets-where-growth-is-going-cm619105

18. Beaver, L. (2016, September 27). *THE SMARTWATCH REPORT: Forecasts, Adoption trends, and why the market isn't living up to the hype.* Retrieved March 18, 2017, from http://www.businessinsider.com/smartwatch-and-wearables-research-forecasts-trends-market-use-cases-2016-9

19. Kontos, E., Blake, K. D., Chou, W. Y. S., & Prestin, A. (2014). Predictors of eHealth usage: Insights on the digital divide from the Health Information National Trends Survey 2012. *Journal of Medical Internet Research, 16*(7), e172.

20. Thackeray, R., Crookston, B. T., & West, J. H. (2013). Correlates of health-related social media use among adults. *Journal of Medical Internet Research, 15*(1), e21.

21. Li, C. & Bernoff, J. (2008). *Groundswell.*, MA: Harvard Business Press.

22. Isaac, B. M. (2017). Notes from the field: Use of social media as a communication tool during a mumps outbreak—New York City, 2015. *Morbidity and Mortality Weekly Report, 66.*

23. Rivas, J. & Bensley, R. J. (2011). *Like Facebook, love your community.* Retrieved June 6, 2017, from http://joinwichealth.org/uploads/docs/Like_Facebook_Love_Your_Community.pdf

24. CMV Action. Retrieved from http://cmvaction.org.uk/

25. Alber, J. M., Paige, S., Stellefson, M., & Bernhardt, J. M. (2016). Social Media self-efficacy of health education specialists: Training and organizational development implications. *Health Promotion Practice, 17*(6), 915–921.

26. Fox, S. & Duggan, M. (2013, January 15). *Health online 2013.* Pew Internet and American Life Project. Retrieved May 19, 2017, from http://www.pewinternet.org/2013/01/15/health-online-2013/

27. Norman C. (2103). *Developing a social media strategy.* Retrieved June 6, 2017, from http://www.ptcc-cfc.on.ca/common/pages/UserFile.aspx?fileId=119863

28. Centers for Disease Control and Prevention. (2011). *The health communicator's social media toolkit.* Retrieved March 18, 2017, from http://www.cdc.gov/healthcommunication/toolstemplates/socialmediatoolkit_bm.pdf

29. Thesis, S. K., Burke, R. M., Cory, J. L., & Fairley, T. L. (2016). Getting beyond impressions: An evaluation of engagement with breast cancer-related Facebook content. *mHealth, 2*, 41.

30. Strekalova, Y. A. & Krieger, J. L. (2017). A picture really is worth a thousand words: Public engagement with the national cancer institute on social media. *Journal of Cancer Education, 32*(1), 155–157.

31. Newbold, K. B., & Campos, S. (2011). *Media and social media in public health messages: A systematic review.* Hamilton, ON: McMaster Institute of Environment and Health. Retrieved May 19, 2017, from http://www .mcmaster.ca/mihe/documents/publications /Social%20Media%20Report.pdf

32. Huh, J., Marmor, R., & Jiang, X. (2016). Lessons learned for online health community moderator roles: A mixed-methods study of moderators resigning from WebMD communities. *Journal of Medical Internet Research, 18*(9).

33. Davies, J., Dhaliwal, M., Brankley, L., McColl, K., Mai, D., & Williams, M. (2014). *Social Media toolkit for Ontario public health units. Wellington-Dufferin-Guelph Public Health, Guelph, ON.* Retrieved May 16, 2017, from http://www.publichealthontario.ca/en /ServicesAndTools/Documents/LDCP /Social-toolkit-public-health-web-final.pdf

34. Centers for Disease Control and Prevention. (2011, September 14). *CDC enterprise social media policy.* Retrieved May 16, 2017, from www.cdc.gov/socialmedia/tools/guidelines /pdf/social-media-policy.pdf

35. Park, A., Hartzler, A. L., Huh, J., Hsieh, G., McDonald, D. W., & Pratt, W. (2016). How did we get here?: Topic drift in online health discussions. *Journal of Medical Internet Research, 18*(11), e284.

36. Li, C. (2013). *The state of social business 2013: The maturing of social media into social business.* Retrieved May 16, 2017, from http:// www.altimetergroup.com/2013/11/research -on-the-state-of-social-business-2013/

37. Johnson N. (2013). *The state of corporate social media.* Retrieved June 6, 2017, from http://events.usefulsocialmedia.com/state -of-csm-2013.pdf

38. Harris, J. K., Choucair, B., Maier, R. C., Jolani, N., & Bernhardt, J. M. (2014). Are public health organizations tweeting to the choir? Understanding local health department Twitter followership. *Journal of Medical Internet Research, 16*(2), e31.

39. Post, S. D., Taylor, S. C., Sanders, A. E., Goldfarb, J. M., Hunt, Y. M., & Augustson, E. M. (2013). If you build (and moderate) it, they will come: The Smokefree Women Facebook page. *Journal of the National Cancer Institute Monographs, 2013*(47), 206–208.

40. Syred, J., Naidoo, C., Woodhall, S. C., & Baraitser, P. (2014). Would you tell everyone this? Facebook conversations as health promotion interventions. *Journal of Medical Internet Research, 16*(4), e108.

41. Neiger, B. L., Thackeray, R., Van Wagenen, S. A., Hanson, C. L., West, J. H., Barnes, M. D., & Fagen, M. C. (2012). Use of social media in health promotion purposes, key performance indicators, and evaluation metrics. *Health Promotion Practice, 13*(2), 159–164.

42. Centers for Disease Control and Prevention. (2012, May 16). *Social media guidelines and best practices.* Retrieved August 3, 2017, from http://www.cdc.gov/SocialMedia/Tools /guidelines/pdf/FacebookGuidelines.pdf

43. Centers for Disease Control and Prevention. (2011). *Introduction to program evaluation for public health programs: A self-study guide.* Retrieved March 18, 2017, from www.cdc .gov/eval/guide/CDCEvalManual.pdf

44. McKenzie, J. F., Neiger, B. L., & Thackeray, R. (2016). *Planning, implementing & evaluating health promotion programs: A primer* (7th ed.). New York: Pearson.

45. Eysenbach, G. (2009). Infodemiology and infoveillance: Framework for an emerging set of public health informatics methods to analyze search, communication and publication behavior on the Internet. *Journal of Medical Internet Research, 11*(1), e11.

46. Glicken, M. D. (2004). *Improving the effectiveness of the helping professions: An evidence-based approach to practice.* Thousand Oaks, CA: Sage Publications.

47. Moorhead, S. A., Hazlet, D. E, Harrison, L., Carroll, J. K., Irwin, A., & Hoving, C. (2013). A new dimension of health care: Systematic review of the uses, benefits, and limitations of

social media for health communication. *Journal of Medical Internet Research, 15*(4), e85.

48. Guidry, J. P. D., Carlyle, K., Messner, M., & Jin, Y. (2015). On pins and needles: How vaccines are portrayed on Pinterest. *Vaccine, 33*(39), 5051–5056.

49. Seltzer, E. K., Jean, N. S., Kramer-Golinkoff, E., Asch, D. A., & Merchant, R. M. (2015). The content of social media's shared images about Ebola: A retrospective study. *Public Health, 129*(9), 1273–1277.

50. Tan, A. S., Lee, C. J., & Chae, J. (2015). Exposure to Health (mis)information: Lagged effects on young adults' health behaviors and potential pathways. *Journal of Communication, 65*(4), 674–698.

51. Gabielkov, M., Ramachandran, A., Chaintreau, A., & Legout, A. (2016, June). Social clicks: What and who gets read on Twitter? In *Proceedings of the 2016 ACM SIGMETRICS International Conference on Measurement and Modeling of Computer Science* (pp. 179–192).

52. Ventola, C. L. (2014). Social media and health care professionals: Benefits, risks, and best practices. *Pharmacy and Therapeutics, 39*(7), 491.

53. Thackeray, R., Neiger, B. L., Smith, A. K., & Van Wagenen, S. B. (2012). Adoption and use of social media among public health departments. *BMC Public Health, 12*, 242.

54. Korda, H. & Itani, Z. (2013). Harnessing social media for health promotion and behavior change. *Health Promotion Practice, 14*(1), 15–23.

55. Hanson, C., West, J., Neiger, B., Thackeray, R., Barnes, M., & McIntyre, E. (2011). Use and acceptance of social media among health educators. *American Journal of Health Education, 42*(4), 197–204.

56. Childs, L. M. & Martin, C. Y. (2012). Social media profiles: Striking the right balance. *American Journal of Health-System Pharmacy, 69*(23), 2044–2050.

57. Farnan, J. M., Snyder Sulmasy, L., Worster, B. K., Chaudhry, H. J., Rhyne, J. A., & Arora, V. M. (2013). American College of Physicians Ethics, Professionalism Human Rights Committee, American College of Physicians Council of Associates, Federation of State Medical Boards Special Committee on Ethics Professionalism. Online medical professionalism: Patient and public relationships: Policy statement from the American College of Physicians and the Federation of State Medical Boards. *Annals of Internal Medicine, 158*(8), 620–627.

58. Bernhardt, M., Alber, J., & Gold, R. S. (2014). A social media primer for professionals: Digital do's and don'ts. *Health Promotion Practice, 15*(2), 168–172.

59. Jones, K., Baldwin, K. A., & Lewis, P. R. (2012). The potential influence of a social media intervention on risky sexual behavior and Chlamydia incidence. *Journal of Community Health Nursing, 29*(2), 106–120.

60. Schenker, M. (2015, May 12). *Former MySpace CEO explains why MySpace lost out to Facebook so badly*. Retrieved June 6, 2017, from http://www.digitaltrends.com/social-media/former-myspace-ceo-reveals-what-facebook-did-right-to-dominate-social-media/

61. Hopwood, S. (2016, June 16). On the rise: Messaging apps may take over social media [Web log post]. Retrieved April 29, 2017, from http://www.apptentive.com/blog/2016/06/16/rise-messaging-apps-may-take-social-media

62. George, D. R., Rovniak, L. S., & Kraschnewski, J. L. (2013). Dangers and opportunities for social media in medicine. *Clinical Obstetrics Gynecology, 56*(3), 453–462.

63. Steel, E. (2014, August 17). "Ice Bucket Challenge" has raised millions for ALS Association. *The New York Times, 17*. Retrieved June 6, 2017, from http://www.nytimes.com/2014/08/18/business/ice-bucket-challenge-has-raised-millions-for-als-association.html?_r=0

64. Williams, D. L. & Duffin, R. (2014). Internet and social media to reach young women with breast cancer: Targeting your message. Annual meeting of the American Public Health Association, November 18, New Orleans.

65. Stone Media Consulting (29 March 2016). *Social Media half life*. Retrieved August 3, 2017, from http://www.stonemediaconsulting.com/2016/03/29/social-media-half-life/

Additional Resources

Print

Bergeron, K., Davies, J., Hahn, S., Brankley, L., Dhaliwal, M., Williams, M., … McColl, K. (2013). Case study: The adoption of social media at three Ontario public health units. Wellington-Dufferin-Guelph Public Health, Guelph, ON.

National Commission for Health Education Credentialing, Inc. (NCHEC), & Society for Public Health Education (SOPHE). (2015). *A Competency-Based Framework for Health Education Specialists-2015*. Whitehall, PA: National Commission for Health Education Credentialing, Inc. (NCHEC) and Society for Public Health Education (SOPHE).

Internet

Overdrive Interactive. (2017). Social media map 2017. Retrieved from http://www.ovrdrv.com/social-media-map/

U.S. National Archives. Social media statistics. Retrieved from http://www.archives.gov/social-media/reports

CHAPTER 9

Working with Media Outlets

David Fouse, BA

▶ Author Comments

I have devoted much of my professional life to improving health. Whether serving as a writer, editor, public information officer, or communications director, I have worked in many environments and across many platforms to educate and engage reporters and the public around health.

I have been interviewed or arranged interviews for spokespeople on many occasions. Sometimes, reporters wanted an interview because my organization had won an award or received some recognition they wanted to publicize. On other occasions, the reporter was looking for an expert to provide background information or commentary on a particular situation. There have also been times when an interviewer wanted to learn about a role my agency played in a controversial situation. Additionally, I have pitched story ideas to reporters to suggest a feature story or to encourage the investigation of a particular concern. On some issues, to get key points across, I have written a letter to the editor or submitted an op-ed for publication on the paper's opinion page. More recently, I have tweeted and blogged to amplify stories through social media. Finally, I have written and issued more news releases than I can remember.

My task in this chapter is to provide you with tips for working with the media. Over the years in my various roles, I have gained unique perspective and hands-on experience, which I am pleased to have the opportunity to share. I hope this chapter will be of benefit to you and your organization as you educate others about health.

🔍 CHES COMPETENCIES

2.4.6	Select methods and/or channels for reaching priority populations.
3.3.7	Use a variety of strategies to deliver plan.
6.1.4	Adapt information for consumer.
6.1.5	Convey health-related information to consumer.
7.1.3	Tailor messages for intended audience.
7.1.6	Assess and select methods and technologies used to deliver messages.
7.1.7	Deliver messages using media and communication strategies.
7.2.5	Use strategies that advance advocacy goals.
7.3.9	Use media advocacy techniques to influence decision makers.

Reprinted by permission of the National Commission for Health Education Credentialing, Inc. (NCHEC) and Society for Public Health Education (SOPHE).

▶ Introduction

Why would a health education specialist want to work with the media? There are numerous reasons such as educating the public about an important health issue, publicizing activities, and encouraging people to take some type of action related to a particular health problem or concern. Sometimes, the information to be shared is mundane such as announcing the place and time a public meeting will be held. At other times, media exposure may be the result of a controversial issue. Regardless of the situation, the media can be powerful allies for furthering a cause.

Other chapters within this text deal with issues associated with social marketing, health communication, social media, and media advocacy. Many of the methods and tools used are the same. This chapter focuses on developing technical skills used to apply these tools. In particular, this chapter addresses skills associated with news releases, fact sheets, interviewing, online media, press kits, and **public service announcements** (PSAs). Also included are tips for working with the different media outlets with examples of what has worked well and what has not.

▶ Steps for Utilizing Media Channels

A number of channels exist for working with the news media—all of which can be useful in a comprehensive health promotion effort. The steps for using each, however, differ. Media channels accessible to health education specialists include newspapers, radio, television, and online. Most traditional news outlets, whether print or broadcast, also have a presence online. While most of these outlets should be interested in what health education specialists have to share, the tools used to share that information vary.

Work with Print and Online Media

Newspapers, radio, television, and online media complement each other, yet differ relative to time and senses used. A newspaper is focused on sight and involves reading, which is a different way of learning than auditory learning. That is not to say the audience is different, but rather the sense used in conveying information differs. As such, a different set of tools is needed for sharing health information.

❓ DID YOU KNOW?

As of early 2016, just 2 out of 10 U.S. adults often get news from print newspapers.

Data from Mitchell et al. (2016, July 7). Pathways to news. *Pew Research Center*. Retrieved from http://www.journalism.org/2016/07/07/pathways-to-news/

News Releases

When an organization has something newsworthy or important to share about its activities, it often issues a news (or press) release. The news release is intended to alert reporters and the public about a special announcement or an urgent message. For example, an organization could use this technique to announce a new board member or staff member, a grant award, or a special activity or event. News releases are often used by organizations to gain community recognition for the organization, its activities, and its members. They may also be used to make position statements, to address controversy, or respond during an emergency.

Effective news releases provide the foundation for good news stories and should include the following elements:

- *Contact information.* Included is the name of a contact person, a phone number and an email address so the reporter knows who to reach out to with questions or to arrange an interview.
- *Headline.* A concise, compelling headline describes the focus of the news release.
- *Body.* The first sentence should identify the location and date of the news release using the following format: city, state, month, day, year. News stories follow the basics of journalism and should be written through the eyes of a reporter. In the first paragraph, they answer the questions who, what, when, and where. The news release should follow an **inverted pyramid** approach, by placing the most important elements early in the story, while saving the least important for later in the story. The body should always include one or more quotes from the primary spokesperson, often a director, president, chair of an organization, or another subject matter expert who has been identified to speak to the news media. Meaningful statistics that support the main point and help sell the story should be included.
- *Boilerplate.* A sentence or two at the end should include information about the agency along with its website address.

A news release generally is no longer than a page or two. It is important to stick to the main points, but include links to the agency's website for additional information a journalist should know. **FIGURE 9.1** is an example news release focusing on breastfeeding rates created by the Colorado Department of Public Health and Environment.

⑦ DID YOU KNOW?

The inverted pyramid—a form of organizing information with the most important information at the top of a story and remaining information following in order of importance—was created during the advent of the telegraph. The form was soon adopted by newspapers and wire service organizations by the early 20th century.

Data from Scanlan, C. (2003, June 20). Writing from the top down: Pros and cons of the inverted pyramid. *Poynter.* Retrieved May 20, 2017, from http://www.poynter.org/news/writing-top-down-pros-and -cons-inverted-pyramid

⑦ DID YOU KNOW?

According to journalism historian David T. Z. Mindich, an Associated Press reporter filed one of the first leads following the inverted pyramid form the night Abraham Lincoln was assassinated:

To The Associated Press

Washington, Friday, April 14, 1865

The President was shot in a theatre tonight and perhaps mortally wounded.

Data from Scanlan, C. (2003, June 20). Writing from the top down: Pros and cons of the inverted pyramid. *Poynter.* Retrieved May 20, 2017, from http://www.poynter.org/news/writing-top-down -pros-and-cons-inverted-pyramid

Letters to the Editor

Writing a letter to the editor of the local newspaper is a good way to raise a concern or share an opinion about an issue. Often the most read section of a newspaper, letters to the editor can help educate the public and raise support around an effort or cause. Letters can be helpful in influencing policy decisions as elected officials monitor them. Letters to the editor are usually submitted in response to a published article. They are typically written and signed by an individual, but may identify the writer's company or organizational affiliation if included (**FIGURE 9.2**).

The following suggestions can help improve the odds of getting a letter published:

- *Responding to an article in the paper.* Letters can support, refute, or offer an additional perspective to something the newspaper published. Citing the headline, date, and author of

FOR IMMEDIATE RELEASE
Colorado breastfeeding rates continue to climb

Denver, Colorado, Aug. 4, 2016—Colorado celebrates World Breastfeeding Week Aug. 1–7 as a national leader in breastfeeding, with the percentage of babies' breastfed from birth through the first six months rising yearly.

According to 2016 data from the Centers for Disease Control, the percentage of babies ever breastfed in Colorado increased from 81 percent for babies born in 2011 to 88.6 percent for those born in 2013. The percentage of babies being breastfed at six months jumped from 55.2 percent for 2011 to 66.2 percent for those born in 2013.

The Colorado Department of Public Health and Environment and all major medical organizations recommend feeding babies only breast milk for the first six months of their lives. Breastfeeding has been shown to reduce the risk of childhood obesity and diabetes, allergies and asthma, ear and respiratory infections, and even Sudden Infant Death Syndrome (SIDs).

"Breastfeeding gives babies a healthy start in life," said Dr. Larry Wolk, health department executive director and chief medical officer. "We've worked with hospitals throughout Colorado to make sure mothers have access to information and resources to help them make healthy choices for themselves and their babies."

In 2013, the health department and 18 hospitals formed the Colorado Baby-Friendly Hospital Collaborative to support hospitals implementing policies and practices to support breastfeeding. The collaborative covers half the babies born in Colorado and is credited with contributing to the rise in breastfeeding rates. Members offer technical assistance, networking and tools to train maternity staff and help new mothers start and continue to breastfeed while bonding with their babies.

Hospitals in the collaborative pay fees and work toward a rigorous "Baby-Friendly" designation by implementing the Ten Steps to Successful Breastfeeding. The designation is monitored for compliance by Baby-Friendly USA. Five hospitals participating in the collaborative recently have achieved the Baby-Friendly designation, bringing the state total to eight.

The health department's Special Supplemental Nutrition Program for Women, Infants and Children (WIC) supports breastfeeding by offering education, mom-to-mom support and breast pumps to low-income women.

The Mothers' Milk Bank supports the collaborative and breastfeeding women by providing donated breast milk to babies who need it.

For more information, go to www.breastfeedcolorado.com.

# # #

Source: Retrieved June 30, 2017, from https://www.colorado.gov/pacific/cdphe/news/colorado-breastfeeding-rates.

FIGURE 9.1 Sample Press Release.
Courtesy of the Colorado Department of Health & Environment.

the story at the beginning lets the editor know to what the letter is responding.

- *Keeping it short*. A focused letter states the main points and why the issue is of concern to the community. Most newspapers have strict limits on length, usually between 150 and 250 words. The newspaper's website will have specific submission guidelines. If

August 9, 2017

Editor
Northport Daily News
Northport, MI 49670

Dear Editor:

To the Editor,
Friday's article, "Sex Encouraged with Comprehensive Education," questioned the effect of comprehensive sex education on sexual activity. Many people worry that giving youth accurate information about sexual health will encourage them to have sex, but this isn't so.

Studies have proven that those of us who receive comprehensive sex education are more likely to delay sexual activity and to use contraceptives when we do become sexually active. Even the Surgeon General has declared that it is "imperative and clear that [youth need] accurate information about contraceptives." Yet, the current administration chooses ideology over science and spends millions of dollars on ineffective and inaccurate abstinence-only programs.

The Responsible Education about Life (REAL) Act would provide states with funding to implement school-based sex education that includes information about *both* abstinence *and also* contraception. It is imperative that we urge Congress to support the REAL Act.

Sincerely,

Timothy Sonnega, MPH
Public Health Director
Leland County, MI

FIGURE 9.2 Sample Letter to the Editor.

Reproduced from Advocates for Youth, Sex Education Resource Center. (2017). Writing a letter to the editor. Retrieved from http://www.advocatesforyouth.org/sercadv/245?task=view

not, a call to the newspaper can be made to find out how best to submit a letter to the editor.

- *Supporting with facts.* Statistics, data, or other evidence can be used to support the main point and ensure accuracy. The more the letter is localized and relevant to readers, the better.[1]
- *Mentioning an elected official by name.* The policymaker's name should be included if the intent is to educate, influence, or thank him or her. This increases the likelihood the official will see the letter.

Op-Eds

Many newspapers provide opportunities to write an **op-ed**, which is a short opinion piece on a specific topic that runs opposite the editorial page. It is another effective way to educate people or mobilize support around an important health concern affecting the community. Given space limitations and competition for space in a newspaper—large newspapers may receive hundreds of op-ed submissions a day—getting an op-ed published requires extra care. Longer than a letter to the editor, an op-ed

COMMUNITY CONNECTIONS 9.1

Jackson was concerned about a new food service program recently adopted by a local school district located within his county. He had expressed his concerns about the lack of healthy food selections by writing to the food service manager and the district superintendent. In his letter, he indicated the program, and although appearing to be a financially sound decision, lacked the appropriate nutrients for promoting healthy growth and preventing obesity. Jackson had extensive experience with nutrition, having developed and implemented guidelines for healthy food promotion within families and children in a variety of settings, and was considered by many to be an expert in the subject. The school district in question, though, had chosen to implement the food service program, based primarily on what the finance director indicated as "food the kids will actually eat, which reduces our cost due to waste." Jackson thought if he could enlist the support of the local paper to do a story on the issue using, in part, factual information he could provide, it might put some pressure on the district to replace this program and install one that provided healthier options to students.

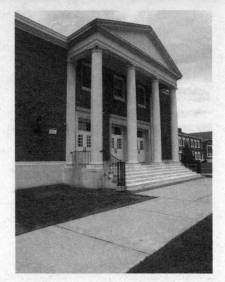

© Cynthia Farmer/Shutterstock.

Jackson called a friend, who also happened to be a newspaper reporter in a different state, who suggested Jackson write a letter to the editor providing factual information about the situation. He also told Jackson to make a phone call or send an email letting the editor know the letter was coming and to make a follow-up call to ensure it was received and see if a reporter would be assigned to cover the story. Jackson wrote a stirring letter, which a reporter then followed up for a feature story.

allows greater opportunity to explain an issue and persuasively develop an argument. Op-eds typically run between 500 and 800 words, but specific guidelines can be found on the newspaper's website.

A **news hook** will make an op-ed timely and relevant to readers. For example, a pending vote in the town council on a smoke-free ordinance can be used to demonstrate its importance to an organization's tobacco cessation work and the health of the community. Another example would be providing a local slant on a national campaign such as breast cancer awareness month in October.

In writing an op-ed, the newspaper should be contacted far in advance in order to introduce the organization to the appropriate newsperson (e.g., the editorial page editor). Newspaper personnel need to be aware there is interest in submitting an op-ed on a topic relevant to their readers, and they can provide advice on any specific guidelines or suggestions that would help ensure placement. Becoming familiar with recent articles, letters, or editorials the paper has published will help in understanding how the op-ed may complement or fill a void in reporting. It is important to follow up about a week after an op-ed has been submitted in order to confirm the submission was received, answer any questions the editor may have, and offer to make revisions if needed.

⑦ DID YOU KNOW?

In addition to inventing the Franklin stove, bifocals, daylight saving time, and electroshock treatment, Ben Franklin also invented newspaper editorials.

Online Comments and Blogging

Most traditional news outlets have a presence online, some of which such as **blogs** only exist online. Similar to submitting a letter to the editor to share perspectives on a story the local newspaper has published, comments can also be submitted online. The comments section of news outlets are often active forums for discussion and debate. Readers' comments might agree or disagree with the premise of the reporting, provide additional perspective and information to the article, suggest a correction to the story, or applaud the reporter for the accuracy portrayed in a story.

Once a news story is published online, the comments section needs to be monitored to make sure it is correct and an accurate perspective is included. Caution must be used, however, when engaging in online comments. Most news outlets have rules of etiquette that encourage civil discourse. While healthy debate and discussion is encouraged, personal attacks are not. If someone expresses a hostile or incorrect position, readers can report the comment to editors for possible deletion. Comments sections, in fact, have occasionally become so hostile that some news organizations have eliminated them from their website.[2]

Blogging is another way to share health news and information. In addition to reporting, many traditional news outlets feature one or more blogs on their website. While a reporter's story may appear in print or on air, it may also be published as a post on a blog or it may exclusively appear on a blog. Blogs allow traditional media outlets to expand their reporting without taking up either print space in a newspaper or airtime.

Blogs also exist in the community. Sometimes, community members take up the call of **citizen journalism** by creating their own blogs. These blogs may feature announcements and observations about local happenings, focus on a specific neighborhood or topic, or provide alternative viewpoints on local news and events. Each blog has its own style. While reporters are trained to objectively write and report based on fact, bloggers often use greater freedom in voicing their own opinion and often in how they conduct their work. Health education specialists should learn about the blogs in the community that are most relevant for sharing health information and whether they are interested in receiving story ideas. All bloggers need content to publish and might be searching for topics and guest posts from experts in the community. Posting to a blog though needs to be met with caution. Every word a health education specialists posts is assumed to represent the views of the agency. Would the agency approve of the content being shared? Is the blog a credible source with which the agency would want to be associated?

Blogs can be started using free platforms such as WordPress, Blogger, or another online app. A health education specialist's blog can provide a forum for sharing short announcements, longer stories, opinions, videos, and photos; for curating content from partner organizations that support and validate messages; and for engaging readers with content they can comment on and share. Other social media tools such as Twitter and Facebook can promote new blog posts and drive readers back to the blog content for the purpose of raising awareness and promoting conversation.

⑦ DID YOU KNOW?

The first blog was created in 1994. Now there are more than 152 million blogs on the Internet, with a new blog created every half a second.

Data from Thompson, C. (2006, February 20). The early years. *New York Magazine*. Retrieved May 20, 2017 from http://www.nymag.com/news/media/15971/

Work with Radio and Television

In contrast to print and online media, which focus on space, the unit of exchange for both radio and television is time. As such, radio and television are limited with respect to offering broad coverage of information with their audiences. Health education specialists most often interact with these media channels through PSAs and interviews.

Public Service Announcement

A PSA is a short informational announcement commonly used by nonprofit, community, and governmental organizations to serve public

COMMUNITY CONNECTIONS 9.2

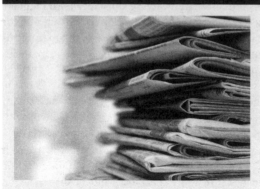

© Billion Photos/Shutterstock.

Jackson's letter to the newspaper resulted in an article that appeared on the front page of the newspaper's education section. Much to his delight, Jackson found the newspaper had done an excellent job investigating the issues he shared and had thoroughly reported them in the paper. Within a week, the letters appearing in the letters to the editor section of the paper were primarily devoted to the food program issue. Comments also appeared in the online version of the paper, with a robust discussion amongst the readers who were leaving comments. It appeared many local citizens were just as concerned as Jackson was with the lack of nutritious options in the food service program. The newspaper had its fair share of supporters for the curriculum, but each such letter seemed to focus on repeating the same argument over and over. Letters from opponents to the newly adopted food service program expressed numerous views as to why the program should be replaced with a healthier solution.

listeners, and are therefore interested in airing information about events and issues that affect the local community and are of interest to listeners or viewers. PSAs that promote positive health and discourage negative health behaviors help stations meet this often unspoken need. Also, a station that airs PSAs designed to promote health may generate community goodwill. The listener views the station as a good citizen of the community that provides a valuable service.

⑦ DID YOU KNOW?

The FCC is an independent U.S. government agency directly responsible to the Congress. The FCC was established by the Communications Act of 1934 and is charged with regulating interstate and international communications by radio, television, wire, satellite, and cable. The FCC's jurisdiction covers the 50 states, the District of Columbia, and U.S. possessions.

One advantage for using a PSA is low cost. Because the airtime is donated, the only real expense is production. However, there is no guarantee that the PSA will be aired or when it will be aired. For instance, it could end up running during the middle of the night when fewer people are listening or watching. Competition for free airtime can also present a challenge, which is dependent on the size of the market and number of nonprofits seeking time on local stations.

Some PSAs are developed and aired nationally. Many of these are made available to community groups, which often add a tagline to identify the local organization. Other PSAs are created by local agencies and intended only for local broadcast.

Whoever is responsible for selecting PSAs for broadcast (e.g., the local station manager, public affairs director) should be able to share information about submission deadlines, format requirements, and preferred length. PSAs are generally submitted as prerecorded digital audio or video files that are ready to air. Some public and community radio stations, however, prefer a script the station's announcers can read live on air.

interests. PSAs are used on radio and television for many reasons, including educating the public, promoting programs or services, and providing resources for behavior and community change.

Radio and television stations are interested in airing PSAs for a number of reasons. The Federal Communications Commission (FCC) reviews a station's public service when deciding whether or not to renew its broadcast license. Stations providing an adequate amount of free airtime are more likely to receive a license renewal. In addition, local stations may feel a responsibility to their

Radio PSAs are easier to develop, cost less, and have a greater likelihood of receiving airtime.[3] The PSA should include the following:

- *Source.* Both the individual and organization should be identified, including mailing address, phone number, and email and website address.
- *Contact person.* The name and contact information of the person responsible for the PSA, which may differ from the person submitting it, should be included.
- *Release date and time.* Is the information ready for immediate release or is there a particular date and time when it should be used? For example, a PSA about Labor Day travel safety should broadcast immediately prior to and throughout the Labor Day weekend. A time range should be included if a PSA is designed to be aired at a specific time of day. For instance, some PSAs may be more appropriate if aired during late afternoon when adolescents are out of school or workers are commuting home.

Television PSAs are either components of a broader state or national campaign or are developed by a local agency. A PSA that has already been developed is much easier and less costly to use than one that needs to be created from scratch. Sometimes, a PSA from a federal agency (e.g., Centers for Disease Control and Prevention) or a national campaign can be tailored to include a message at the end identifying local contacts and action. In contrast, locally developing a PSA allows the issue to be customized for specific community needs, populations, and problems. Often, local personalities will give their time to appear in a television PSA, which can provide a professional quality to the product and greater recognition within the community.

Audio and video PSAs can also reach online audiences. Files can be uploaded to an agency website, YouTube channel, or other video sharing platforms and promoted across the organization's social media channels. **FIGURE 9.3** provides an example PSA created and used by the Alabama Department of Public Health.

Community Calendars

Many local radio and television stations maintain a calendar of community events. The station may announce upcoming events on air or feature a calendar on its website. Submitting an event such as a 5K walk or run, a flu immunization fair, or farmers market to a community calendar helps alert community members about how they can participate. The station's website should have information on how to submit an event, or the

---

FOR RELEASE: June 2017
CONTACT: Connor Sharp, Alabama Department of Public Health,
Connor. Sharp@adph.gov or (517) 773-5238
TIME: 30 seconds

SKIN CANCER

SUMMER'S HERE — TEMPERATURES ARE SOARING — AND UNFORTUNATELY SO IS YOUR RISK FOR DEVELOPING SKIN CANCER ...

THIS IS STATE HEALTH OFFICER DOCTOR TOM MILLER ... THE SUN'S HARMFUL ULTRAVIOLET RAYS CAN DAMAGE YOUR SKIN IF IT'S NOT PROPERLY PROTECTED — SO WHEN YOU'RE OUT IN THE SUN THIS SUMMER MAKE SURE YOU WEAR PROTECTIVE CLOTHING LIKE HATS AND LONG SLEEVES AND BY ALL MEANS PUT ON SUNSCREEN...

FOR MORE INFORMATION, VISIT OUR WEBSITE AT ADPH—DOT—ORG—SLASH—SKINCANCER.

FIGURE 9.3 Sample Public Service Announcement.

Data from Alabama Public Health. (2017). Radio PSAs. Retrieved June 30, 2017 from http://www.alabamapublichealth.gov/news/radio.html

public affairs director or station manager can share deadlines and submission criteria.

Conduct Interviews

Media personnel may contact health education specialists to obtain further information about a topic, to answer questions about a controversial issue, or as a follow-up to information that was sent to them. This contact may be in the form of an interview, which can be either formal or informal, and conducted over the phone, onsite at the radio, or television station at the interviewee's agency or some off-site location or online.

Maintaining a good relationship with the media requires being flexible and accommodating to their schedule. In many cases, reporters work on tight deadlines, so promptly returning calls and doing what is necessary to assist them will improve relations. Cooperatively working with the media may result in future interviews. Many agencies, however, have a designated spokesperson for such interviews and the health education specialist should not interview with a reporter unless the agency's procedure for such is known.

Telephone and Radio

A reporter who calls requesting an interview or a statement related to a particular news item usually initiates a telephone interview. Sometimes, an initial call is made to arrange a time for an interview, which provides the interviewee with time to prepare. The interview may be recorded so the reporter will have an accurate account or, if it is for radio or television, to broadcast later. Also, the telephone interview may be one that is conducted as part of a live radio show, perhaps with call-in questions from listeners. While an interview may be conducted on a cell phone, a reporter may prefer use of a landline to ensure a higher quality recording or guarantee the connection will not be lost during a live broadcast. Promoting the organization and providing the website address is acceptable to share within the interview.

Television

Like telephone interviews, television interviews are sometimes arranged in advance such as being a guest on a local talk show devoted to community events, while at other times there is little notice. The interview may be part of a story or series that has been developed over a period of time, or it may be an attempt to determine local response to a breaking news story.

It is important to remember television, especially a news program, broadcasts video clips and sound bites that are measured in seconds. Often, television reporters will record an interview in the field to be aired later. Instead of showing the entire interview, the television producer determines which segments to broadcast. The interviewee should prepare several main points to communicate during an interview and reinforce those points when possible to increase the likelihood the intended key messages are included in the final broadcast. A short, prepared statement can be beneficial in the event the interview focuses on a controversial issue.

The most obvious difference between television and other types of interviews is the viewing audience. Many television interviews are requested at the spur of the moment, and some professionals who are often called upon for interviews keep a change of clothes at their office for such occasions. It is important to look nice, even on short notice.

Online

Television news requires video. When an in-person on-camera interview is not possible, the reporter may ask to conduct the interview online as part of a podcast or webcast from a remote location. Additional care needs to be taken prior to conducting an interview online, including checking equipment to make sure connections work, ensuring the background for the interview is appropriate and free of clutter or distractions, and making sure there will be no interruptions during the interview.

Last-Minute Interviews

Last-minute interviews often require an expert in a subject area to respond to questions. In these situations, time may not allow for background research. If contacted for an interview on short notice, it is important to have a clear understanding of the topic and inquire as to the length of the interview. It is acceptable to decline the interview if

COMMUNITY CONNECTIONS 9.3

Jackson was amazed at the amount of newspaper and television coverage of the food program issue. In fact, he had been called by three local radio stations and the local television station, all of whom wanted to interview him. Two of the three radio interviews were conducted over the telephone and one took place via an online podcast. In preparing for the telephone interviews, Jackson double-checked all his facts and had available copies of published research papers associated with the issue. During the interview, Jackson made certain to only express that which he knew to be true rather than dabble in anything that could be misconstrued as a false "alternative fact," and was careful not to express opinions that he could not back up. His answers were short and succinct. Each interviewer appreciated his comments and aired exactly what he said. Although he was prepared, none of the interviews involved call-in questions from listeners.

the reporter is looking for information and expert opinion on a topic that is unfamiliar to the interviewee. Declining an interview should include affirming the invitation was appreciated, sharing topics that may be more suitable based on level of expertise, and making a referral to someone who can better meet the reporter's needs.

Conduct a News Conference

A news conference is sometimes held in conjunction with a major announcement such as a new building, organization, or services provided in the area. News conferences could also be held to announce major projects, fundraising, the latest statistics on health or safety issues, in response to an emergency, or for sharing any other newsworthy item. News organizations in the area are invited to attend news conferences.

A prepared statement, background about the news item, and supporting material is provided during the news conference. The media might ask for additional information to help them build an interesting news story, so it is important to have a thorough base of knowledge pertaining to the issue. A press kit is distributed to the media at news conference events, and typically includes a news release, speaker bios, statements, and background information about the issue.

▶ Tips and Techniques for Effectively Working with the Media

Create a Media List

Engaging the media to benefit a cause involves becoming familiar with the people reporting the news in the community. This can be accomplished by finding out what reporters and media outlets in the community cover stories similar to the proposed story, and identify the reporters, editors, and producers responsible for health news. Depending on the focus of the issue, other reporters might be identified, for example, the reporter covering city hall if the desire is to advance health policies, the environment reporter if concern is in relation to smog and rates of asthma, or the business reporter if focus is on sharing trends regarding bullying at the workplace.

What is the best way to find media contacts? Some ideas include calling the newspaper, radio station, or television station and asking for media contact names, following the **bylines** or the names of the reporters who write relevant stories, searching the websites of news outlets for relevant stories and learning who is reporting them, attending community events reporters may cover and introducing self in person, and following news personnel on social media. Creating a list of media contacts make it easier for outreach, as these are the people who should need to receive relevant news releases.

Build Relationships with Reporters

Getting to know and following local news outlet reporters and their bylines is important, but it is even better if they know and view health education specialists as reliable and trustworthy sources of information—individuals they can call when information about an issue is needed. Establishing rapport provides an avenue for contact with the news media, and cultivating such relationships can create a win-win situation for both parties. Becoming a trusted resource for news personnel fosters strong working relationships. Reporters and editors need to be aware of a multitude of topics and issues, and trying to keep on top of all the constantly occurring changes can be overwhelming. In many cases, the media rely on trusted sources for up-to-date information and late-breaking news. Emailing new findings or resource information to media contacts reduces the need for them to spend time searching for it. Critically important though is to make sure what is given to the media is correct and pertinent, because misleading, inaccurate, or irrelevant information can be detrimental to fostering the desired relationship.

Pitch Story Ideas

A first step in reaching out to a reporter when seeking media coverage is to prepare a **pitch**. Why would the reporter be interested in writing the story? What elements of the story are most compelling? Is this a new story that has never been reported, or is it an old story with a different slant that needs to be told anew? In general, being prepared before picking up the phone, sending an email, writing a letter, or replying to a tweet builds good rapport. Reporters do not have a lot of time, as they may receive dozens of pitches a day and are often on deadline. The following basic guidelines can help sell a story:

- *Know the publication and reporter.* Taking time to know which media outlets are interested in the story and which reporters at those outlets are most likely to cover the story is a critical first step before sharing any newsworthy items.
- *Target each pitch for each outlet and consider the elements available to offer the news organizations.* A daily newspaper may cover the release of new data on alcohol use among teens, but television news likely would prefer a video or an on-camera interview with an expert in order to tell the story.
- *Contact the reporter.* This can be done by email, phone call, letter, text, social media, or making a pitch in person if a relationship has already been established.
- *Open with an intriguing introduction or otherwise have a good hook.* Why the reporter should be interested and, more importantly, why the readers or viewers would be interested needs to be made known. To respect the reporter's time, any contact should be kept brief.

Increase Chances of a PSA Being Aired

Ways to increase a PSA being aired include adhering to a defined time element, being concisely written, and following station protocols:

- *Keep the PSA short.* Most PSAs are less than 30 seconds long. Time is a precious commodity in broadcasting where every second is tracked, which means carefully selecting material to be included in the PSA. Time blocks typically are available in 10-, 15-, 20-, 30-, 45-, and 60-second lengths.
- *Write the PSA in a concise manner.* Colleagues and members of the focus audience should proofread the PSA prior to submission. Reading the copy aloud at a deliberate pace can help determine approximate length. Timing does not have to be exact though as the station may trim the copy to fit the time slot.
- *Call targeted stations.* It is helpful to find out who the person is who deals with PSAs and let him or her know about the PSA, explain why the PSA is important, ask the best way to get a PSA on the air at the station, and follow the advice given are all good strategies to employ. Sometimes, stations will work with organizations to help produce a PSA.

⑦ DID YOU KNOW?

Modern-day radio broadcasting was pioneered by Frank Conrad in the backyard garage of his home in Wilkinsburg, Pennsylvania, from 1919 to 1920. Conrad was the first person to ever air an advertisement over a radio.

Increase Chances of a News Release Being Used

Thinking like a newspaper and considering what would appeal to their readers can help guide in writing a news release. In particular, **TABLE 9.1** lists a number of tips for ensuring a news release is seen by and useful to the news media.

Enhance Interviewing Skills

There are ways for increasing the likelihood of a successful interview. Many of these tips might seem like common sense, but applied collectively will result in a more polished and professional interview. At the same time, it will ensure the message being conveyed is both accurate and relevant to the intended audience (**TABLE 9.2**).

Follow up After an Interview

After the interview, the interviewee should check to see if what appeared in the newspaper, online, on television, or on radio accurately reflected the statements made. Sometimes, reporters take what they hear and put together a news story that represents all aspects of a situation. Other times though they simply make errors. The quote taken from the interview may not be close to an individual's or agency's true position on an issue. The reporter may not have understood all that is involved and, working on a tight deadline, might have made an honest mistake. In other cases, the portions of the article based on an interview, or the short segment of video or audio aired, may not be at all representative of the entire interview.

If reporters do a good job, they should be provided with positive feedback. If there are problems

---

TABLE 9.1 Tips for Writing a News Release

- *Keep the news release short.* Suggested length is no more than one or two pages double spaced. Each sentence should be concise and free from jargon.

- *Write a compelling headline.* This will help the reporter or editor understand at a glance what the news release is about in a way that is relevant to their readers or listeners.

- *Write the news release as though it were a news story.* Some community newspapers with limited reporting staff may run the news release as is and appreciate having a finished product to publish.

- *Include quotes from the agency's spokesperson.* While the news outlet likely will not print the news release in full, the reporter may directly use a quote from the news release in the story.

- *Include contact information.* Providing a phone number and email address allows the reporter to follow up with questions.

- *Email news releases to the relevant reporters and editors.* When possible, editors should be given ample lead time—up to a week—before requested publication.

- *Follow up with a phone call or text message.* Newsrooms are very busy and reporters receive many emails a day. A quick phone call or text can help make sure the news release was received and noticed.

- *Share the news release and link it to the organization's website.* Social media can be used to share the news release with followers and reporters with a link back to the website.

TABLE 9.2 Interviewing Tips

- *Prepare for the interview.* If requested for an interview, it is important to know who is calling, the organization represented, and the purpose of the interview. Some agencies have a public relations policy that states only specific individuals may speak with the press, which may impact who can engage in the interview. When preparing for the interview, taking a moment to gather background information and offering to call back can provide needed focus prior to responding to questions. The first few times doing an interview may be stressful, which is typical. Being able to relax and act normal is important, as anything said may be heard on the air or printed in the paper.

- *Provide the reporter with appropriate background information.* Often, reporters may have only a small amount of information on a topic. Most reporters will appreciate assistance, especially if the information provided is relevant.

- *Know in advance who will conduct the interview.* If not familiar with the interviewer, listening or watching the show or reading newspaper articles written by the interviewer prior can help in preparing for the interview. It is important to become familiar with and understand the format and interview style. For example, if for broadcast, is it a live interview or will it be recorded and aired at a later time?

- *Identify the intended audience.* Is the audience primarily teens? Older populations? The business community? Understanding the focus audience matters. Audience information may be available from the marketing department of the news organization or from discussions with people who are familiar with the program outlet.

- *Prepare to answer as many questions as possible.* Some interviewers will provide sample questions that may be asked. Other questions, however, may come up during the interview or from outside callers.

- *Prepare a few key messages in advance to share during the interview.* The message can be made more compelling and understandable by supplementing and supporting each message point with a fact, statistic, or anecdote.[4] Information can be added to the conversation if the interviewer does not ask for it. Using questions can help bridge to key messages.

- *If necessary, have organized reference material available.* The key word is organized—shuffling papers is not a positive image and sends a message of uncertainty. Being able to quickly locate information is a benefit.

- *Consider speaking from a prepared statement, and do not stray from it.* Staying focused on the topic that is of concern prevents being led into answering loaded questions or talking about issues that would be better left alone. Also, it may happen that a question might be asked that was not part of the interview preparation. It may be helpful to work out a few ground rules with the reporter before anything is recorded. The reporter should be made aware of issues to avoid prior to the actual interview. If the reporter agrees to conditions but asks the questions on camera anyway, it is acceptable to politely indicate the interview is over. The poorly answered question or least desirable response to a statement may be what ends up being aired.

- *Provide honest answers.* If an answer to a question is not known, it is acceptable to say something like, "That is a good question. I do not have the answer for that at this moment. I will have to do some additional research and get back to you." Admitting lack of knowledge is much better than providing inaccurate or incorrect information.

(continues)

TABLE 9.2   *(Continued)*

- *Have a final statement prepared.* The interviewer might ask if there is anything else to add. This is where key points can be succinctly restated in order to drive home the main message.

- *Do not be late to a scheduled interview.* Time is a precious commodity for media, so being late needs to be avoided.

- *Dress for success.* Professional clothing in solid colors is the preferred attire for an on-camera interview. White or patterned clothes such as pin stripes or checkered designs should be avoided. Accessories should be limited to prevent noise, distractions, and reflections from studio lights.

- *Maintain good posture.* This includes comfortably sitting in the chair, not slouching, keeping legs crossed or feet flat on the floor, and slightly leaning forward toward the interviewer. Keeping gestures to a minimum is also important, as too much movement can be distracting on television.

- *Remain calm and professional.* Nervous reactions might be recognized over the telephone, radio, or online.

with the story, they also should be made aware. It is important that views are correctly represented and the information provided to the public is factual. Reporters want to represent their sources and run good stories, and they may never know there was a problem unless they are informed.

Develop a Press Kit

A press, or media, kit is a packet of information prepared by an organization about the organization

COMMUNITY CONNECTIONS 9.4

After he listened to his interviews, Jackson sent a thank you note to each reporter, expressing his appreciation for being able to share information and for their willingness to accurately address the topic. He even received a call back from one of the reporters, who said, "I received your letter and hope you don't mind if I keep you on my list for any future programs I develop that have to do with nutrition-related issues." Jackson was pleased his efforts paid off and glad to serve as a future source for providing research-based guidance regarding healthy eating.

or about a particular topic, story, or event provided to the media and other interested agencies. **Press kits** include basic background such as the history and mission of the organization or its work, leadership biographies, and financial information. Press kits are prepared when a press conference or special event is planned such as a political rally or other public news event. For instance, a press kit could be developed for the opening of a new facility (e.g., laboratory or community recreation center) or in conjunction with the release of the latest local statistics on rates of immunizations or influenza transmission by the local health department. A press kit ensures the same information is disseminated to interested parties and, to a large degree, eliminates the need for individual interviews or routine requests for information. By providing the material to the media, the organization can assure accuracy by having control over what is released.

There are no specific rules as to what can or cannot be included in a press kit. Included are fact sheets or other documents that provide answers to questions about the organization, the topic, and key personnel. For example, a press kit for special events can include a copy of the program or schedule of events, a list of speakers with a brief bio for each, copies of the speakers' remarks, and the news release prepared for the event. Catalogs or other organizational materials such as an annual report, calendar of events, or copies of the organization's newsletter can also be included. Digital media press kits can include an easily downloadable logo, photos, or video files saved in multiple sizes and formats. Having a press kit available can avoid the extra work of preparing responses and fulfilling individual requests for information.

Press kits can be presented in hard copy with printed pages inserted into a pocket folder, on a jump drive, or via a website. Well-organized information that provides answers to most of the questions reporters might have conveys a positive image of the organization. Elaborate presentation style, however, cannot substitute for quality content. Reporters are interested in the value of the information presented and its ease of use.

Use Media Fact Sheets

A fact sheet is another tool to help reach the media and encourage reporting about health education and promotion efforts. Like a news release, it presents important information in a concise, organized format. But unlike a news release—and as the name implies—it sticks just to the facts. A fact sheet provides answers to some basic questions about the agency or issue. The source of all facts should be cited. For instance, a childhood immunization fact sheet could provide community immunization rates, when and where immunizations are provided, and the benefits to the community in terms of costs and lives saved if every child were immunized.

A fact sheet provides a structured format of information to the editor to assist in developing a story idea. It does not provide all the details of the story, but does provide an idea and supporting information that can be expanded into a longer, more detailed article. The editor may make a decision to assign a reporter the task of developing a story idea based on the information provided in the fact sheet.

The fact sheet can be shared with the news media via email with a brief note providing a summary of a basic concept, giving a description of the problem, and identifying possible solutions. It can be included in a press kit, distributed with a news release, or used in lieu of a brochure. The goal of the fact sheet is to make it easier for a writer to report a newsworthy piece about an organization's work.

Fact sheets are not complicated. They are usually one or two pages and they provide the reader with some general but important information about an agency's business. Most fact sheets include:

- *The name and address of the business.* If using standard letterhead for the organization, this information probably is already included. If not, it needs to be added.
- *Relevant contact information.* Readers need a way to get in touch with the agency contact. This can be accomplished by listing the name of the contact person, job title, phone number, and email.
- *The subject or title of the fact sheet.* It is all about easy access to information, so the title needs to be clear and descriptive. There should be no question what topic the fact sheet covers.
- *Sticking to the facts.* The fact sheet is not a sales piece, even though the urge to make it one might exist. The purpose of the fact sheet is to give bloggers, journalists, and writers clear, useful information.

It is important to follow up the submitted fact sheet with a phone call to the news editor. For example, "Last week, I sent you information about the food deserts existing in lower income neighborhoods in our community. The data we have found shows a clear relationship between food deserts and childhood obesity. What can I do to encourage you to do a story concerning this issue?"

⑦ DID YOU KNOW?

Journalists and media outlets are the most active group on Twitter. Among the more than 300 million active users, reporters and media organizations account for about 25 percent of all verified users on the social media platform and tweet more often than any other group of Twitter users—more than professional actors, athletes, and musicians.

Data from Kamps, H. J. (2015, May 25). Who are Twitter's verified users? *Medium.* Retrieved May 20, 2017 from http://www.medium.com/@Haje/who-are-twitter-s-verified-users-af976fc1b032

Use Online Channels for Rapid Dissemination of Information

Other dissemination channels exist that can be used as part of a health education campaign. These methods offer an alternative to sending a news release or working through traditional media outlets, and can be just as effective in promoting the work of an agency or calling attention to an important issue.

- *Blog post.* Announcements needing to be shared can be done so through a blog post. It is simple and effective as long as the intended audience reads the blog.
- *Online video streaming.* Many people carry a smartphone, which is an easy way for receiving a variety of media. Instead of hoping the newspaper runs a statement from the board chair or president of an organization, a message from the organization's spokesperson can be recorded and uploaded to an online video streaming platform such as Facebook Live or YouTube. It can then be, for example, shared on a blog, tweeted via Twitter, posted to Facebook, or shared via some other social media channels. Sending it to media contacts may result in the video being **embedded** along with a related story published on the outlet's website.
- *Tweet or initiate a Twitter chat.* If the organization has developed a large following on Twitter or has influential followers, a tweet quickly disseminates new information. Hosting a Twitter chat can offer an opportunity to engage stakeholders, the media, and others in an online conversation organized by a predetermined hashtag. As a result, the chat can get a lot of people and organizations tweeting about an important topic.

▶ Overcoming Challenges in Working with Media Outlets

As with any of the other methods described in this text, there are many barriers or problems health education specialists routinely encounter in working with the media. Anticipating these problems and understanding how to overcome them are as important as mastering the techniques associated with media tools described in this chapter.

Ensure Media Coverage

What happens if PSAs are rarely used, if ever, or news releases never wind up as news stories? Unfortunately, this may be the case. The media are bombarded with many groups vying for airtime and print space, so at times there is great competition for media attention. Taking time to develop personal relationships with people at the media outlets who make the decisions regarding airtime for PSAs and who decide which stories to cover can increase the likelihood of success. It is alright to engage in open and honest communication if the media coverage is not forthcoming. This can help in determining what needs to be changed in material development to increase the likelihood of airtime or making it to print.

Limit Statements Taken Out of Context

Many times, only a fraction of what an interviewee says is aired or printed. Unfortunately, statements used may then be taken out of context or include that which the interviewee had said but hoped would not be disseminated. Media sources have limited time or print space in which to fit a whole host of competing stories. Providing interviewers with much more information than can be used gives them the opportunity to choose what is important and what is not, and subsequently what appears in the story. When a controversial issue is involved, operating from a brief, prepared statement is wise. Taking few, if any, questions and when answering questions staying close to the prepared statement will reduce statements being taken out of context. This strategy provides editors with the bulk of what is intended to be shared, reducing the probability of misrepresentative statements being aired or printed.

Make Time for Fostering Media Contacts

One of the biggest payoffs when seeking media coverage is to develop relationships with reporters, which includes being regarded as a trusted resource and knowing when they prefer to be called. For example, it is usually best to call newspaper reporters midday, as mornings often require editorial meetings and late afternoons bring deadlines for filing a story. At the same time, it is important to be considerate of their time. Contacting reporters with new information is fine, while making sure not to demand too much of their time. Rather it may be best to share a little information and let them know how best to contact you if they have further questions.

▶ Expected Outcomes

What outcomes can one expect from working with the media? It is reasonable to expect attempts to publicize an event or to disseminate a message will receive some airtime or print space. It is unreasonable to expect the station or newspaper will take on the cause as its own and provide free daily publicity. Airtime and newsprint space are valuable commodities and, as such, competition is high. The better the relationships built with news reporters, the greater the likelihood of being seen as a valuable source of information.

It is also reasonable to expect the media can be used as a means for providing health information to the public. But it is unreasonable to expect use of the media to substantially change individual health behaviors. As part of a more comprehensive approach, however, consistent use of the media and the development of positive working relationships with newspaper, radio, television,

and online reporters and writers increase the likelihood of creating positive change.

Finally, it is reasonable to expect that media coverage will increase community interest in the issue at hand. In contrast, it is unreasonable to expect media coverage to always be favorable to particular positions. Media are bound to provide broad coverage of what they deem as being newsworthy to the community while, at the same time, maintaining their right to hold diverse opinions. Thus, it is essential to ensure any information shared with the media is both reliable and valid.

▶ Conclusion

Working with the media provides individuals and organizations with opportunities to share information with others on a broader scale than would otherwise be possible. The information provided might be directed toward an awareness of healthy and unhealthy behaviors, address controversial issues, or promote a particular organization, cause, or event. Each of the tools presented in this chapter may be used in any community health education agency, with some more applicable than others. The tools assist in making audiences aware of inappropriate social behavior that should be changed in order to ensure a safer and healthier life. Typically, attitudes are not changed as a result of media tools, because most attitudes and behaviors are deeply rooted in social culture and social and environmental determinants of health. An effective PSA or news release, however, may increase awareness and initiate a questioning process with individuals. Both legislators and the public can be influenced through the use of appropriate media tools, and the consistent use of these tools and development of positive working relations with the press and news media increase the likelihood of affecting change.

Key Terms

Blog A shortened form of the words web log, a blog is a website that features informal posts that are published in reverse chronological order, much like an online journal.

Citizen journalism The reporting of news and information by the general public or members of the community that is published and distributed online such as by a blog post, video, or podcast.

Byline A line in a newspaper or magazine that names the writer of the story.

Embed To place text, images, video, or sound in a document, device, or web page.

Inverted pyramid A journalistic style of storytelling that leads with the most important or newsworthy information, followed by less important information, and ending with the least important.

News hook An event, activity, or milestones that can help make a story more newsworthy in the eyes of the news media. Examples: The start of hurricane season may be a news hook for a story about preparing for emergencies. The opening of a new WIC clinic may be a news hook for a story about the importance of providing prenatal care in your community. The release of the governor's budget may be a news hook for a story on the importance of health funding.

Op-ed A guest editorial written by someone outside of the news organization that often runs opposite the editorial page in a newspaper.

Pitch An idea for a news story organized in a concise, compelling way and often shared with a reporter over the phone, in an email, in a letter, or in person.

Press kit A packet of information prepared by an organization about the organization or about a particular topic, story or event provided to the media and other interested agencies.

Public service announcement A short, informational announcement that serves the public interest shared on radio and television stations for free using donated airtime.

References

1. Stop Diabetes. *Tips for writing a letter to the editor.* Retrieved June 12, 2017, from http://www.stopdiabetes.com/advocacy-center/activist-toolkit/tips-for-writing-a-letter-to-the-editor.html?referrer=http%3A%2F%2Fctb.ku.edu%2Fen%2Ftable-of-contents%2Fadvocacy%2Fdirect-action%2Fletters-to-editor%2Fmain

2. Gross, D. (2014, November 21). *Online comments are being phased out.* Retrieved July 6, 2017, from http://www.cnn.com/2014/11/21/tech/web/online-comment-sections/index.html

3. Hampton, C. Section 7. *Community Toolbox: Preparing public service announcements.* Retrieved June 30, 2017, from http://ctb.ku.edu/en/table-of-contents/participation/promoting-interest/public-service-announcements/main

4. American College of Emergency Physicians. *Effective media interview techniques.* Retrieved June 18, 2017, from http://www.acep.org/Advocacy/Effective-Media-Interview-Techniques/

Additional Resources

Print

Bonk, K., Tynes, E., Griggs, H., & Sparks, G. (2008). *Strategic communications for nonprofits: A step-by-step guide to working with the media (2nd ed.).* Hoboken, NJ: Jossey-Bass.

National Commission for Health Education Credentialing, Inc. (NCHEC), & Society for Public Health Education (SOPHE). (2015). *A Competency-Based Framework for Health Education Specialists-2015.* Whitehall, PA: National Commission for Health Education Credentialing, Inc. (NCHEC) and Society for Public Health Education (SOPHE).

Scott, D. M. (2017). *The New rules of marketing and PR: How to use social media, online video, mobile applications, blogs, news releases, and viral marketing to reach buyers directly.* Hoboken, NJ: Wiley.

Internet

Community Toolbox: Media advocacy. Retrieved from http://ctb.ku.edu/en/table-of-contents /advocacy/media-advocacy

Media guide for SOPHE Chapters. Retrieved from http://www.sophe.org/resources/media -guide-sophe-chapters/

National health education week 2016 toolkit. Retrieved from http://www.sophe.org/wp -content/uploads/2016/12/NHEW-2016 -Toolkit-10516-Reformated.pdf

The OpEd Project. Retrieved from http://www .theopedproject.org/

Applying Community and Public Health Education Methods and Strategies at the Community and Policy Level

CHAPTER 10

Facilitating Groups

Kathleen M. Roe, DrPH, MPH

Kevin Roe, MPH

Frank V. Strona, MPH

▶ Author Comments

Throughout our careers, in different settings and with diverse groups, we have each had the pleasure of developing the art and skills of facilitation. This aspect of our health education practice is always interesting, sometimes challenging, and definitely rewarding. We have been impressed by the ways that skilled facilitators can guide a group through a complex process, even on a seemingly impossible time-line or with daunting objectives. We have witnessed facilitation that moved groups from frustration and conflict to communication and productivity. We have noted how culturally responsive facilitation can assist people to find their voices in a large group, engage with others in new ways, and contribute to participatory democracy. We have enjoyed discovering facilitation styles that draw upon the best of our own personalities and professional commitments, working with groups brought together by chance, assignment, or shared interests. In short, we have seen how disciplined and sentient facilitation strengthens our common wealth.

⌕ CHES COMPETENCIES

2.1.2	Use strategies to convene priority populations, partners, and other stakeholders.
2.1.3	Facilitate collaborative efforts among priority populations, partners, and other stakeholders.
2.2.2	Develop vision statement.
2.2.3	Develop mission statement.
2.3.5	Address diversity within priority populations in selecting and/or designing strategies/interventions.
2.5.2	Develop plans and processes to overcome potential barriers to implementation.
3.1.1	Create an environment conducive for learning.
3.1.6	Comply with legal standards that apply to implementation.
4.1.8	Develop data collection procedures for evaluation.*
5.3.5	Elicit feedback from partners and other stakeholders.*
5.5.1	Facilitate efforts to achieve organizational mission.*
5.5.5	Conduct strategic planning.*
5.6.10	Employ conflict resolution techniques.*

*Advanced level competency

▶ Introduction

Facilitation is one of the basic tools in the health education specialist's toolbox, regardless of practice setting, content area, or populations. Health education specialists are always involved with groups. Traditionally, groups met face to face, but 21st-century groups also meet over the phone or Internet. While group settings, players, purposes, and politics may vary, facilitation principles remain the same.

Facilitation can be defined as "making something easier,"[1] and is a set of skills that crosscut all seven areas of responsibility of the Certified Health Education Specialist (CHES).[2] Health education specialists' facilitation skills promote communication and collaboration in groups as small as a support group or as large as a national coalition. A facilitator's skills help group members conceptualize and organize tasks and procedures so they are accessible and achievable, and to course correct as needed. Following ethical principles of integrity, dignity, and respect for all persons,[3] artful facilitation creates settings and nurtures interactions that are meaningful, rewarding, and productive for all participants. If the purpose of health education is an open society, health education specialists are particularly good facilitators because of commitments to participation and inclusion, respect for dissent, and proactive embrace of diversity.[4]

Effective facilitation is developed through keen observation and reflective practice. Fortunately, health education specialists have many opportunities to refine these skills, as they often facilitate groups they create, convene, or even lead. Health education specialists are often elected or persuaded to serve as facilitators of groups of which they were once only members. They may be invited to serve as "outside" facilitators, bringing a neutral voice to a complex group process. Regardless of role or relationship, facilitating has a skill set and orientation that is different from directing, leading, advocating, or persuading. Effective facilitators focus on process rather than content. In fact, facilitators often have to separate themselves from the issues under discussion in order to attend to group communication and progress. This is not always easy. To an effective facilitator, however, *how* the group works together is often more important than the content of *what* they do or decide.

COMMUNITY CONNECTIONS 10.1

Jade Smith has been a community health education specialist for nearly 20 years. One day, she received a call from her colleague Valerie, who had just been named project director of a large, multiyear community health initiative. This project required all kinds of group work—a community advisory group, a planning council, working groups, and ongoing meetings of the staff supporting the work over the next three years. Although most of the meetings would be in person, up to 25% would be conducted "live online."

"Jade, this has got to be a participatory process, and the timeline is tight. I need someone to help me with facilitation. We've been in so many meetings together and I've always admired the way you handle group dynamics. Any chance you'd like to take this on as a consultant?" asked Valerie.

Jade was surprised. It was true that she had been in a lot of meetings with Valerie and often served as an informal facilitator; however, the extent of her formal training in facilitation was a group dynamics course in college and occasional continuing education workshops. But Valerie made the opportunity sound so interesting, and Jade had time to take on one more project —so, taking a deep breath and wondering what she was getting herself into, she said, "Sure, Valerie. I'd love to help."

Types of Groups

Much of what is done in health education is done so through groups—all kinds of groups. Health education specialists are likely to be involved in a variety of different groups, depending on need, purpose, and function. For instance, health education specialists frequently form groups in order to accomplish specific program objectives or mobilize community involvement. Groups may be required by funding mandate or employed as best practice by an organization as a way to achieve their mission and vision. They may be organized by formal charter or bylaws, workplace protocols, or underlying cultural norms. Groups can be large or small, and can stay together for years or disband when a specific task is accomplished. Group members can be elected, appointed, or volunteers. They can have oversight responsibilities, advisory roles, specific tasks to accomplish or products to develop by a designated deadline, or be formed merely to explore and share ideas and experiences. This diversity of group function keeps group facilitation fresh and exciting, even for seasoned practitioners. The following sections describe different kinds of groups and their respective facilitation opportunities.

Communication and Decision-Making Groups

Groups established for communication and decision-making are often the backbone of organizational units, partnerships, community, or professional groups. They work well when the purpose, scope, priorities, and communication modes are clearly established and comfortable for all. Effective facilitation addresses each of these elements.

Partnership and Staff Groups

This type of group is composed of people who work together through formal arrangements or organizations. While their structures and locations may be quite varied, both tend to operate through regular meetings of key members. Department meetings, staff meetings, faculty meetings, and partnership meetings all benefit from facilitation that utilizes the diversity of perspectives and interests while nurturing communication and shared priorities to achieve the unit's objectives. A unique challenge of effective staff or partnership facilitation lies in preexisting alliances and personal interests. An effective facilitator finds ways to engage participants despite differences in position, investment, and status, using those differences to strengthen the group's capacity to serve its mission. Facilitators must be mindful of differences and the ways they can marginalize participants, as well as skilled in the art of creating spaces and processes that are inviting and inclusive when working with partnerships or staff groups.[5]

Standing Committees

Standing committees are subgroups that contribute to the overall work and productivity of the organization or effort. For example, a community-based youth development organization might establish standing committees for resource development, outreach and recruitment, and after-school programs. The focus and composition of the standing committees may change over time as new group priorities or work demands emerge. Standing committees should have a charge, specific objectives, and scope of work. The facilitator supports a standing committee by establishing and managing group processes that help the group meet the charge, while allowing adequate time and support for the work to be accomplished. Standing committee facilitators are usually members of the committee.

Subcommittees

Like standing committees, subcommittees are smaller groups formed from a larger group. For example, a standing outreach and recruitment committee might have a subcommittee to focus on social media and another to organize tabling at community events. Subcommittees take on a specific segment of the larger committee's charge. Effective facilitation helps the members stay focused and relate their work to that of the larger committee.

Task-Specific Groups

Ad hoc committees, task forces, and coalitions are groups that are formed for a defined period of time to explore and/or take action on a particular issue or emerging situation. Once the task has been completed or the designated time elapsed, the group can either be dissolved, extended, reconfigured, or recommissioned.

Ad Hoc Committees

Ad hoc committees have a charge and a relatively short timeframe. This type of committee is often formed to give issues a "quick study," explore options, and formulate recommendations for a larger body. For example, a health education unit of a college health service may decide to review its promotional materials to determine whether they should be merely updated or completely revised. An ad hoc group, composed of two staff members, the summer intern, a clinician, and two students could be formed to look at the materials, research what other campuses are doing, solicit opinions from clients and marketing experts, and make a recommendation to the full staff within two months. An ad hoc committee's membership is usually open to anyone in the larger group who wants to participate and may include others with interest or useful perspective. Its facilitator, usually a member of the ad hoc committee, keeps members task oriented and productive.

Task Forces

A task force is formed for a slightly longer time to complete a specific activity or task. Task force membership begins with individuals from an existing group and is almost always supplemented by participation from others with expertise, perspectives, resources, or energy that will contribute to the task. For example, a task force might be formed to expand the number of farmers markets in a city, develop a plan to replace drinking fountains with hydration stations in a district's public schools, or explore options for a profession-wide accreditation system. Task force members contribute the human power and do the work; the facilitator tends to the process. Similar to ad hoc groups, once the defined objective is achieved, the task force is discontinued. The parent group, however, may convene a new task force—or reconvene the first one—should a similar need arise in the future. Depending on the scope of its charge and supporting resources, task force facilitation may come from within the group itself or an outside consultant.

Coalitions

A coalition is a large group, formed from other groups, with the specific purpose of sharing information, raising awareness, producing an event, developing community capacity, or advocating for an issue.[6] Coalitions tend to be formal relationships between individuals and agencies with goals that cannot be accomplished without collaborative effort. Some coalitions disband once the founding objective is achieved such as a community-wide 5K race and fitness fair. Others, such as the Coalition of National Health Education Organizations, work productively together for decades. A coalition's facilitator may be elected, drafted from participating organizations, or provided by the convening agent such as the funder or parent organization. The facilitator's primary task is to work with the leadership to make sure group meetings are energized, productive, and adequately supported so the coalition makes progress toward its goals.

> ### ⑦ DID YOU KNOW?
>
> The International Association of Facilitators (IAF) promotes the value of facilitation around the world. The IAF develops industry-accepted professional standards, provides accreditation, has established a code of ethics, and works to "advocate and educate on the power of facilitation and embrace the diversity of facilitators."

Source: Data from International Association of Facilitators. *IAF World*. Retrieved from http://www.iaf-world.org

The decision to create a committee, task force, or coalition is usually made when specific work needs to be done outside the structures, scope, or capacity of an existing group. The "work" can be exploration, thinking, discussion, deliberation, or actual physical labor. The facilitator plays a key role in the group's success by understanding the entire process from forming the group to achieving the end product; making sure the charge, resources, and timeline are SMART (strategic, manageable, achievable, realistic, and time-specific)[7]; creating and maintaining group focus and productivity;

celebrating the group's effort and accomplishment when the task is completed; encouraging ongoing evaluation of the group's performance; and making recommendations for future group structure and support.

> ### ⑦ DID YOU KNOW?
>
> One of famous anthropologist Margaret Mead's most well-known statements is about the power of groups: "Never doubt that a small group of thoughtful, committed citizens can change the world. Indeed, it's the only thing that ever has." Although the source of this statement is not known, it is one of the most frequently cited statements about the power of groups.

Oversight, Planning, and Advisory Groups

Community health efforts often rely on information and guidance from experts. For example, the local health department may be named the lead agency for a new oral health initiative for an underserved part of the county, or a community mental health coalition may decide that they need to study isolation among rural elders. In both cases, insight and advice beyond the regular group may be needed.

Advisory Groups

Advisory groups enable health education specialists to obtain direction and guidance from people who understand the key issues and dynamics of a community-based program or initiative. Advisory groups are often central to community-based participatory research projects.[8] An advisory committee might be created, for example, to discuss the implementation of a school wellness policy, advice on a community-based assessment of the health needs of refugee families, or comment on planned revisions to a community college health education curriculum.

Advisory group members are selected for the perspectives they bring to a project or organization. Typically, they include content experts and members of a priority population. For example, the advisory group for a community clinic's new Vietnamese breast and cervical cancer screening outreach program might include Vietnamese community leaders, staff of local agencies serving Vietnamese clients, and cultural competency guides. The advisory committee for a prominent foundation's social marketing campaign might include media advocacy experts, content specialists, and members of the priority population. A health education unit's strategic planning process might engage an advisory group of outside experts to provide insight into emerging population needs and workplace trends.

Because advisory groups do not make decisions, facilitation may use a less formal style than used with other kinds of groups. This is particularly important when community members are invited to participate in new ways or in venues that might be intimidating. The facilitator is key to creating an environment conducive to full participation and dialogue, and to help a diverse group move their ideas to useful recommendations.[9]

Planning Councils and Commissions

Planning councils are a specific kind of advisory group, often sponsored by government agencies, as a way of soliciting broad participation in program priorities and public resource allocation. For example, the Centers for Disease Control and Prevention (CDC) requires directly funded jurisdictions to convene HIV planning councils that bring together a broad range of stakeholders to develop an evidence-based integrated plan for HIV prevention and care services for their area.[10] Planning councils have a specific charge, formal operating procedures, and clear objectives. Some have decision-making authority, whereas others are advisory to policymakers such as a mayor or health department director. Inclusive facilitation is key to productive planning councils and other groups that bring "unequal partners" to the table.[11] For example, CDC specifies parity, inclusion, and representation as core processes of effective HIV planning councils. Principles of facilitating these

core processes can be applied to other priority health education topics and initiatives.[12]

Commissions are another type of deliberative body, usually appointed by an organizational or government leader, charged with making recommendations on a specific issue or problem. For example, the leader of a professional organization might want guidance on how the organization can be more inclusive and welcoming in order to increase the diversity of its membership. In that case, the leader could appoint a commission of experts—individuals within and outside the organization—with complementary expertise and insight into the organization, diversity, and the professional field. While similar to advisory groups in many ways, commissions are more formal and bring a level of gravitas to an issue or exploration. Commissioners meet periodically over a designated time frame, hear evidence, discuss the issues, and develop recommendations. Resources for a commission are provided by the sponsoring organization. The designated head of the commission usually provides the meeting facilitation, often with staff support, to organize the scope of the inquiry and manage communication between commission meetings. Some commissions are short term, whereas others such as county health commissions are part of ongoing resource allocation processes in communities or local governments. Facilitation of this type of group requires disciplined and artful management of competing interests, passionate advocacy, and deliberative decision-making within a specified time frame.

? DID YOU KNOW?

Groups that make decisions about use of public funds are subject to "open meeting" laws as established at federal, state, county, and sometimes city levels. These laws mandate that all deliberations contributing to government resource allocation be open to the public, including meetings, minutes, and email communication. Facilitators of open meetings have a particularly important obligation to participants and the public.

Data from Ballotpedia. Open meeting laws. Retrieved from https://ballotpedia.org/Open_Meeting_Law.

Steering Committees

Steering committees oversee the implementation of programs or initiatives. Some are involved for short term projects such as launching a series of worksite wellness focus groups. Others may be convened for the duration of a grant-funded program such as implementation of a chronic disease self-management study. Steering committees can even assist with the responsible and ethical end of a program, such as the necessary closure of a health education community center or transition of a neighborhood walking program from a city health department to parks and recreation. Steering committees may be made up of members of the larger group or complemented by the addition of at-large members from the community. Their primary task is to make sure that program-related activities are true to the mission and goals of the organization, follow the commitments of the grant or work plan, and be responsive to the priority population.

Members of effective advisory groups, planning councils, commissions, and steering committees serve specified terms, meet periodically, and commit to the specific and significant responsibilities of their positions prior to joining the group. They benefit from facilitation that establishes a climate of inclusion and active participation, maintains the group's focus, and reinforces the importance and boundaries of their respective roles. Effective facilitation of steering committees, advisory groups, and planning

councils and commissions is one of the ways that health education specialists and other stakeholders can ensure that community health programs reflect and serve community priorities, capacities, and imagination.

▶ Steps for Effective Group Facilitation

Meetings are the heart of group facilitation, because that is where a group's work gets done. Exemplary facilitators are able to plan effective meetings, develop productive agendas, decide on meeting procedures and arrange for minutes, attend to other meeting details, plan the beginning and end of the meeting, establish a climate of inclusion, keep group discussions on task and on time, and evaluate the meeting. The facilitator may also be involved with organizational staff or broader leadership outside the meetings for various tasks, including establishing group membership, outreach and recruitment, publicizing meetings, recording key decisions, collaborating on the minutes, and conducting process evaluation. The facilitator's overarching goal is to nurture the group's confidence and capacity to effectively work together to achieve its vision, charge, or tasks. Seven steps of effective meeting facilitation are discussed in this section, followed by a brief discussion of other considerations when meeting participants are not all in the room together.

COMMUNITY CONNECTIONS 10.2

Over the next few weeks, Jade and Valerie met with various groups and individuals who would be involved in the project. It quickly became clear that Valerie's facilitation needs covered everything from a formal group of highly experienced advisors to informal groups of youths, community workers, and the general public. Jade felt fairly confident about her ability to facilitate many of the groups, but realized she did not have the experience or skills for some of them. With Valerie's agreement, she invited her colleague Justin to join her as an additional consultant. She had worked with Justin in the past and always enjoyed his sense of humor, ability to get along with almost anyone, professionalism, and integrity—all important qualities in a facilitation partner. Justin agreed to come on board. Together, they felt they could help this process meet its goals and objectives, as well as contribute to community capacity and leadership. With their team in place and group membership established, it was time to plan the first meeting!

Plan Effective Meetings

The following questions can help the facilitator begin to plan a useful and productive meeting:

- What is the purpose of the meeting?
- Where does this meeting fit in the ongoing or future work of the group?
- Who should attend?
- Will the meeting be in person, by conference call, online, or some combination?
- If in person, where should the meeting take place?
- What happens if everyone cannot attend?
- When should the meeting be held and how long should it last?
- Do any meeting plans inadvertently and/or unfairly challenge or limit participation of any participants?

Groups will differ in their preferred meeting mode, times and location, meeting length, and optimal composition. Even within a group, each of its meetings may be slightly different due to group development, geographic challenges, or progress on its charge. Effective facilitation helps ensure there is a purpose for every meeting and meetings are set for a time and mode that work for its members.

Develop Productive Agendas

The meeting **agenda** is one of the facilitator's most important tools. The agenda's four basic purposes during the meeting include (1) establishing the order of events, (2) providing a road map for the facilitator while the meeting is in progress, (3) helping participants prepare in advance, and (4) limiting and focuses discussions to deal with the crucial **action items**. Even before the meeting, an interesting and relevant agenda can generate interest and enthusiasm for participation.

The facilitator is ultimately responsible for the agenda, although input from others is critical. Project leadership, group members, and a steering or staff committee could be consulted for big picture planning or specific agenda item development. This guarantees the agenda's relevance to group priorities and contributes to group investment in the meeting's success. Agenda planning should begin well before the scheduled meeting.

Most groups function best with a relatively formal agenda (**TABLE 10.1**). Once the overall approach is determined, it is helpful to use the same broad outline for each subsequent meeting. This consistency serves three purposes: (1) Committee members and the public are assured all meetings will follow a definite plan of order; (2) the facilitator has a predetermined outline to follow for each regular meeting; and (3) ongoing participants become familiar and comfortable with the flow, pace, and momentum of the meetings.

The less controversial, easy to handle, and informational items are often placed early in the agenda in order of increasing difficulty. Once a welcoming and efficient rapport has been established, participants may feel ready to deal with more difficult issues. The most important part of the agenda (e.g., specific presentations, action items) is strategically placed in the middle. This provides time for latecomers to arrive before key issues are discussed and allows space for the facilitator to adjust the allocated time if a discussion is particularly important. After difficult items have been resolved, the group can move on to lighter items for discussion, new business, input into future agendas, and meeting closure.

Specified time allotments can be an important addition to the printed agenda. Allocating time in advance allows the facilitator to be confident that

---

TABLE 10.1 Key Agenda Elements

Call to order
Welcome and introductions
Consideration and approval of minutes
Committee reports and announcements
   (written or oral)
Discussion and action items (itemized separately)
New business (for this meeting or for future
   consideration)
Closure (review of upcoming tasks or meeting
   evaluation)
Adjournment

the group's business can be conducted within the time set aside for the meeting. In order to reconcile all the potential agenda items with the total available minutes, some items may need to be handled more quickly than others, some may need to be addressed through brief written reports, and some may be moved to a future meeting. Specified time allotments also let group members know what to expect. They help members make focused presentations, pace the discussion, and understand why the facilitator may move an item to closure or limit discussion (**TABLE 10.2**).

The agenda should be broadly distributed prior to the meeting, optimally one week in advance (required if the meeting falls under open meeting laws). Advance distribution alerts participants of the issues to be covered, particularly votes or action items. It also allows participants to come prepared for their own presentations or important discussions.

The agenda may be slightly modified during the meeting, but this is unlikely if it has been carefully prepared and is sensitive to pressing deadlines, group dynamics, and events in the broader organizational or community context. Members have a vested interest in items listed on the agenda because of the time spent prior to the meeting preparing to discuss them. Moreover, visitors or guests may have organized their own schedules to be at the meeting for only specific items. If the agenda is modified, particularly if items are deleted or the schedule is significantly altered,

participants or the broader public may lose confidence in the group's leadership and facilitation. A clear and functional agenda, created with stakeholder input and managed with discipline and good humor during the meeting, is one of the facilitator's most important assets.

Decide on Meeting Procedures and Arrange for Minutes

The meeting procedures establish ground rules for group discussion and decision-making. The **minutes** of a meeting are the impartial, written record of who participated and what happened.

Meeting Procedures

Two of the most important protocols to establish with any group are the guidelines for discussion and way in which decisions will be made. Some groups function well with open- and free-form discussions, relying on the facilitator to look for emerging consensus and bring the group to closure as decisions begin to take shape. This is rare, however, and gives extraordinary power to either the facilitator or dominant members of the group. Far better is to have a plan for orderly discussion and an agreed upon process for making formal decisions.

Most groups rely on some form of parliamentary procedure; the most formal and most commonly adopted is known as **Robert's Rules of Order**. This set of meeting procedures, originally developed in 1876 and regularly updated, is designed to ensure there are enough people present for decisions to be made (**quorum**), everyone has a chance to be heard, and decisions are made clearly and without confusion.[13] Following Robert's Rules brings structure to what can otherwise be confusing or contentious group experiences. Some groups, however, feel these rules are based on cultural assumptions that promote argument over consensus, individual expression over group dialogue, and forceful persuasion over understanding. Groups often adapt Robert's Rules to fit their own objectives or cultural styles (and then refer to them as "**Bobby's Rules**").

TABLE 10.2 Partial Agenda with Time Allotments	
Welcome and introductions	2:00 pm
Agenda Review	2:15 pm
Review and approval of minutes	2:25 pm
Budget review	2:35 pm

Whatever procedures are decided upon, it is critical the facilitator understands the rules and consistently and proactively applies them. This can be a little intimidating for new facilitators, but there are many reference guides and cheat sheets available in print or online.[14-16] Once a health education specialist has facilitated several meetings, the rules and procedures become not only much clearer, but also extremely helpful in guiding the group through respectful deliberation and decision-making.

---

⑦ DID YOU KNOW?

The National Association of Parliamentarians (NAP) was established in 1930 and is the largest professional nonprofit association of parliamentarians in the world. The group has a global membership of over 4,000 parliamentarians. Their website, http://www .parliamentarians.org, offers information on parliamentary procedure, online training and continuing education opportunities, a resource catalog, and a calendar of upcoming events.

Minutes

The written record of what happened at a meeting is called "the minutes." Most groups are well served by even brief minutes that document the meeting occurred, the date and location, who attended, what was covered, any decisions, and who recorded the minutes. Accurate minutes require active and attentive listening during the meeting, making notes throughout, and careful attention to wording and detail when writing them up to ensure that the text and tone are brief, unbiased, and accurate.

Most facilitators find it too difficult to monitor group process and take the minutes during the meeting. A formal group may have a secretary or historian with this specific responsibility. Some groups have support staff responsible for minutes. Less formal groups may decide to rotate responsibility for minutes among participants. Most important is someone is designated as the recorder

and there is **consensus** on the type of minutes to be produced. If a more detailed account of discussions is necessary, an audio recording can be helpful to the person developing the minutes. If more concise, action-only minutes are preferred, however, the designated recorder will most likely be able to get all the necessary information through notes taken during the meeting.

There are several styles of written minutes. A formal style is particularly useful for decision-making groups. If important organizational priorities or resource allocations are being decided, the group may need minutes that provide detailed summaries of the discussions and record the decision-making process. If the group is following Robert's Rules of Order, the names of individuals who moved and seconded all motions, and the numbers voting for, against, and abstaining may need to be recorded. Some groups will not require the details of their discussions, preferring shorter or action-only minutes. New facilitators can draw from numerous examples and templates online to determine the type of minutes appropriate for their groups.[17-19]

Selecting the appropriate minutes style is an important part of meeting planning. The **facilitator**, meeting staff, and/or chair (who may all be the same person) should think about the meeting's overall objectives, legal or organizational requirements, the interested parties and stakeholders who will want to know what transpired, and the nature of the record that group participants want or need to leave behind.

Once the meeting is over, the recorder should prepare the draft minutes and circulate them to the chair and facilitator for review. Reviewing the draft minutes is very important because it ensures the accuracy of the public record. Minutes, particularly action minutes, should be circulated to all group members within a few days of the meeting so that participants can refer to them as a reminder of actions they promised to take before the next meeting. Regardless of when the minutes are distributed, one of the first actions of the next meeting should be to review, correct if needed, and formally approval minutes of the previous meeting.

Attend to the Details

Once the meeting is planned, the agenda developed, and the minutes arranged, the effective facilitator can attend to other meeting details. This step is critical to the group dynamics of even a very carefully planned agenda.

Setting

Whether virtual or in person, the setting of the meeting is important. Meetings should be held in places accessible to all potential participants. This may require attention to transportation options, distance, acoustics, and accessibility. In-person meetings benefit from an attractive and comfortable space that encourages attendance and invites participation. The room, lighting, and furniture arrangement can promote a positive atmosphere—one in which participants feel relaxed and focused, can see each other and the facilitator, and are inspired to be productive. Sometimes, it is important to hold the meeting in a formal setting such as city hall or the health department. Other times, it is important to hold the meeting where people work or in community venues where the public can easily attend as observers. Working meetings need tables and appropriate work space. Presentation meetings require visibility and proximity to the speaker. Discussion meetings may be best held around a conference room table or with chairs in a circle. Most often, facilitators have to work with what they have, and so thoughtful attention to ways to make the space and furniture work can be important to what happens once people are there. It may seem obvious to a well-prepared health education specialist, but the facilitator should be sure to set up and double check any equipment that will be used during the meeting such as projectors, microphones, or WiFi connections.

Attention to the "setting" of meetings where people phone or login is as important as it is for in-person meetings. Will the meeting use a platform accessible to all potential or invited participants? Will there be designated technology support for the inevitable login or connection problems? If participants are distributed across time zones, is the meeting scheduled at a time that is reasonable for everyone (not too early, not too late)? If a meeting is going to have people both in person and remotely participating, is the equipment reliable? Will all participants be able to hear each other, whether or not they are in the room?

Refreshments

The decision regarding whether or not to serve refreshments—and if so, what they will be—can be complicated! Some groups have a tradition of refreshments at all meetings, others do not have interest or budget for providing food or beverages. There may be organizational rules regarding bringing in outside snacks or requiring preapproved vendors. Evening or lunchtime meetings may benefit from a catered meal, if budget allows, or even water, coffee/tea, and fruit. Facilitators need to be mindful of dietary restrictions and allergies, cultural preferences, and other sensibilities among group members, such as recyclable utensils or local vendors. As more and more agencies adopt healthy food policies, a facilitating health education specialist can help the group find healthy refreshments that everyone will enjoy. Whatever is decided, it is important participants know in advance so their unique needs are considered.

⑦ DID YOU KNOW?

The Center for Science in the Public Interest has a website devoted to healthy meetings. The site offers information about healthy meeting guidelines, including healthy snacks. Your organization can even join over 50 others across the country that have signed on to the healthy meeting pledge.

Data from Center for Science in the Public Interest. Healthy meetings. Retrieved from http://www.cspinet.org/protecting-our-health/nutrition/healthy-meetings.

Participant Identification

Nametags, nameplates, the wording on the roster— these details matter. How participants are identified may seem a minor detail but can have a major impact on the way group members interact. The format of everything printed on an online roster, a nametag, or name card should be specifically chosen.

The facilitator can help staff or other stake-holders make decisions that will establish the tone and reinforce the relationships desired for the meeting. For example, will listing degrees on the nametags positively establish the credentials of group members or create imbalances of prestige and presumed authority? Will emphasizing first names in bold font facilitate conversation between members or appear uncomfortably familiar and disrespectful in a culturally diverse group? Will preprinted nameplates communicate inclusion or spotlight and embarrass those who were not expected but are still welcome? Does the roster and its contact information establish parity within the group or identify status and resource differences that will affect members' comfort with each other? Will participants be asked to state their preferred gender pronouns? Will virtual participants be asked to identify themselves by name before they speak and, if so, throughout the meeting or only the first time? There is no formula for getting this right—the best decisions will be based on the culture, purpose, and experience of the group.

Plan the Beginning of the Meeting

The tone of a meeting—formal, informal, warm, inviting, serious, urgent, focused, or scattered—is communicated by the facilitator's behavior and opening words as the meeting gets under way. Arriving early (to the physical or virtual space), making sure everything is set and ready to go, being calm and focused, and perhaps greeting people as they arrive, all communicate important messages to participants about the focus and dynamics of the meeting. When the facilitator is rushed, anxious, or distracted before the meeting, the group process gets off to an awkward start. Conversely, a calm and engaging facilitator is ready for participants and begins facilitating the group process when the very first participant arrives or logs in.

Whether to begin exactly at the appointed time is a matter of culture and meeting needs. Some groups have developed a punctual tradition, beginning and ending exactly on time. Other groups have a more relaxed attitude, either starting when the majority of expected participants are present or at a commonly understood "real" start time (e.g., 10 minutes after the published time). Introductions are important and some groups benefit from carefully chosen icebreakers. Because of formal training in interpersonal communication, health education specialists often find this part of facilitation to be natural and common sense.

Plan the End of the Meeting

The facilitator is responsible for watching the time and alerting the group throughout the meeting when they need to move along in order to meet their objectives during the time remaining. Ending a meeting on time is extremely important to most people. Running overtime may make individuals late for their next commitments or require them to leave before the meeting officially adjourns, and perhaps before agenda items they are very interested in are discussed. In addition to the *time* at which the meeting ends, the *way* in which it ends is important. The facilitator can bring closure to the meeting by summarizing what has been accomplished, reminding people of the next meeting time and location (if another meeting is scheduled), and thanking the group for their attendance and participation. If time permits, this can be an opportunity for team building and affirmation through participatory process evaluation.

Establish a Climate of Inclusion

The facilitator is (perhaps) the most visible group participant, particularly during meetings. This visibility may be challenging in diverse groups, groups with different vested interests, or groups with an unhappy history. Sometimes, the facilitator's power is in the "little" things, such as learning people's names, correctly pronouncing them, and remembering individuals from one meeting to the next. Inclusion is enhanced by the facilitator's attention to who has spoken and who has not, and then active solicitation (during the meeting or on break) of perspectives from people who have not yet been heard. Facilitators may need to be both vigilant and courageous in the face of subtle, professionally condoned microaggressions that effectively marginalize voices and perspectives such as interrupting, talking over, or disregarding previous speakers. Indeed, the power of an inclusive embrace is transformative, particularly when backed by fair and understandable operating procedures and consistent facilitation. These are all dependent on the foresight, leadership, and skill of the facilitator. Health education specialists are particularly well suited to these challenges, as they know how to make individuals comfortable, demystify procedures, stimulate interest, and nurture the stages of change. Inclusive facilitation is the same concept, but with groups instead of individuals.

Keep Group Discussions on Task and on Time

An effective facilitator thinks through all the details of the meeting in advance and is thus prepared for an intentional beginning, a productive middle, and a calm, affirming end. Once the meeting is underway, the facilitator needs to fully concentrate on the group's discussions and deliberations (as well as the content), attending to an inclusive and productive process that keeps the group focused on its task and working towards successfully completing agenda items. The facilitator can help the group stay focused, particularly if the discussion starts to wander. For example, the facilitator can introduce each item, highlighting its relation to the group's charge, and specifying the time allotted and the desired end result (e.g., discussion or decision). The facilitator can periodically summarize what has been said, as items are being discussed, thus helping group members avoid repetition, and gently moving the group toward closure. The facilitator who loses track of the group's direction or conversation should not be evasive or defensive, but rather use keen facilitation skills to remind everyone of the discussion directions by asking questions such as, "Where are we going with this?" or "Who can summarize where we've been?" A short break is often useful,

even if not on the agenda, so that the facilitator can consult a colleague or the group's recorder. A summary of the discussion, after the break, is an effective way to refocus the group and align it with the conversations and actions that need to happen.

Evaluate the Meeting

The facilitator can learn a tremendous amount by taking a few minutes at the end of a meeting for evaluation. The formal way to do this is to distribute a written evaluation form to each participant. In-person meetings can be structured to allow time for participants to complete the survey before leaving; surveys can be emailed to participants immediately following online or conference call meetings, with instructions to complete and return the survey within 48 hours.

The specific questions on an evaluation survey should be derived from the meeting's goals and objectives. In addition to providing guidance to the facilitator, survey results help participants view their own experience in context. Results should be made available to all participants as soon as possible, optimally within a few days of the meeting. The facilitator might also want to review the results with group leaders or the sponsoring agency in preparation for the next meeting. Comparing the results of selected indicators over time helps the facilitator understand the way the group or its meetings are trending and provides valuable data for reinforcement or change.

Less formal evaluation methods can bring warmth and closure to a meeting, while also providing the facilitator with invaluable process insight. For example, a facilitator who knows a meeting has gone particularly well might invite each person to share one word that describes his or her experiences. Sessions that involved a presentation might end with participants sharing something they learned that will be particularly useful in their work. Even a meeting that was difficult might benefit from this sort of one-minute evaluation, asking members to each say or write down details that worked well for them at the meeting as well as items that would help them more fully participate next time. Asking for "three words to describe your experience of the meeting" is a wonderfully evocative evaluation question. Brief process evaluation techniques such as this provide the facilitator with important information about participants' experiences and are rich with suggestions to maintain or improve the quality of future meetings.

Considerations When Participants Are Not in the Same Physical Space

It is now quite common for groups to meet together, in real time, without being in the same place. Various technologies allow remote participants to hear each other, view presentations, share screens, and participate in group discussions. Internet conferences and teleconferences increase access to meetings for many people, particularly professionals with office equipment and settings conducive to extended phone or computer use. These technologies also allow people to participate from far distances, decrease meeting costs, and enhance attendance and participation by eliminating travel time and expense. It should be noted that, even now, not everyone has access to the equipment or contexts that make Internet meetings and teleconferences possible. Facilitating health education specialists need to work with their groups or leadership to determine what is lost and what is gained by not meeting in person.

Group facilitation by conference call or the Internet follows many of the same guidelines of in-person facilitation. There are, however, a few additional considerations:

- Include login information or call numbers and passwords when sending out meeting materials. Include this information with all reminder notices.
- Organize introductions at the beginning of the meeting. Periodically check to see if anyone else has joined the call.
- Remind participants to clearly and slowly speak into their microphones.
- Ask that people listen with their phone or computer on mute. People often multitask on teleconference calls or online meetings, which can be disruptive or disheartening when everyone else can hear them typing, talking to their kids, or ordering coffee.

- Have a plan for what to do when the technology fails! This will help a facilitator stay calm and make decisions for the good of the group if connections are lost, calls are dropped, or participants cannot see a shared screen.
- Become comfortable with the idea that participants may be communicating with each other or other people during the meeting in ways that you cannot see (e.g., real-time texting or posting to social media). This can be unnerving at first to a facilitator who relies on body language cues during meetings to gauge interest and participation. However, with time and practice, the new etiquette will emerge and facilitators will find other ways to gather vital information that used to be so easy to discern when everyone was in the same room.

---

⑦ DID YOU KNOW?

The *Community Tool Box* is an online resource for facilitators of all kinds of groups. Based out of the University of Kansas, this free and easily navigated website is loaded with tips, examples, and background information on almost anything you might need regarding group facilitation and more. The full site is now available in English, Spanish, and Arabic.

Data from Community Tool Box. www.http://ctb.ku.edu/en.

▶ Tips and Techniques for Effective Group Facilitation

Group facilitation can be extremely challenging. It requires the facilitator to be relaxed yet alert, confident yet open to change, disciplined yet warm and inviting, consistent yet adaptable. Facilitators must keep their "eyes on the prize" while fiercely guarding group process. Most important, a facilitator must learn to be productive with each new group, focused on nurturing the group's capacity to address its charge, learn from each other, and contribute to the broader effort of which they all are a part. The way a facilitator responds to the group, specific individuals, tasks at hand, or unanticipated events directly affects the group's effectiveness. Artful facilitation thus requires the ability to quickly think, see the big picture, be sensitive to nuance, and act with confidence. Indeed, a confident, responsive facilitator sends a steady nonverbal message to the group and invites similarly calm and responsive participation.

Several basic health education orientations support this kind of effective, engaging, and rewarding facilitation. Among the most important of these orientations are genuine belief in the power of groups, interest in others and an attitude of inquiry, an open and respectful interaction style, commitment to capacity development, and a sense of humor.

Have a Genuine Belief in the Power of Groups

Facilitators are often leaders in their own right, but the strategies and techniques they use while in a facilitation role are very different. Effective facilitators, like leaders, often have a clear vision of the future, passion for the issues they care about, personal commitment to a cause, and persuasive advocacy skills. These must be carefully held in check, however, when facilitating! Facilitators place their faith in the power and wisdom of the group. That does not mean they have no influence on the group's vision, strategies, decisions, or subsequent advocacy; however, the facilitator must be willing to give more attention to the *process* of the group than the *outcome*. This is really only possible when the facilitating health education specialist truly believes in what people can do when they work together and is willing to support that process over any specific outcome. Facilitators who wish to offer content to the discussion should state that they are "stepping out of the facilitator role" to make the comment, and then return to facilitation duties. Stepping out in this way, however, should be reserved for extraordinary circumstances. A facilitator who does this too often will be seen as distorting the role and privilege of facilitation.

Have a Genuine Interest in Others and an Attitude of Inquiry

Effective facilitators know good group decisions require active input and participation from all members. The facilitator needs to be genuinely interested in the attitudes and perspectives of all participants. This can be challenging, particularly when a group includes individuals or perspectives the facilitator has found troubling in previous contexts. As facilitators, however, health education specialists need to shift their frame of reference from past experiences to the potential for positive participation that always exists with new groups. One of the best ways to learn about the perspectives and potential contributions of both new and familiar participants is to ask questions. An attitude of inquiry on the part of the facilitator establishes a group tone of engagement, interest, and potential. By asking questions and listening to the responses, both facilitator and participants can visualize from new perspectives, work together in new ways, and imagine new strategies for community health. One particularly effective technique is the written process tool referred to as "dialogue boxes", in which participants get to comment to each other about what is working well or what they would like to change about the group process.[20] Interest and inquiry also help avoid misunderstandings and a false feeling of agreement regarding decisions being made by the group. The facilitator's genuine interest in each participant's contribution, and consistent outreach to all participants and points of view, protects the integrity and potential of the group process.

Exhibit an Open and Respectful Interaction Style

Integrity and authenticity are two of the most important aspects of a facilitator's reputation. Health education specialists' ethical commitments to honesty and informed participation provide a familiar foundation for this aspect of facilitation.[3] Even in the most trying circumstances, facilitators should not resort to deception or coercion to obtain involvement. Participants will quickly see through each. Insincerity is counterproductive because individuals will either anticipate it or be irritated by it. Manipulation leads to a lack of confidence and low levels of trust between members of any group, which then results in an inability to function. Remaining neutral while facilitating a group, both during and outside of meetings, is also crucial to the facilitator's integrity. This means avoiding gossip, judgmental small talk, or other forms of divisive group noise. As any health education specialist knows, the greater the trust between group members, the higher the capacity for learning—and thus the greater the level of group effectiveness.

Maintain a Commitment to Capacity Development

Effective facilitators support and assist group members in accomplishing their tasks. When the tasks are relatively simple, interest is high, adequate support is available, and capacity development is easy. In this case, the facilitator can play a key role in capacity development by helping participants see what felt easy was actually the result of very specific skills, responsibility, and group work. Not all group activities, however, are so simple. Facilitators perform their most important work when problems arise. This is not to say that the facilitating health education specialist "helps" the group by solving its problems. As in other helping relationships, facilitators have to be extremely careful in the way in which they offer assistance. Appropriate facilitator support includes helping a group learn from both its successes and its missteps. For example, if a news release was sent out too late to be effective, the facilitator can help the group move from blaming the individual who missed the deadline to understanding the process, analyzing the organizational or social context that failed to prevent the problem, and planning so that it does not happen again.

Have a Sense of Humor

Effective facilitators enjoy the process, the people, the challenges, and the rewards of groups, all of

---

COMMUNITY CONNECTIONS 10.3

Jade and Justin spent time together, brainstorming and discussing the commitments they were about to make to this project, to the communities with which they would be working, and to their colleague, Valerie.

"I want to make sure people aren't being used just because the funder specifies *community involvement*," said Justin.

"I agree. And I want to make sure people get something out of each group meeting they attend," added Jade, "whether it be new contacts, new information, reassurance and encouragement, or a sense of what's really possible when people work together."

"I want to ensure full participation by everyone, not just the ones who are the loudest or the most assertive," said Justin. "And I want to make sure everything we do, from the little details to the big decisions, strengthens community capacity."

"I'll need to make sure that I don't get frustrated by the pace of group process," noted Jade, "and I'm excited to see how it works when we meet online instead of in person."

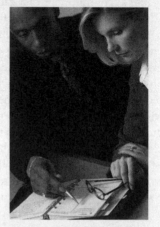

© Hemera Technologies/PHOTOS.com/Getty.

Justin thought for a moment and then said, "Jade, I'm going to need you to help me with some of the politics of this project."

Jade replied with a smile, "And I'm going to need you and your sense of humor to help me keep it all in perspective."

which is bolstered by a healthy sense of humor. Being able to see the humor in situations, laugh at ourselves, heartily relish the unpredictable, and find the fun in even mundane situations prepares health education specialists to facilitate almost any group under almost any condition. A facilitator who enjoys life, people, and groups is a flexible, grounded, and effective vanguard of group process and productivity.

Effective and artful facilitation requires an alert, honest, and adaptable facilitator. A genuine belief in the power of groups, interest in others, and an attitude of inquiry, an open and respectful interaction style, commitment to capacity development, and a sense of humor all well serve a facilitator.

▶ Overcoming Challenges to Group Facilitation

Group facilitation is as much about the skills and capacity of the group as it is about the work of the facilitator. Most groups will face challenges as they learn to communicate and work together, meet their objectives, and reconcile internal differences. Even the most successful groups exist within broader contexts (e.g., personal, cultural, organizational, social, political) that place demands on members that will affect group dynamics and may present facilitation challenges. Among the most common challenges are uneven participation, poor group attendance, disruptions caused by technology, conflict, and burnout.

COMMUNITY CONNECTIONS 10.4

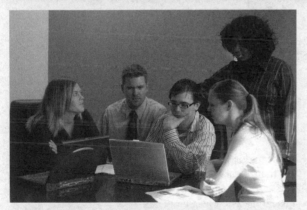
© ArrowStudio/Shutterstock.

Six months into the project, Justin and Jade found themselves loving the work. They were challenged, excited, and learning every day. They met regularly with Valerie and her staff leader, Tracey, to debrief past meetings and plan for those ahead. They dedicated considerable time to preparing for group meetings and always found the investment paid off. Their agendas were workable, the groups were engaging, the tasks were clear, and people kept coming back. That is not to say, however, the work was easy.

"I have the hardest time keeping the Clinic Directors group on task," exclaimed Jade one day. "They go off on so many tangents. I'm nothing but a timekeeper and a grouch in that group!"

"Have you considered listing the two or three primary objectives of the meeting at the top of the agenda?" asked Justin. "That might help them see what absolutely must be accomplished in the coming hour, no matter how excited and off-topic they get about other things."

"That's a good idea," said Jade. "Another issue that is really distracting is the way some advisory group members constantly rustle through the handouts I pass out for each item. I think I'll ask our assistant AJ to help me make meeting binders containing the necessary handouts for the next meeting. At the end, they can take home the handouts and leave the binders for the next meeting."

Brainstorming about a group that had trouble completing the agenda, Justin suggested, "You might consider asking one of them to be the timekeeper next time. If you're too focused on time management, they're not getting all they could get out of a good facilitator. Having someone else watch the time might allow you to watch and nurture other aspects of the group process—including helping those youngest members find their voices and start speaking up."

Encourage Participation

It is not uncommon for meeting participants to have different levels of comfort speaking in groups. Some members may feel intimidated by the expertise, position, age, or style of other members. Other participants may be more or less prepared. Cultural differences might exist in interpersonal communication, the use of silence, deference, and respect that are not understood by all. Some members may be eager to participate in the group process, while others might be there because they were told to attend. Last, others might experience dynamics between their lives and jobs. The most important participation concerns for the facilitator are: (1) establishing a process that honors differences and encourages communication, (2) monitoring the emerging dynamics to encourage all members to participate in the manner in which they are most comfortable, and (3) ensuring that the group process benefits from as much participation and group input as possible. Strategies to help the facilitator overcome uneven participation in a group meeting can help the facilitator deal with uneven participation at individual meetings, while establishing and reinforcing a norm of full and respectful communication over the longer life of the group (**TABLE 10.3**).

TABLE 10.3 Strategies for Encouraging Participation

- Establish full participation as an explicit goal when opening the meeting.
- Include a round of introductions or a brief icebreaker at the beginning of the meeting, so each participant gets a chance to hear his or her own voice—and be heard by others—within the first minutes of the meeting.
- List "full participation" as an indicator in the meeting evaluation tool, both as a way of reinforcing its importance and in order to gather information on participants' perspectives and needs.
- Periodically remind the group of the importance of full participation, inviting members who have not yet spoken to comment or share their perspectives.
- Track the number of people who have spoken and the number who have not, as the discussion progresses. Share observations with the group before calling on the next person. As facilitator, it is appropriate to say, "I'd like to hear first from those who haven't yet offered their opinion. Then, I'll call on those who have already spoken."
- Try small group discussions for 5 or 10 minutes in the middle of a larger discussion, as some people will be more comfortable talking with two or three others than speaking before an entire group.
- Consider adding a co-facilitator who brings additional insights into the participation dynamics of this particular group and who might be able to bring out greater participation.
- Privately check in with participants, both those who do not participate and those who may be dominating the discussions. The latter may not realize their own patterns or their effects on others. People who do not speak up may feel honored and surprised at the facilitator's interest in their perspective and thus encouraged to join the group dialogue. In both cases, ask for recommendations on how to balance group participation.
- Offer to facilitate or coordinate training on multicultural communication, group dynamics, or decision-making for the group, an orientation for those who are feeling behind, or a social event to allow participants to interact in a less formal way. Sometimes, merely adding a working lunch to a regularly scheduled meeting or hosting a drop-in gathering with light snacks 30 minutes before the scheduled starting time changes the dynamics and allows participants to warm up to each other outside the roles and structures of the meeting.
- Report on the "full participation" evaluation results as a way of stimulating discussion of ways to make group discussions more inclusive. Seeing in print that the group gave "I was able to participate as I wanted" an average low rating of "2" on a scale of 1–5 can be informative as to the group process.

Maintain Attendance

Groups that meet on a regular basis often encounter attendance problems. Sometimes, this is due to structural issues such as where the meeting is held or the time of day. Other times, poor attendance is purely personal, the result of busy people having too much going on and the meeting not being their primary or pressing priority. Health problems, family responsibilities, car trouble, or work crises can all interfere with a group member's intention to attend a meeting, even one carefully planned and eagerly anticipated by the facilitator.

Facilitators should not only be prepared for uneven attendance from time to time, but also be alert to the meaning of persistent absences. Applying techniques for understanding, improving, and maintaining meeting attendance can help enhance the effectiveness of meetings (**TABLE 10.4**).

Minimize Technology Disruptions

In the past, skilled facilitators could create a meeting space with limited outside interruptions. The proliferation of mobile technology has changed the meeting atmosphere. Participants may come to an in-person meeting with smart phones, tablets, electronic calendars, and social media just a click away. Time pressures, multitasking, and the desire to be always in touch have made these technologies a "must have" for many, and a unique facilitation challenge. The following are suggestions for dealing with the reality of communications technologies and meeting facilitation:

- Make sure the opening remarks include the instruction that cell phones and other devices be placed on vibrate or, better yet, switched off until the break or completion of the meeting.
- Pay attention to whether texting or social media distraction is creating a disturbance to the group process. Many people use text messaging to communicate with others when talking by phone is not possible or appropriate such as in a meeting. On most occasions, this is not a problem. In some circumstances and with some groups, however, use of text messaging can create the appearance of a silent "cross talk" that can be chilling to full participation. Effective facilitators are familiar with the technologies used by group members and not afraid to request that "essential"

TABLE 10.4 Techniques for Strong Attendance

- Send reminder notices well in advance, even if the next meeting date and time have been well publicized.
- Make sure that the meeting time and location work for participants. Sometimes, a change in time or venue makes all the difference in a member's ability to regularly attend, whether in person or online.
- Consider making personal calls or email contact to ensure everyone feels welcome prior to the meeting.
- Check in with people who have not been attending. Find out why and see if there is anything that can be done to make it easier for them to regularly participate.
- Conduct a survey to gather opinions and recommendations for enhancing meeting attendance and share the results with the group.
- Review meeting procedures and meeting formalities to make sure all members encourage and honor participation.
- Make sure all participants have meaningful roles. No one wants to go to a meeting in which they have no role or feel ignored. Similarly, people do not want to waste their time at meetings that do not really make a difference.
- Do not take it personally. Things happen, the office gets busy, childcare falls apart, people get overwhelmed, the Internet fails, a storm is on the way—there are many reasons why people may miss a meeting here or there. It is best to just check in to see what happened, let them know they were missed, and welcome them back when they return.

texting, posting, and email be kept to a minimum. Carefully review organizational rules regarding recording, photos, and posting what goes on during the meeting. Some entities require that proceedings be public, others will protect privacy of participants. Be sure that everyone understands the rules, the reasoning behind them, and any permissions necessary before recording, taking photos, or posting meeting participants, content, process dynamics, or decisions.

Resolve Conflict

Facilitators work with groups of individuals from different backgrounds, multiple perspectives and motivations, varying degrees of comfort and commitment to group process, and sometimes history that together predates the new committee or task force. This can be a source of stimulating exchange and invigorated group action. It can also be the source of both minor and profound conflict. It is the facilitator's responsibility to ensure that conflict enriches the group's explorations, decisions, and actions.

Avoiding *all* conflict is not an effective facilitator's goal. A vigorous exchange of even heated opinions helps a group better understand the issues, gather new information, and explore the potential consequences of even seemingly minor decisions. Conflict generated from outside the group can forge group identity in ways that might not have happened without the external threat. Generally speaking, when the facilitator is afraid of conflict and the group tries to please each other at all costs, the group arrives at lower quality decisions compared with groups in which controversy and disagreement are properly facilitated.

Effective facilitators have a number of specific techniques they can try when a group is being disrupted or paralyzed by conflict (**TABLE 10.5**). Facilitators vary in their own personal experience with conflict, which results in various approaches to facilitating groups when conflict arises. In general, the facilitator who withdraws from disagreement

out of personal discomfort adds another burden to an already stressed group. The emergence of conflict requires quiet and consistent leadership on the part of the facilitator, for he or she is now modeling respectful engagement under trying circumstances. The confidence to facilitate in the presence of conflict comes from experience, the ability to "breathe" through dissonance, and an active commitment to the group's ability to be enriched by appropriate use and resolution of the conflict that has emerged.

In order to optimally deal with conflict, facilitators need to believe there are a number of strategies that can be used and adapted to fit the group, and that conflict can be an opportunity for growth. The facilitator's attitude of inquiry can make the conflict inherently interesting rather than frightening or destructive. Exploring the various perspectives represented in the conflict, being willing to listen and learn, promoting the integrity of those who have differing opinions, and above all, protecting the integrity of the group and its process will lead the facilitator to the strategies and tactics that appropriately manage any conflict that emerges.

❓ DID YOU KNOW?

The American Psychological Association publishes a quarterly journal entitled *Group Dynamics: Theory, Practice, and Research,* which is a very helpful resource for facilitators.

Source: http://www.apa.org/pubs/journals/gdn/.

Avoid Burnout

Both facilitators and group members get tired. Too many meetings, too many discussions, and too many challenges can exhaust even the most committed participant. Effective facilitators understand the emotional demands of the art of facilitation and proactively nourish their own hearts and minds. A facilitator cannot facilitate well when tired, stressed, or burned out. A few

TABLE 10.5 Techniques to Resolve Group Conflict

- *Help the group articulate its ground rules, proactively defining its own norms and standards for group interaction.* Ground rules should specify the importance of mutual respect, the unacceptability of personal attacks, the validity of multiple perspectives, and the centrality of personal safety and mutual trust. Once adopted, the group's ground rules can be made into a banner or colorful poster that is displayed at each meeting, included with the agenda, and articulated at the beginning of each meeting.

- *Hold firm to the ground rules.* Once the rules have been established, it is the facilitator's responsibility to keep them visible and fairly enforce them. This is much easier when the ground rules are known to all, formally adopted by the group, and reinforced by the facilitator and group leaders.

- *Explore what the conflict is really about.* It is not uncommon for persistent conflict to be about something other than the subject at hand. An effective facilitator watches, listens, and explores with key individuals the concerns. Getting to the real issue will help the facilitator and members approach the conflict and the individual(s) involved, with greater insight and compassion. It will also suggest strategies that might not have been thought of before understanding the issues at that deeper level.

- *Check in with key individuals.* Sometimes, the facilitator's best process ally is the person "causing" the conflict. Quietly and nonjudgmental talking outside the meeting can often change the dynamics of an angry or hostile participant. An effective facilitator also checks in with others who observe or participate in the meeting, looking for insight and perspective to help defuse or reframe interpersonal conflicts when they again emerge.

- *Have a plan for what can be done the next time conflict arises in the group.* The response, what might be said to the group, and the range of reactions to draw from (depending on the degree and timing of the conflict) should be contemplated. A good facilitator might even role play possible responses with colleagues or key group members (e.g., opinion leaders, staff) in order to be calm and confident at the next meeting.

- *Use good judgment.* Some conflicts are healthy and move the group to new levels of awareness and response. But nonconstructive conflict can cause real harm. Physical and emotional safety are basic needs that must be met if a group is to be able to work together. The effective facilitator needs to listen carefully to participants' expressions of fear or vulnerability. Even if a facilitator does not feel threatened, proactively responding to the felt needs of group members may lead to important logistical changes such as moving the meetings to a different location, changing meeting times, arranging for security, or rearranging seating.

simple techniques help a facilitating health education specialist keep the batteries charged:

- *Try not to rush.* Allowing adequate time to get to the location, get to the room, assemble the materials, and settle in before others arrive can make all the difference. Taking a few minutes at the end of the meeting to make notes about what went well and what one might try differently next time, similarly helps calmly end the facilitation. This kind of beginning and ending well serves a facilitator.

- *Remember why this kind of work is done.* Most health education specialists do these jobs because of deeply held values. Consciously remembering those values helps to see the bigger picture when the details are trying. Facilitation is an art—a set of skills that are applied to an emerging and creative process. Consciously linking the day-to-day experience of facilitation to a deeper purpose and commitment to life can be a powerfully grounding experience.

- *Talk with others.* When enthusiasm for the task is lost or the expectations feel like a burden, talking with others can help cast the experience in a new light. Colleagues who are not part of the group may be able to offer important perspectives. Trusted friends can help put a facilitation challenge in a larger context. Sometimes, just expressing feelings of exhaustion, frustration, or stress helps relieve the pressure and reawakens one's more hopeful energies.

COMMUNITY CONNECTIONS 10.5

Near the middle of the second year, Jade and Justin encountered a kind of group conflict they were not sure how to handle. A group of activists in the community had been increasingly critical and vocal of the health department—one of the project's primary sponsors. They disrupted public meetings, staged demonstrations at government buildings, lobbied the media, and generally stopped work for a variety of county-sponsored projects. By the time their attention turned to the project with which Jade and Justin were working, the agitating group was fairly well discredited in the community, but their actions were increasingly unpredictable and their demeanor aggressive and threatening. Members of several of the project groups were concerned about their safety or comfort if they came to meetings—and yet the meetings had to continue if they were to make progress on the project. This posed a significant facilitation challenge.

"I knew I might be nervous when facilitating, but I never thought I'd be downright scared," exclaimed Jade after a particularly hostile encounter with one of the activists during a public meeting. "I think I'm in over my head. Maybe we should think about giving notice."

"I know what you mean," Justin responded. "But facilitation is really all about helping groups find their voice, articulate their visions, and organize themselves to make the things happen that they believe in. What message would we be giving if we back out when it gets rough?"

"Good point. But what are we going to do?" replied Jade. "This is some pretty serious stuff, and it's getting so bad that people aren't coming to meetings anymore. When they do, they just sit there in silence, afraid to say anything for fear of being jumped on by the activists."

"I think you need some help," said their friend Cameron, who had been listening in. "Just because the group looks to you for process expertise doesn't mean you have to know it all."

Over the next week, Justin and Jade spoke with Valerie, Tracey, and Cameron—people who had experience with this particular group of activists—and others they knew who were experienced at conflict management and communication. They checked in with key group members and they pulled out their old group process texts. Cameron offered to do an online literature review for them. Justin consulted his friend, Ed, an organizational development expert. All these different perspectives gave them ideas and insight into the situation they were facing and the unique roles and responsibilities of the facilitators.

In the end, they decided to try the following: At the request of many group members, they recommended the meetings be held in a secure building. This would allow Jade and Justin to return to the role of facilitation and not be responsible for group safety and security. They reviewed the group's participation ground rules and made them into a large banner easily read by all in the room. They adjusted the agenda to allow a few moments at the beginning of each meeting to clearly state the ground rules and the consequences of breaking them. They developed a carefully worded introduction to the meeting that welcomed all who were there and articulated the importance of an open, participatory process, and brainstormed and prioritized their responses to a wide range of disruptive actions that might occur at the next meeting. And although they were still pretty nervous, they agreed to come to the meeting rested, refreshed, and relaxed, for, as Ed reminded them, "If you don't take care of yourselves, you won't be able to do the work the way you want to."

COMMUNITY CONNECTIONS 10.6

As Jade and Justin entered the last quarter of the project, they decided to take a look back at all the meeting evaluations they received over the three years. Early on, Valerie had hired Juan and Christina, two process evaluation consultants, to develop a method of evaluating the short- and long-term effectiveness of the group meetings, including facilitation. Their monthly reports and process memos provided Jade and Justin with a wealth of information from which to continuously analyze and improve their facilitation skills.

"Look at how excited participants were in the first months," exclaimed Jade, as she flipped through surveys from the early meetings. "People really had a lot of hope for this project."

"They sure did. I think it really helped to have the goals and objectives of the project, each working group, and each meeting clearly defined. Look at how the average ratings went up once we made that standard procedure," said Justin. "Ratings and attendance also went up last year when we moved the meetings to a location that felt safer."

"That was a really hard time. I was scared, but I'm glad we stuck with it," said Jade.

"Look at these ratings, Jade—they really like your color visuals and the way you begin and end the meetings," exclaimed Justin.

"And they appreciate the way you really listen," said Jade, looking over some comments from the past year.

The evaluations also showed that participants appreciated the snacks, valued getting the agenda in advance, felt comfortable with the decisions that were made, and were proud of being part of the project.

"But you know what seems to make the most difference?" Jade asked. "That what happened in the groups made a difference in their community. Vince, an experienced community activist and leader in the group, even reports that his experience in our group has strengthened his facilitation style and effectiveness in his own work. Groups working together, learning together, and making changes that support community health—that's what this was all about!"

- *Seek out experts.* Resources and learning opportunities abound for facilitators. In addition to the books, journals, and websites already noted, workshops, conferences, continuing education, and professional development events may provide opportunities to observe, consult with, or learn from experts in the art and skills of facilitation. The proliferation of blogs and online forums on this, like every other topic, means that facilitators never need to feel alone or at a loss.

- *Take care of yourself.* It is crucial to get adequate rest, eat well, exercise, remember what is important, and live life in balance. These basic self-care techniques help a facilitator remain grounded, flexible, focused, and creative.

▶ Expected Outcomes

There are many characteristics that make attending meetings meaningful for group members (**TABLE 10.6**). Although having satisfied group members is important, satisfaction alone does not ensure group success. An effective group collectively and productively works to meet a common goal. This common goal should always be the forefront of planning, deliberating, and evaluating the group's efforts.

TABLE 10.6 Characteristics of Effective Group Meetings

- *Careful time management.* Time is a vital and carefully guarded commodity. Some facilitators designate a timekeeper to help with this or rotate timekeeping responsibilities among members.
- *The facilitator and members are respectfully engaged.* All members listen to and respect others' opinions. The environment is safe for expression, exploration, and multiple realities.
- *Goals and objectives are clearly defined.* All members understand the group's agenda, time frame, budget, planning, and evaluation procedures.
- *Interruptions at meetings are not allowed or are held to a minimum.* When the meeting is in progress, it has priority.
- *The facilitator is prepared.* Materials are ready and available, both prior to and at the meeting.
- *The atmosphere is engaging.* Even when the format is formal, there is a welcoming ambiance.
- *Members are qualified and have a vested interest in the group's purpose.* People who are there want to be there.
- *Accurate minutes or records are maintained.* The printed record of decisions and actions is quickly available and provides direction for action between meetings.
- *Members feel validated.* Recognition and appreciation are given for contributions. Everyone has a role and everyone's participation is acknowledged.
- *The group's decisions or recommendations are actually used.* Members' work made a difference in something that matters.

▶ Conclusion

Health education specialists make great facilitators. Both formal training and on-the-job experiences prepare them to participate in the work of individual, group, and community change. The profession's core competencies and unified code of ethics provide the tools for group work. The inherent belief in the power of groups, commitments to capacity development, and genuine interest in others are the northern stars that guide all actions. As facilitators, health education specialists are able to serve as stewards of individual hopes, weavers of context,[21] and agents of community change.

Key Terms

Action items Items on a meeting's agenda that require a decision or action by the group.

Agenda A meeting's blueprint, indicating, at a minimum, the items to be covered and the order of events.

Bobby's Rules A more relaxed version of Robert's Rules of Order, in which questions are asked more informally and discussion flows more freely; however, decisions are still made through formal procedures and majority vote.

Consensus Agreement within a group on an action or principle that allows the group to go forward, even though there may be differences of opinion on some aspects of the issue.

Facilitation The act of making a meeting easier.

Facilitator The individual accepting the role of facilitation.

Minutes A brief, impartial account of what happened at a meeting. At a minimum, minutes record the date and location of the meeting, participants, topics covered, and decisions.

Quorum The minimum number of members who must be present for a group to conduct business or make decisions.

Robert's Rules of Order The most typically used parliamentary protocol in the United States, involving a structured set of rules and a process for majority vote decision-making. Booklets describing Robert's Rules can be found at most bookstores and libraries.

References

1. Facilitate. (n.d.). Retrieved March 4, 2017, from http://www.merriam- webster.com/dictionary /facilitate

2. National Commission for Health Education Credentialing. (2015). *Responsibilities and competencies for health education specialists.* Retrieved March 1, 2017, from http://www .nchec.org/responsibilities-and-competencies

3. Coalition of National Health Education Organizations. (2000). *A code of ethics for the health education profession.* Retrieved March 4, 2017, from http://cnheo.org/ethics .html

4. Nyswander, D. B. (1967). The open society: Its implications for health education specialists. *Health Education Monographs, 1*(22), 3–15.

5. Becker, A. B., Israel, B. A., Gustat, J., Reyes, A. G., & Allen, A. J. III (2013). Strategies and techniques for effective group process in CBPR partnerships. In B. A. Israel, E. Eng, A. J. Schulz, & E. A. Parker (Eds.), *Methods for community-based participatory research* (2nd ed., pp. 70–96). San Francisco, CA: Jossey-Bass.

6. Butterfoss, F. (2007). *Coalitions and partnerships in community health.* San Francisco, CA: Jossey-Bass.

7. Public Health Quality Improvement Exchange. (n.d.). *Developing and using SMART objectives.* Retrieved March 1, 2017, from http://www.phqix.org/content /developing-and-using-smart-objectives

8. Minkler, M., & Roe, K. M. (1993). *Grandmothers as caregivers: Raising children of the crack cocaine epidemic.* Thousand Oaks, CA: Sage.

9. Cohen, L. & Wolfe, A. (2010). Working collaboratively to advance prevention. In L. Cohen, V. Chavez, & S. Chehimi (Eds.), *Prevention is primary: Strategies for community well-being* (2nd ed., pp. 114–136). San Francisco, CA: Jossey-Bass.

10. Centers for Disease Control and Prevention (2012). *HIV planning guidance.* Retrieved March 4, 2017, from http://www.cdc.gov /hiv/pdf/p/cdc-hiv-planning-guidance.pdf

11. Fetterman, D. M., Kaftarian, S. J., & Wandersman, A. (1996). *Empowerment evaluation: Knowledge and tools for self-assessment and accountability.* Thousand Oaks, CA: Sage Publications.

12. Roe, K. M., Montes, J. H., & Roe, K. T. (2008). Parity, inclusion, and representation: Lessons from a decade of HIV prevention community planning for the movement to eliminate health disparities. Presented at the annual meeting of the American Public Health Association, October 25–29, 2008.

13. *Introduction to Robert's rules of order.* Retrieved March 1, 2017, from http://www .robertsrules.org/rulesintro.htm

14. *Robert's rules cheat sheet.* Retrieved March 1, 2017, from http://diphi.web.unc.edu/files /2012/02/MSG-ROBERTS_RULES_ CHEAT_SHEET.pdf

15. *Robert's rules of order basics.* Retrieved March 1, 2017, from http://www.youtube .com/watch?v=Tqs-RcphzdA

16. Jennings, C. A. (2016). *Robert's rules for dummies* (3rd ed.). Hoboken, NJ: John Wiley & Sons.

17. *How to take minutes (with sample minutes).* Retrieved March 1, 2017, from http://www .wikihow.com/Take-Minutes

18. *How to take meeting minutes—a crash course.* Retrieved March 1, 2017, from http://www .youtube.com/watch?v=0GV_w8nQJpE

19. *Meeting minutes—Office templates.* Retrieved March 1, 2017, from http://templates.office .com/en-us/Meeting-minutes-TM00002073

20. Roe, K. M. & Roe, K. T. (2004). Dialogue boxes: A tool for collaborative process evaluation. *Health Promotion Practice, 5*(3), 199–208.

21. Casey, C. (1998). *Making the gods work for you.* New York, NY: Harmony Books.

Additional Resources

Print

Berkowitz, B. & Wolff, T. (2000). *The spirit of the coalition.* Washington, DC: American Public Health Association.

Brown, C. R. & Mazza, G. J. (2005). *Leading diverse communities: A how-to guide for moving from healing into action.* San Francisco, CA: Jossey-Bass.

Hogan, C. (2007). *Facilitating multicultural groups: A practical guide.* Philadelphia, PA: Kogan Page Ltd.

International Association of Facilitators. *Group facilitation: A research and applications journal.*

International Association of Facilitators. (2005). *The IAF handbook of group facilitation: Best practices from the leading organization in facilitation.* San Francisco, CA: Jossey-Bass.

Landreman, L. M. (2013). *The art of effective facilitation: Perspectives from social justice educators.* Sterling, VA: Stylus Publishing, LLC.

National Commission for Health Education Credentialing, Inc. (NCHEC), & Society for Public Health Education (SOPHE). (2015). *A Competency-Based Framework for Health Education Specialists-2015.* Whitehall, PA: National Commission for Health Education Credentialing, Inc. (NCHEC) and Society for Public Health Education (SOPHE).

Wilkinson, M. (2012). *The secrets of facilitation: The smart guide to getting results with groups* (2nd ed.). New York, NY: Wiley.

Internet

Facilitator guides. Retrieved from http://www.cdc.gov/diabetes/ndep/training-tech-assistance/facilitator-guides.html

Facilitation tip sheet. Retrieved from http://www.cdc.gov/phcommunities/docs/plan_facilitation_tip_sheet.doc

Facilitator tool kit: A guide for helping groups get results office of quality improvement. University of Wisconsin-Madison. Retrieved from http://oqi.wisc.edu/resourcelibrary/uploads/resources/Facilitator%20Tool%20Kit.pdf

Facilitation tools for meetings and workshops. Retrieved from http://www.seedsforchange.org.uk/tools.pdf

Group facilitation and management. Retrieved from http://effectiveinterventions.cdc.gov/docs/default-source/street-smart-implementation-materials/Group_Facilitation_Handout.pdf?sfvrsn=0

Mahal, A. (September 2015). *Facilitator's and trainer's toolkit: Engage and energize participants for success in meetings, classes, and workshops.* Technics publications. Retrieved from http://play.google.com/books/reader?id=pozX-BgAAQBAJ&printsec=frontcover&output=reader&hl=en&pg=GBS.PP1 (e-book)

CHAPTER 11

Building and Sustaining Coalitions

Frances D. Butterfoss, PhD, MSEd

▶ Author Comments

Developing and sustaining coalitions for health promotion is both challenging and rewarding. Working with local- and state-level coalitions over the past 25 years has enabled me to forge new insights about community organizing, local and state politics, and interagency collaboration. By collaborating with individuals and organizations in coalitions, I have expanded and enriched my professional networks. I have learned firsthand that coalition efforts reach more people and reap much greater benefits than health education specialists could hope to achieve by working alone.

My past personal experiences, ideas from coalition practitioners, research findings, and the wisdom and advice of national experts help inform this chapter. I hope this information will help guide you in your efforts to develop and sustain productive community coalitions. I have not developed a static formula for building and sustaining the ideal coalition. Each community provides a unique context in which a coalition can grow and realize its potential. Some ideas herein are designed to help newcomers mobilize community partners to focus on a specific health issue, whereas others are designed for seasoned activists who are concerned with keeping existing coalitions on track. No matter what stage you are in, I expect you will discover tips that make sense for your coalition.

Nurturing coalitions to achieve their aims is a long-term endeavor. Invite diverse groups and individuals to join your coalition effort and create daring visions about what the coalition might accomplish. Above all, remember that coalition work is demanding—keeping a good sense of humor and celebrating every "win" along the way is essential.

⌕ *CHES COMPETENCIES*

2.1.1   Identify priority populations, partners, and other stakeholders.
2.1.2   Use strategies to convene priority populations, partners, and other stakeholders.
2.1.3   Facilitate collaborative efforts among priority populations, partners, and other stakeholders
5.3.1   Assess capacity of partners and other stakeholders to meet program goals.
5.3.2   Facilitate discussions with partners and other stakeholders regarding program resource needs.*
5.3.3   Create agreements (e.g., memoranda of understanding) with partners and other stakeholders.
5.3.4   Monitor relationships with partners and other stakeholders.
5.3.5   Elicit feedback from partners and other stakeholders.*
5.3.6   Evaluate relationships with partners and other stakeholders.
5.5.1   Facilitate efforts to achieve organizational mission.*
5.6.10   Employ conflict resolution techniques.*
5.6.11   Facilitate team development.*

*Advanced level competency

Reprinted by permission of the National Commission for Health Education Credentialing, Inc. (NCHEC) and Society for Public Health Education (SOPHE).

▶ Introduction

There is no doubt that strategic relationships are fundamental to modern society. Organizations, businesses, and even nations form alliances, joint ventures, and public-private partnerships. One specific type of partnership, coalitions, develops when different sectors of the community, state, or nation collaborate to create opportunities that will benefit the entire locality. A **community coalition** is defined as a group of individuals representing diverse organizations, factions, or constituencies within the community who agree to work together to achieve a common goal.[1] Coalitions are characterized as formal, multipurpose, and long-term alliances.[2] The size of its membership may vary, but a community coalition usually involves both professional and grassroots organizations. A coalition is different from other types of groups in that a structured arrangement for collaboration between organizations exists in which all members work together toward a common purpose. If the group is composed solely of individuals and not groups, then it is probably an organization or network and not a "coalition" in its truest form.

As an action-oriented group, a coalition focuses on reducing or preventing a community problem by (1) analyzing the problem, (2) identifying and implementing solutions, and (3) creating social change. More specifically, coalition functions include planning, advocating, promoting public awareness, promoting risk reduction, conducting professional education, networking, building partnerships, and creating community change.[3]

Coalitions promote community change by serving as effective and efficient forums for the exchange of knowledge, ideas, and strategies. Through coalitions, individuals and organizations may become involved in new, broader issues without being solely responsible for them. Additional benefits of a coalition include[3]:

- Demonstrating and developing community support or concern for issues.
- Maximizing the power of individuals and groups through collective action.
- Preventing duplication and reducing competition.
- Improving trust and communication among community agencies.
- Mobilizing talents, resources, and strategies.
- Building strength and cohesiveness by connecting individual activists.
- Building a constituency.

A coalition can be a very effective means of instituting social change. Central to this effectiveness is the ability for many organizations to work on a problem from many perspectives. No single approach for community change is as effective as a broad-based coalition effort that provides the means for multiple strategies and involves key community stakeholders.[4] Coalition building is a process that involves a long-term investment of time and resources; however, a coalition is not ideal if a simpler, less complex structure will get the job done or if the community opposes the concept.

This chapter is intended for those who are called to develop or manage coalitions for health promotion and disease prevention. It focuses on issues regarding community organizing and development of coalitions, qualities and characteristics of successful coalitions, steps to building effective coalitions, tips and techniques for managing and sustaining coalitions, strategies for overcoming barriers, and expected outcomes for coalitions.

Community Organizing and Involvement

Traditional health education is just one piece of a comprehensive community campaign. The focus of health education often has been on health education specialists as teachers and agents of change for individual health behaviors. Such efforts involve organizing educational events, teaching classes, and counseling individuals within schools, health departments, community-based organizations, and healthcare systems.

In contrast, coalitions attempt to alleviate community problems by organizing the community to bring about change. The general focus of **community organizing** is on changing systems, rules, social norms, policies, and environments to ultimately change the legality and social acceptability of behaviors. The venue for community organizing is the policy arena and often involves elected officials, businesses, community groups, media, and local and state legislatures. As such, community organizing is an ongoing process that involves identifying the many facets of a problem in a community and implementing a comprehensive plan to address the issue through community channels and systems.

Although coalitions usually operate in community settings, not all of them take advantage of communities' inherent power. When real community engagement exists, coalitions can address community health concerns while empowering or developing **capacity** in those very communities.[5] In particular, health-related coalitions can foster local involvement and ownership that emphasize local assets and advocate for fair distribution of public resources and complementary activities to meet community health needs and issues.

Development of Coalitions

The development of coalitions has escalated over the past 30 years, and they form for many reasons. For instance, local health organizations may form or join coalitions to augment their limited resources of staff, time, talent, equipment, materials, contacts, and influence. Joining with other agencies and individuals can benefit an organization by providing expanded access to printing and postage services, media coverage, social media, marketing services, meeting space, community residents, influential people, personnel, community and professional networks, and expertise.[3]

For example, health, civic, and faith-based groups develop coalitions to ensure adequate housing for the elderly and health insurance for the poor. Coalitions of health-related agencies, school districts, and community-based action groups may form in response to an opportunity, such as new funding (e.g., tobacco settlement funds helped support coalitions in their efforts to eliminate tobacco use among youth). Coalitions may also form because of a threat, such as a national story about rising obesity prevalence or a local event like an outbreak of meningitis on a college campus. Thus, concerned advocates rally to highlight their issue or enable favorable policies and legislation.

The best of these coalitions are vehicles that bring people together, expand available resources, focus on a problem of community concern, and achieve better results than any single group or agency could have achieved alone.[2] Not every coalition has been successful, however, and not every successful coalition has achieved its results without having its organizations pay a rather high price.[6] Even though coalitions are usually built from unselfish motives to better communities, they may experience the same challenges that are common among other voluntary organizations. With the initiation of a new coalition, new frustrations arise, such as promised resources may not be made available, conflicting interests may prevent the coalition from having its desired effect in the community, and recognition for accomplishments may be slow in coming.

TABLE 11.1 Characteristics of Successful Coalitions

- Continuity of coalition staff, particularly the coordinator position
- Ownership of the problem by coalition members and community
- Support of the coalition and its efforts by community leaders
- Actively involving community volunteer agencies
- High level of trust and reciprocity among members
- Frequent and ongoing training for coalition members and staff
- Benefits of membership outweigh the costs
- Active involvement of members in developing coalition goals, objectives, and strategies
- Developing a strategic action plan rather than a project-by-project approach
- Reaching decisions more by consensus rather than by voting
- Productive coalition meetings
- Deconstructing large problems into smaller, solvable ones
- Guidance of coalition by steering committee of elected leaders and staff
- Design and implementation of strategies by task or workgroups of members
- Formalization of roles, rules, and procedures
- Active involvement of local media
- Continuous evaluation of coalition and its activities

② DID YOU KNOW?

Community coalitions are usually easier to build than they are to sustain over time. Coalitions should begin to think about sustainability relatively soon after they form to ensure they exist long enough to achieve their goals.

Successful coalitions display certain qualities that allow them to accomplish difficult tasks. They tend to be diverse, both in their organizational membership and in individual activists; formal in their working relationships and role expectations; flexible in considering new approaches to health issues; efficient in their group response to

community issues; and collaborative in working toward a common goal by sharing risks, responsibilities, and rewards.[6] Regardless of their reason(s) for formation or focus, effective coalitions have certain factors in common (**TABLE 11.1**).[3,7]

▶ Steps for Building Effective Coalitions

No two coalitions are alike or operate in the same way, and not every coalition needs to be community based. A coalition can be composed and take direction from a state agency, hospital, or nonprofit organization, and the structure of the coalition should fit the goals and resources of the organization. A statewide organization with a considerable budget might develop a formalized structure with bylaws, multiple committees, and a professionally developed communication plan. In contrast, a local coalition with minimal funding and part-time staff can be effective with less structure.

Even though developing innovative strategies is more exciting than focusing on internal coalition development, this aspect of coalition building cannot be ignored. It has been found that one of every three organizations or activities based on partnership fail, and up to half of all coalitions fail within their first year of operation.[8,9] Thus, whatever structure is created should be logical, simple, and help members accomplish their goals[7]. Steps for building an effective coalition provide a basic overview to the process, but local circumstances must be considered so that coalitions respond to community needs (**TABLE 11.2**).

Analyze the Issue

The first step in forming a coalition is to analyze the issue or problem in the community, which can be accomplished by identifying and studying resource documents and collecting data (both local and state) relative to the issue. Many local health departments have conducted in-depth analyses, surveys, focus groups, and community assessments of health-related issues, which are available for

---

COMMUNITY CONNECTIONS 11.1

Natasha is a health education specialist who works in a local health department. Her supervisor has tasked her to develop a regional childhood obesity prevention program. She has a minimal budget and resources, a part-time administrative aide, and a constituency that includes several rural communities and a high migrant farming population. Considering the paucity of resources and magnitude of the problem, Natasha realizes that the best way to develop strategies that will prevent overweight and obesity in pre- and school-aged children is to collaborate with other community agencies and groups. She decides to investigate the possibility of forming a community coalition to address this issue.

---

public use. City, university, and state health department libraries have excellent resources, including books, journals, and other documents. Many health-related statistics are available through state vital statistics offices, state agencies, community-based organizations, and community and state websites. Centers for health promotion and chronic disease prevention at state health departments also offer free resources, statistics, and consultation on health-related issues. Interactive websites such as the *Community Commons*, *America's Health Rankings*, and *County Health Rankings and Roadmaps* can be very useful in assessing the community (see Additional Resources).

Develop a Rationale

Once the available data related to the priority public health issue(s) has been reviewed, a rationale must be developed for why a specific health or social issue has been chosen. Selection of an appropriate rationale and criteria on which to judge the merit of potential focus areas is important to avoid selection based on bias or hidden agendas and ensure that everyone is "on the same page." This rationale should address the following key elements[10]:

- Cost and/or return on investment.
- Availability of solutions.

TABLE 11.2 Steps for Building an Effective Coalition

1. Analyze the issue or problem on which the coalition will focus
2. Develop a rationale
3. Create awareness of the issue
4. Conduct initial coalition planning and recruitment
5. Develop resources and funding for the coalition
6. Create coalition infrastructure
7. Elect coalition leadership
8. Create an action plan

- Impact of the issue.
- Availability of resources (e.g., staff, time, money, equipment) to solve the issue.
- Urgency of solving the issue.
- Size of the problem (e.g., percentage of population affected).

Further, in thinking through the rationale for using a coalition-based approach, the following questions should be considered[10]:

- Is there available expertise to build and sustain a coalition?
- Is a coalition likely to implement effective solutions to the issue?
- How feasible will it be to implement coalition-based strategies?
- Are there any potential negative consequences?
- What are the legal considerations?
- What impact will these strategies have on policies, systems, and environments?

Once these questions have been fully answered, building awareness and support for the issue(s) and the coalition can begin.

Create Awareness of the Issue

Creating public awareness of an issue helps to raise public concern and support for the coalition and its strategies, recruit coalition members, and obtain funds. Making the public aware of a health issue can be accomplished by providing information to the local media, including newspapers, radio, television, and web media like blog posts, department webpages, and social media pages. A relationship with the media can be established by introducing one's self to local health reporters, newspaper editors, and other media personnel. Networking with the media as well as social media may help maximize coverage on the issue and increase the likelihood the coalition may become a future resource for the media. Providing presentations to community groups and local officials on an issue and how it affects community members can also create awareness, garner support for coalition development, and secure funding. Coalitions members should be aware

that promoting community awareness of an issue is an ongoing process.

Some coalitions emerge because public awareness and concern about an issue already exists and funding is made available to help alleviate the problem. For instance, local government often will designate funding to allow for community prevention and control efforts on specific issues such as violence, tobacco, and diabetes.

Conduct Initial Coalition Planning and Recruitment

Coalition planning can be conducted in different ways. In most communities, an initial planning meeting is organized, where local voluntary agencies (such as the American Heart Association), health departments, medical personnel, and elected officials are invited to participate. The purpose of this meeting is to discuss the feasibility of developing a coalition, addressing the following[1]:

- *Establish the coalition.* Is it worth the effort? Do other established human service coalitions or groups exist that might consider either broadening their interests to include the issue or establishing a subcommittee that functions like a mini coalition? Some effective community coalitions are subcommittees of established broader human service collaborating bodies.
- *Brainstorm who should be invited to participate.* Potential coalition members should be identified by using member contacts; phone books; local government listings; web searches; appropriate social media outlets; and human service agency, business, school, and other community directories. Agencies and other groups that currently focus their efforts on the same or similar issue as that of the proposed coalition should be included in the list of potential members. Parent groups, local voluntary associations, religious associations, youth groups, personal acquaintances, representatives of the priority population(s), and the media also might be recruited. Coalitions

with diverse memberships that reflect their communities are more likely to be effective.

- *Choose a date, time, and place for the first coalition meeting.* The initial meeting should be scheduled at least one month in advance to reduce scheduling conflicts. If possible, this meeting should coincide with another meeting at which some of the potential members are likely to be in attendance (e.g., a human service coordinating council meeting). The best ways to invite potential members (e.g., phone, email, mail, media, social media, or personal visits) needs to be determined. Follow-up phone calls or other personal contacts are likely to increase the numbers who attend.

- *Decide who should lead the coalition.* A lead agency or individual needs to be identified who will continue to take responsibility for initiating the coalition effort. After the coalition is well established and funding has been secured for the group, leadership should be elected.

- *Develop an agenda for the first coalition meeting.* The first coalition meeting is crucial. Individuals will likely decide at the first meeting if they will become members or if their time could be better spent elsewhere. The agenda should include an overview of the issue, formation of mission, goals, work or task groups, meeting dates/times, and an opportunity for networking.

- *Contact the media.* Someone who has prior experience in dealing with the media or is well versed on the issue and coalition plans should contact the media regarding the establishment of the coalition. Press releases should be developed and distributed prior to the first meeting.

- *Develop funding for the coalition.* Attendees at the initial meeting should explore all potential funding sources that may exist in their professional and personal networks.

Develop Resources and Funding for the Coalition

Coalitions must have or obtain the human and financial resources to do collaborative work.

COMMUNITY CONNECTIONS 11.2

Natasha's immediate focus is on the community groups that might be interested in this health issue and how to engage them. Sector by sector, she contacts agencies, groups and individuals who might have an interest in childhood overweight and obesity. She asks each responder to suggest other groups that might be interested. In this way, she recruits an active core of participants that includes the hospital, government, and social services, including WIC, public schools, pediatric/family practices and clinics, nutritionists, a parent advocacy group, YMCA, parks and recreation programs, school PTA groups, American Red Cross, Kiwanis and Rotary Clubs, a nondenominational minister's group, and the mayor's Health Council. They agree to hold a meeting to plan their approach.

Funding itself, however, does not ensure longevity and effectiveness. Some coalitions have succeeded in accomplishing their goals with little or no outside funding, while other well-funded coalitions have failed. A coalition must constantly ensure its agenda is driven by its mission and goals, and not by its funding. A coalition can do some activities with minimal funding, if member organizations are willing and committed to its vision and work, but a diverse funding portfolio is the key to coalition stability. Funds can come from membership dues, line items in the lead agency's budget that pay for staff and basic operating expenses, donations from civic groups and businesses, partner financial and in-kind contributions, grants, contracts, and fundraisers.[7]

Generally, coalitions do not need substantial funding to be effective, because coalitions often succeed when they work through established community events rather than spending time and money initiating new ones. For example, many communities hold regular events such as health fairs and breast cancer screenings. By capitalizing on these events to disseminate educational messages, coalitions can contribute with minimal cost. In fact, a large budget can cause problems such as focusing too much time and energy on encumbering funds, debating how to spend the money, and paying bills. If one agency contributes most of the funds for the coalition (through a grant or other source), contributions from other member organizations may decrease, which could ultimately diminish teamwork, involvement, and support from other members. In addition, if one agency contributes the bulk of the funding for the coalition, it may feel the need to control the agenda, which can be caustic, as a lack of shared input can be detrimental to the development of the coalition as a true partnership. Coalitions that involve a broad spectrum of people from the community as equal partners are most successful at building support and locating funding sources within their communities.

Grants to support activities that may involve a coalition are often available through state and federal agencies, private foundations, local community agencies, and businesses. They usually have very specific guidelines for activities, may involve significant reporting requirements and other paperwork, and come with certain restrictions on how the money can and cannot be spent, which may force a coalition to narrow or broaden its focus to qualify. Before applying for a grant, coalition members need to consider whether the benefits of receiving a grant outweigh the responsibilities and requirements.

Effective coalitions are usually successful at seeking and securing donations from local businesses and community organizations due to their visibility and public awareness of their accomplishments. Many businesses and community groups look for opportunities to be associated with a positive venture and may give money in exchange for their business' name being listed as a sponsor. Businesses that may contribute services to coalitions in exchange for recognition include printers, office supply stores, public relation firms, hospitals and other healthcare organizations, and restaurants, to name a few. Community groups that would be likely to contribute funds to community coalition efforts include service groups, such as the Lions Club, Rotary Club, Kiwanis International, Junior League, and Urban League, or a local community foundation.

Requests for funding involve delegating specific coalition members to make phone calls, send emails, attend meetings, and conduct presentations about the coalition, its goals, and needs for financial assistance.

Other funding methods may include membership dues and fundraising events. Some coalitions collect annual membership dues from individuals and organizations. Dues should be no more than needed to cover expenses, and because they may discourage people from participating, should be cautiously used. Similarly, fundraisers (e.g., golf tournaments and fun runs) can be time-consuming, divert the coalition from its mission, and have low rates of returns on time invested.

Coalitions should be supported and maintained by the communities they serve. When grant funding ends, the coalition is more likely to sustain itself if it is independent of outside funding. Similarly, if the organizational members of the coalition feel that they own the coalition and are responsible for its success, they are likely to support its meetings and activities. The exception here is funding for staff, research positions, and infrastructure (rental of space, office equipment, and supplies), which is costlier than most organizations can support. For example, coalition meetings may be sponsored by member organizations, with different ones providing meeting space, parking, and lunch. In this way, the meeting site rotates, which gives the sponsoring agency visibility, educates coalition members about their peer organizations, and makes travel time to sites fair for all. Thus, each organization gives what it can in terms of cash, in-kind material support, or volunteers to implement activities.

A resource development team may be formed to obtain resources to help the coalition thrive, ease the transition from one source of funding to another, and find money or goods from various sources. This group generally creates a development plan of objectives, strategies, and action steps to obtain financial resources for the coalition.

Sometimes, coalitions decide they need more autonomy from their lead agencies or independence to pursue other goals. They may

COMMUNITY CONNECTIONS 11.3

Because funds and resources are low, the newly formed *Coalition for Food and Fitness* agrees that each member organization must contribute to enact their action plan. The health department offers part of Natasha's time and clerical support, the hospital agrees to provide media and marketing expertise to develop a website and social media presence, the ministers provide refreshments and meeting space, the Kiwanis and Rotary Clubs agree to raise funds for prevention strategies, and the school PTA groups offer volunteers to work sharing information through schools. WIC and the pediatric and family practices agree to assess promising parent education methods and strategies that might be offered in their clinical settings to change eating and exercising behaviors. The social services representative agrees to help Natasha write a grant to obtain more funds for the coalition.

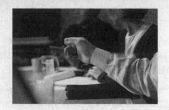
© Duncan Smith/Photodisc/Getty.

decide to apply for tax-exempt status as a 501c (3) organization, but prior consideration of the pros and cons of such a move is recommended.

Create Coalition Infrastructure

The infrastructure of an effective coalition should be formalized and supported by bylaws that are regularly reviewed and revised. The **bylaws** include rules of governance as well as descriptions of the roles of officers and coalition members. Organizational structure is critical to coalition management, especially because many coalitions are large and have members who are not necessarily active. Therefore, the work of the coalition is conducted through smaller committees rather than large membership meetings. Such subgroups are often called work, action, or task groups to connote their action orientation.

A sample workgroup structure and its functions are presented in the following list. All workgroups serve the priority population as identified by the coalition. For each workgroup, task subgroups are developed as needed to carry out specific activities.

- *Assessment and Evaluation.* Provides needs assessment and evaluation as the basis for community planning and action to promote health and prevent disease and injury.
- *Community Empowerment and Education.* Reaches out to communities through public awareness to ensure appropriate education and access to health services and programs to improve health outcomes.
- *Healthcare Providers.* Improves the knowledge, attitudes, and practices of healthcare providers to reduce barriers in the healthcare delivery system that contribute to the health problem under consideration.
- *Special Support Team.* Develops as the need arises. For example, a media advocacy team may develop to provide technical expertise and assistance in promoting newsworthy coalition activities.
- *Resource Development.* Provides expertise in identifying and securing in-kind and other resources and materials for the coalition and its workgroups.

In addition to workgroups and task subgroups, a **steering committee** should be established to set the coalition agenda, coordinate the activities of all committees, and serve as a fast response team for the coalition when immediate action is required. The elected coalition leadership, coalition coordinator, and other honorary representatives from the lead and key agencies make up the steering committee. This committee ensures representative decision-making and coordination among all components of the coalition. The steering committee meets three to four times per year, usually prior to regularly scheduled membership meetings.

Elect Coalition Leadership

Capable leadership is integral to the success of a coalition. Leadership can be elected or appointed, formal or informal. The key to successful coalition leadership is the ability to delegate tasks to the membership, negotiate when differences of opinion arise, and openly and effectively communicate with members and the community. Coalition leaders should know how to motivate members but not overwork them. Effective leaders give their time and expertise, share credit for successes, focus on member talents, know which members can provide extra support, realize that coalition members' time is valuable, and recognize community assets as well as needs.[3]

Coalition leadership generally consists of a coalition chairperson and vice-chairperson, workgroup chairperson and vice-chairperson, and coalition coordinator, as described in the following subsections. A nominating committee may be appointed by the chair to present a slate of officers for the steering committee to consider prior to the first coalition meeting of the year. Qualifications and statements from the candidates are distributed to coalition members, who are given the opportunity to add names to the slate. Election of workgroup chairs occurs at their first regular meeting by nominations from the floor and consensus voting. The term of office for all positions should be decided as well as whether consecutive terms are allowed.

Coalition Chairperson

Many coalitions opt to elect a chairperson for a one- or two-year period. The chairperson's responsibilities include facilitating meetings, representing the coalition to the public, and guiding strategies. The chairperson works closely with the coalition coordinator to[1]:

- Set meeting agendas.
- Ensure that each meeting is well organized.
- Encourage member discussion and input.
- Delegate responsibilities to members.
- Bring the coalition to consensus on issues.
- Conduct follow-up with members.

- Recruit and recognize members for accomplishments.
- Appoint a media spokesperson.
- Deal with difficult people and personalities.
- Set up training for members.

Coalition Vice-Chairperson

Given the busy schedules of health professionals and community volunteers, the vice-chairperson represents the chairperson during his or her absence. In addition, the vice-chairperson is mentored by the chairperson to promote development of leadership skills and future transition of leadership.

Workgroup Chairperson and Vice-Chairperson

The workgroup members elect these leaders from within the group. Leader characteristics and responsibilities are like those described for the coalition chair and vice-chair. Workgroups are smaller, more focused, and good training grounds for those who will later assume greater responsibility for the coalition. Meeting facilitation and task delegation are critical skills at this level.

Coalition Coordinator

Coalition coordinating, a job that can often be demanding and time-consuming, is integral to coalition success. The coalition coordinator works behind the scenes to organize meetings, complete necessary paperwork, recruit members, organize orientation and training, and coordinate membership recognition. Accomplishment of coalition outcomes hinges on the coordinator's experience, energy, commitment, persistence, and credibility.

The lead agency of the coalition generally is responsible for selecting or hiring the coalition coordinator. This individual should not serve as coalition chair, but is responsible for coalition management. A health education specialist with community organizing interests and experience would be a natural fit for the coordinator role.

Create an Action Plan

After the coalition forms, a mission statement, goals, objectives, and strategies need to be developed. Coalitions begin by formulating their vision statement, which is one sentence that describes what the coalition hopes to achieve in the ideal. The mission statement describes how the coalition plans to accomplish its vision and for whose benefit the coalition exists. A sample mission statement might read: "The Food and Fitness Coalition will reduce the incidence of childhood obesity among county residents by implementing policies, systems, and environmental change strategies."

The coalition should also develop short- and long-term goals, which are broad statements of purpose. For each goal, objectives (which are short range, specific outcomes of a program or project) should be written. Objectives can be either process oriented (e.g., outlining who will perform the activity, what will be done, and when the activity will take place) or outcome based (e.g., providing quantifiable, measurable courses of action that can be evaluated).

Involving members in creating **action plans** builds coalition capacity. For example, one coalition reported that after planning together, 76% of members rated their planning ability as high and 71% agreed that the resulting action plan accurately reflected their earlier needs assessment.[11] The same members reported that their capacity to plan in other arenas was increased because of their coalition experience. To increase effective implementation and evaluation phases, the action plan must resonate with the concerns of the people that will be served. Having a coalition plan that represents the community makes this outcome more likely.

Strategic plans can help focus a coalition's limited resources and time on developing strategies that affect outcomes. Strategies for achieving coalition objectives should be realistic, built on the experience of others, flexible, respectful of organizational cultures, and designed to enhance coalition unity. Effective educational strategies must consider that people learn as much from the process as from the result.[12] Several ongoing strategies may be simultaneously implemented by the coalition. Examples of successful strategies include organizing a cardiovascular disease conference for healthcare providers that focuses on developing a standard system to counsel patients on heart disease risk reduction, and conducting a media event that highlights how the community walking project helped participants decrease body fat and blood pressure.

Initially, coalitions should pursue strategies that are both noncontroversial and "easy wins." These strategies could include booths at community events to promote community awareness about an issue, youth poster contests in community schools to promote health behaviors, and awards to individuals and businesses that have made a positive impact. Small successes are critical to building confidence and unity among members. Even the best-planned strategy, however, is not guaranteed to work. As coalitions mature, members will learn from their mistakes and successes, resulting in easier and more effective strategizing.[12]

▶ Tips and Techniques for Managing and Sustaining Coalitions

The previous section on the steps for building an effective coalition should serve as a road map to get communities started in the coalition-building process. As multifaceted as this process is, nurturing and sustaining the coalition beyond its first year can be even more challenging. Government agencies, nonprofit organizations, and grassroots groups usually are enthusiastic in their support of coalitions that form to address a common need, threat, or opportunity. The real challenge lies in harnessing that enthusiasm and participation over the long haul. The following section provides suggestions on how to effectively manage and sustain coalitions by paying attention to stages of development, cultural competency, criteria for membership, recruitment, internal and external communication, relationships, marketing, and evaluation.

Understand Coalition Stages of Development

Coalitions move through a sequence of stages as they work toward their goals. In general, these conform to the chronological stages of formation, implementation, maintenance, and accomplishment of goals or outcomes.[2] Understanding the developmental stages of coalitions gives practitioners critical insight to make strategic decisions (**TABLE 11.3**).[11] Coalitions are dynamic organizations; they may cycle through formation, implementation, and maintenance stages as new members are recruited and as old strategies are revised or new ones initiated.

Sometimes, coalitions that form in response to the availability of outside funding engage in a *preformation stage*, in which needs assessments and other planning tasks are accomplished. *Healthy Start* infant mortality initiatives, *Allies Against Asthma* initiatives, and *ASSIST* tobacco control coalitions had the advantage of this early stage of preparation. Most coalitions, however, begin with the formation stage. Key tasks during formation include clarifying the mission, recruiting members, and creating rules, roles, and operating procedures for the coalition.

During the *implementation stage*, coalitions move from formation tasks to planning the strategies designed to achieve the coalition's goal(s). Raising community awareness about the problem and the coalition, assessing needs, and planning action are central to this stage.

Implementing, refining, and expanding coalition strategies take place during the *maintenance stage*. During this time, generating coalition funds and resources is essential.

In the *outcome stage*, coalitions begin to measure accomplishment of goals and objectives. Further community actions and community change should result in positive health outcomes, and coalitions need to work with funders to develop realistic expectations about the time needed to reach these outcomes. The lifespan of a coalition should be tied to the accomplishment of its goals and objectives. When goals are measurable, an end date tied to accomplishing those goals is implied. If goals are broad or indefinite, the coalition should revisit long-term goals at least every three to five years and decide whether to disband or to add more time or expand goals.

TABLE 11.3 Stages of Coalition Development

Stage	Time Estimate	Tasks
Formation	3–6 months	■ Identify community problem ■ Recruit members ■ Set vision and mission ■ Create rules and roles ■ Train on goals and issues
Implementation	9–12 months	■ Assess needs ■ Collect, analyze, and feedback data ■ Develop action plan
Maintenance	12–18 months	■ Initiate and monitor strategies ■ Support and evaluate coalition process
Outcome	18 months to 3 years	■ Begin to accomplish goals ■ Achieve results or impact from community-wide strategies

Consider Cultural Competency

To be most effective, coalitions need to be culturally competent. Effective coalitions tend to consist of members who represent the diversity of the community under consideration, cite more benefits than costs of membership, and participate often in coalition meetings and activities.[13] Diversity in coalitions refers not only to race and ethnicity, but also to age, gender, sexual orientation, education, and socioeconomic and work status. Members should be actively recruited from all sectors of the community, including individuals who either directly or indirectly suffer from disease or hardship relative to the issue, as they are excellent resources for better understanding the issue. A multicultural coalition allows diverse social and cultural groups the ability to interact in order to shape the coalition by planning, making decisions, creating a unique organizational culture, and guiding all actions. It defines itself by the interaction of people with diverse values, perspectives, and experiences and celebrates the contributions of culture. Coalitions also must ensure their strategies and activities are multiculturally competent.

Coalition members should be involved from the start in planning, implementing, and evaluating interventions with a focus on cultural competency. Then, members will appreciate that organizational and personal styles and communication and language differences must be accommodated. For example, planning must proceed at a pace that is comfortable for all, with enough time for members to question decisions. In meetings and activities, coalitions must be sensitive and aware of the different religious/cultural holidays, customs, and food preferences of the members and priority groups they are trying to reach. Finally, during intervention and evaluation phases, materials and communications must reflect the language, reading levels, and content for the priority populations.

ⓘ DID YOU KNOW?

The average meeting attendance rate for coalitions is about 50%.

Create Criteria for Membership

Coalitions should develop written criteria for participation to determine membership. This approach is not intended to exclude members, but rather to build a goal-oriented coalition. Potential coalition members can be asked to share volunteer and communications networks and demonstrate organizational support for the coalition's issues. Ties to the media and relationships with elected and appointed officials are also valuable member resources. Specific criteria for member organizations include the following[14]:

- Designate a specific individual as liaison to the coalition.
- Participate in meetings and activities.
- Place key coalition issues on agendas of their respective organizations.
- Communicate information to their members through newsletters, mailings, and other methods.
- Take formal, organizational positions on issues consistent with coalition policies.
- Provide in-kind contributions of time, and financial and material resources to the coalition.

Both organizations and individuals representing those organizations should be recruited to join the coalition. However, even though an organization may be admired for its community work, it may not be the best partner for a coalition. An individual may not reflect the strong characteristics of the organization, and a marginal organization may be chosen because of a specific, strong individual. Good coalition partners have certain traits in common: They usually follow a plan, make and fulfill commitments, act in an egalitarian manner and support all coalition members, communicate well, and provide and respond to leadership.[6]

Recruit Partners

The most critical component of any health promotion coalition is its membership, as the ultimate success of the coalition depends on how well its members are invested in and committed to collaboration. While a loyal core of member organizations is enough to start a coalition, more members are usually needed to effect real change. From the outset, core members must be involved to expand and strengthen membership. To that end, a few principles of recruitment stand out: (1) recruit about twice as many volunteers as needed; (2) develop specific criteria for members, with "job descriptions" that outline duties; and (3) find out why volunteers want to be involved while stressing the benefits the coalition offers to them and their organizations.

Turnover of coalition members, new arrivals to the community, changing needs, and new ideas for including groups and individuals in the coalition make membership recruitment a constant process. Encouraging people to join the coalition and invest their time and energy will take some effort, especially because many potential members participate in other community groups.

Some coalitions have had success recruiting members by organizing membership drives. Other approaches include staging a well-publicized special event or meeting; conducting phone or in-person interviews to identify interested persons and organizations; marketing the coalition at community events; placing ads in local newspapers or online outlets; requesting businesses and human service organizations appoint a person to represent their organization on the coalition; presenting information to religious groups, PTA groups, and community associations about the issue and coalition plans to alleviate the problem; appealing to area schools for students who need community service opportunities; and approaching other volunteer groups for assistance on projects.

Personal contacts are generally more successful in recruiting members than mass efforts such as emails or mailings. Members also may be recruited through invitation letters from administrators of lead organizations involved in the coalition planning group. Each organization that accepts an invitation should appoint a representative to the coalition. A follow-up phone call or email may be needed to confirm the representative.

Local chapters of associations related to the coalition issue are likely prospects for membership. For example, relevant organizations for a tobacco prevention coalition might include the American Heart Association, American Lung Association, and American Cancer Society. Staff and volunteers associated with these organizations work to improve the health of their community and may be interested in serving on relevant coalitions.

Local policymakers and other influential individuals in the local community may seek membership because of their commitment to the community and the coalition's potential to provide personal recognition and visibility. Coalitions should try to achieve a balance, however, between the "doers" and those who lend only their names and voices to the effort.

Coalitions also may enlist the support of volunteers interested in providing community service. Volunteers may be located through a local volunteer action center, university or community college, high school, or voluntary association. In addition, offering potential members something tangible in return for participating is helpful in recruiting. For example, an organization may need assistance with media training or contacts to attract attention to its cause. A media expert from the coalition could assist in return for their commitment to work on a coalition project.[15]

⊘ DID YOU KNOW?

Approximately one-third of coalition members on the roster form the active core of the coalition.

Organized youth groups such as 4-H Clubs, church groups, peer-to-peer counselors, local chapters of Students Against Destructive Decisions (SADD), environmental youth clubs, and athletic clubs can be enlisted to join the coalition or support specific coalition strategies. Other youth groups may be willing to adapt their mission statements to include the coalition issue. For example, a SADD chapter might consider including other drugs such as tobacco in its mission and work on specific tobacco use prevention strategies.

No matter which sector of the population is recruited to the coalition, personal motivation for why they want to join the coalition should be considered. Generally, individuals will participate in coalitions because of their commitment to alleviating a problem, while other members may participate because they gain a sense of satisfaction from volunteering and working with other professionals. Becoming active in a coalition can help individuals to overcome the sense of powerlessness that can discourage even the most committed advocates. Experience shows that individuals are motivated to participate based on the need to[1]: fulfill a shared interest; improve community services and the health of community members; share resources, including money, staff, and materials; and be visible in the community and demonstrate civic responsibility.

Marketing efforts that consider why potential members might be motivated to join the coalition will likely improve recruitment and retention. A six-step member recruitment process called the *buddy program* has proved helpful for many coalitions (**TABLE 11.4**). Implementing this process results in new members attending their first coalition meeting after reviewing relevant coalition documents, and leaving knowing at least two members of the group and feeling more engaged. The goal with this strategy is for them to return to the next meeting and fully participate.

Promote Internal and External Communication

Coalitions are valued because they bring different people and organizations together in a collaborative relationship. This strength in diversity, however, is often a challenge to communication. Communication at every level between staff and members is beneficial, and clear and frequent communication concerning the action plan and its level of implementation is especially crucial. Coalitions can take the following concrete actions to promote communication[16]:

- Create an environment where people can have open discussion and input.

TABLE 11.4 The Buddy Program for Coalition Member Recruitment	
Step 1	Each time a new strategy is introduced, the chair asks members to consider this question: "Who is not at the table that might help us enact this strategy or idea?"
Step 2	For each identified organization, a member who has the best connection to that organization is asked to begin the recruitment process and volunteer to be the "buddy."
Step 3	The buddy contacts the prospective member about joining the coalition. The buddy encourages the recruit and answers any immediate questions about the coalition. Successful contact information is forwarded to the chair and coordinator.
Step 4	The coordinator follows up with a phone call or email and sends an orientation packet to the prospective member which contains the coalition brochure, roster, bylaws, recent coalition minutes, event calendar, recent program materials, and press coverage.
Step 5	After receiving the meeting notice, the buddy contacts the recruit, ensures that the notice was received, and encourages the recruit to attend. Childcare or transportation needs are also considered.
Step 6	At the meeting, the buddy meets the new member, helps acclimate the member to the surroundings and meeting protocol, and introduces the new member to others. The member introduces himself or herself to the group. A personal welcome and offer of assistance by the Chair occurs at some point during the meeting.

Reproduced from Coalitions Work LLC. Buddy program for member recruitment. Retrieved from http://www.coalitionswork.com/wp-content/uploads/Buddy-Program-for-Member-Recruitment.pdf

- Distribute member rosters and meeting minutes in timely fashion.
- Use many communication channels such as telephone, fax, email, or social media alerts about meetings and events.
- Follow up by telephone/email if members miss meetings.
- Expect members and staff to report on completed tasks.
- Set up expectations about how communications will take place and evaluate their effectiveness.
- Use newsletters, mailings, and email to keep organizations' leaders involved, even if program staff usually attend the coalition meetings.

Coalitions also must learn how to communicate with the world outside the coalition. Materials should be developed that explain the coalition and its position on relevant issues in order to produce open, positive external communication. Then, every organization likely to be involved should be regularly contacted, especially those that have a real stake in the issue.

Monitor Relationships with Partners and Stakeholders

When coalition partners and stakeholders do not meet agreed-upon expectations, the coalition should know how to improve their performance and accountability considering they are not being paid for their services. The best way to approach this issue is to shift perspective to expect the same quality of service and provide the same support and guidance an agency would receive from or provide to an employee. The following guidance may help increase engagement and commitment of partners:

- *Be realistic when recruiting partners.* Partners' commitment to the coalition is often minimized to make participation more attractive. Clearly defined roles and responsibilities help them make a sound decision about whether to commit to the coalition. A time should be set to follow up with partners and let them know their choice will be respected either

way, as participating in a coalition is a serious decision and commitment.

- *Provide job descriptions, task checklists, and timelines for partners.* These tools create accountability and the basis for future performance discussions. The job description and checklist will reinforce expectations and allow partners to reselect the "job" based on current expectations.
- *Schedule periodic phone or in-person meetings with partners.* These meetings can be used to review their roles and responsibilities, offer support, and provide opportunities for feedback. Partners should be asked if their expectations for partnership are being met and be assured that the coalition leadership is open to discussing concerns at any time. If volunteers are unable to fulfill their roles due to personal or professional demands, they should feel comfortable approaching leadership to minimize or withdraw their commitment.
- *Agree on actionable tasks, measurable outcomes, and specific target dates.* If deadlines are not met, partners should be contacted about the missed date and agree to a new date for the expected deliverable. A prompt response from the coalition leadership sets a clear standard for meeting future deadlines. Meeting with key stakeholders on a quarterly or semi-annual basis to discuss progress toward shared outcomes increases the likelihood coalition goals and objectives will be accomplished. More importantly, partners and community stakeholders will stay involved with coalition work if they see fruits from their labors.

Market the Coalition

A coalition is affected by the same dynamics as every other for-profit or nonprofit organization. To sustain its momentum, a coalition needs to engage in marketing. Marketing is not directed at sales promotion, but rather at making someone desire the service or product being offered. Marketing can help build a positive image, recruit members, promote awareness, obtain funding, build morale, and gain support from influential people.[6] Additionally, marketing helps a coalition present itself as valuable so that other organizations and individuals are willing to make an exchange of time, material goods, or services to be a part of it.

Evaluate Coalition Success

Evaluation is critical to a coalition's development and maintenance. Evaluation helps provide accountability to members and funders (Did the program achieve results?) and improves programs or develops better approaches (What programs work well?). Linking coalition efforts to empirical endpoints is complicated because coalitions often work on long-term projects (e.g., changing community policies) that may ultimately affect personal behaviors. An extended time may pass before the behavior change takes place and can be measured. For instance, assessing if a coalition project designed to encourage parents to quit smoking affects whether children will initiate smoking is difficult. Evaluation may be compromised because the data needed to evaluate coalition efforts often are not collected. Funds are usually spent on intervention rather than evaluation, making it difficult to evaluate coalition effectiveness.

Given these challenges, three types of evaluation are appropriate for coalitions[7]:

- *Process evaluation* documents what was done and how many people were reached by coalition interventions. With this form of evaluation, record keeping of coalition efforts is essential. An annual report that highlights coalition accomplishments and the number of people served can be used to report process results. Process evaluation also can document whether the coalition itself is optimally functioning and as originally intended. Attendance records, types of organizations that make up the membership, meeting minutes, satisfaction and participation of members in coalition activities, and costs and benefits of membership are examples of process measures that may be used to document the coalition's structure and function.

- *Impact evaluation* documents accomplishments of specific objectives. This type of evaluation determines the extent to which the coalition efforts were effective. These measures can be determined by recording whether action plan objectives were achieved, partly achieved, or not achieved. Impact evaluation results can be helpful for recruiting organizations and fundraising for coalition activities.

- *Outcome evaluation* assesses long-term results and measures the changes brought about by the coalition and its activities. This type of evaluation involves measuring the effect coalition efforts have had on key community indicators such as obesity rates, teen pregnancy, and drug and alcohol use. An outcome evaluation focuses on all changes (positive and negative) brought about by coalition activities, not just those that were intended. Because of the inability to control extraneous variables, however, accurately determining the long-term effect of coalition efforts is challenging.

Coalitions must conduct regular evaluation to justify refunding, gain additional support, demonstrate the effectiveness of various programs, and provide a basis for future planning.[6] The coalition and its member organizations implement activities that are developed through the planning process. Each of these activities is related to specific educational or behavioral outcomes and, ultimately, to health status outcomes. Without participation and significant effort by members and member organizations, these activities will not be achieved.

The data that measure the participation of coalition members and efforts of the coalition itself are generated by (1) self-report in member surveys (e.g., role and number of hours devoted to specific coalition activities); (2) structured interviews with key stakeholders outside the coalition regarding specific contributions of the coalition in addressing the health problem; (3) process evaluation data about the participation of the intended priority groups in planned activities and concomitant changes in knowledge, attitudes, behaviors, and health status of those groups; and (4) pre- and post-intervention data on outcomes from agencies such as emergency rooms, inpatient facilities, clinics, schools, and other community settings. The first two types of data are obtained and managed by coalition staff with developmental input and feedback from coalition members. Process and outcome data are gathered by coalition member organizations (e.g., childcare centers, health departments, hospitals, schools). Data from state agencies (e.g., health departments) are managed by those institutions and shared with the coalition by permission. Numerous web sources contain state or county data that can be very useful for determining the community's strengths and challenges (see Additional Resources).

▶ Overcoming Challenges to Coalition Success

All coalitions face problems or barriers that hinder their ability to achieve goals and objectives. These problems could seriously impact the effectiveness of the coalition and set back community efforts to address the issue (**TABLE 11.5**).

TABLE 11.5 Common Problems That Coalitions Experience

- Too many planners and not enough "doers"
- Difficulty engaging local policymakers in the cause
- Not enough upper management support from coalition organizations
- Lack of funding or inadequate funding from local sources
- Difficulty coming to a consensus about what should be done
- Failure to plan or failure to act
- Membership burnout and turnover
- Lack of training among coalition members and staff
- Inadequate time allocated for coordinator to effectively manage the coalition

The following sections detail suggestions that help coalitions to avoid barriers known to impede success. These suggestions encourage coalition coordinators and leaders to recognize member efforts, obtain member organization commitment, link with other coalitions, maintain equal member representation, address expectations of staff and members, delegate tasks, and manage conflict.[12]

Recognize Member Efforts

Member recognition and retention should be high priorities. Attention should be paid to the "six Rs of participation": recognition, role, respect, reward, relationship, and results.[17] According to the six Rs, members need to:

- Be publicly *recognized* for their coalition efforts.
- Have clear expectations of the *role* they will play in coalition operations and strategies.
- Be *respected* for their culture, religion, race, and educational level.
- Be *rewarded* for their contributions.
- Develop meaningful *relationships* with other members and leaders.
- Find that their efforts will lead to measurable *results*.

Paying tribute to members for their efforts in the coalition is paramount. Through public and personal recognition, members feel their efforts are worthwhile and appreciated. Activities for member recognition may include hosting a recognition breakfast, sending letters of appreciation to members and their supervisors at work, publishing a program newsletter that includes highlights of members' involvement, presenting certificates of service, and soliciting area businesses to provide complimentary tickets for community events.

Obtain Member Organizational Commitment

Top administrators of lead organizations should demonstrate their commitment by communicating regularly to the coalition and the public. An annual letter of commitment or **memorandum**

of understanding (MOU) that outlines the expectations of membership regarding participation in coalition meetings and activities and contribution of time, talent, and resources (monetary or in-kind) should be signed by members. MOUs are not legally binding, but they carry a degree of seriousness and mutual respect that is stronger than a handshake or verbal commitment. Often, MOUs are the first steps toward a legal contract, such as when a coalition has grant or foundation funding and is expected to obtain MOUs from each coalition partner. Groups that remain uncertain and uncommitted to the coalition's mission or are unwilling to sign an MOU can be asked to assume a less formal type of commitment such as remaining on a mailing list or being part of a "friend of the coalition" network.

Link with Other Community Coalitions

A coalition that advances the work of its partners and sister coalitions gains community credibility. The coalition must constantly define and redefine its mission and the role it plays in promoting community health. A fine line must be drawn between promoting a coalition's self-interest and letting go to enhance the work of other groups. For example, by agreeing to contribute volunteers and resources to established events such as the American Heart Association's *Great American Smokeout*, the March of Dimes' *Walk America*, and the American Cancer Society's *Relay for Life*, all coalitions and collaborating agencies win. Such collaboration and selflessness will eventually pay dividends by building a respectable coalition image. When community members outside of the coalition seek the opinions, advice, and contributions of coalition members, the coalition's future is further assured.

Maintain Equal Member Representation

The coalition coordinator must discover and respond to the hidden agendas of its members. While coalitions should attempt to meet individual agendas, the overall common mission must not be lost. Domination by one or more powerful groups in the coalition might deprive other groups of their sense of equal participation. This can be addressed by promoting more open communication and a "one-vote rule" for each organization, regardless of its size or financial contribution.

Address Expectations of Staff and Members

Because of the diverse nature of coalitions, both staff and members approach coalitions with different expectations. Members want to know how much time away from job and family duties will be required and their role and how their time and talents can best be used. Staff are concerned about whether they will be able to handle the demands of a job where most of the work is done by volunteers, as well as how to motivate volunteers who have varying degrees of understanding and commitment to the coalition. They may be concerned about their ability to obtain funds and resources for the coalition. Finally, they are most certainly likely concerned about how to coordinate the many activities the coalition engages in a timely manner.

To encourage realistic expectations, coalitions should develop job descriptions for volunteers and staff that carefully outline the prerequisite skills, time commitments, and expected duties. Both staff and volunteer leaders should have formal performance appraisals that show whether they are exceeding, meeting, or not meeting expectations as outlined in their job descriptions. Biannual staff and member surveys can help determine whether personal expectations are being met by coalition work. Providing varied opportunities for training, technical assistance, and networking with other coalitions can also increase satisfaction and commitment.

Delegate Tasks

Delegation is the process of transferring the following to coalition members:

- *Responsibility*. The obligation to carry out an assignment.

- *Authority*. The power necessary to ensure that results are achieved.
- *Accountability*. The responsibility for results.

Delegation is essential because the coalition staff cannot and should not do all the coalition work. Delegating tasks promotes a sense of coalition ownership among its members—the coalition is not one agency's initiative but one that is shared by all members. Engaging many members in coalition efforts will have more impact than utilizing the energy of only a few people.

To effectively delegate tasks, the coalition goals and strategies should be clearly stated and volunteer workers actively recruited and trained in skills needed to accomplish objectives. Members should be provided with tasks that fit their area of interest or expertise, as working on issues in which members are interested increases ownership and commitment. The key is to get to know each of the members and find common interests that will benefit individual members and the coalition. Additionally, leaders must be able to release control of the process and details associated with coalition activities and encourage mutual input on strategies and expected outcomes. Finally, an environment that fosters initiative and rewards should be cultivated.[18]

In contrast, certain characteristics are likely to hinder the coalition leader's successful delegation of tasks and should be addressed by leaders (**TABLE 11.6**).

Manage Conflict

Conflict is inevitable when working with people who are trying to agree on and achieve mutual goals. Conflicts are frequently the basis for defensiveness, reduced communication, and strained relationships among group members. Sources of conflict include differences in values and goals; allocation of scarce resources such as money, facilities, and time; perceived threats to autonomy, rights, or identity; and differences in relation to how desired ends should be achieved. If not addressed and minimized, conflict can cripple a coalition. Conflict can be resolved in constructive ways that will likely enhance future collaboration and creativity (**TABLE 11.7**).[1]

TABLE 11.6 Characteristics That Hinder Task Delegation

- Unclear goals and objectives
- Attitude of "doer"—doing tasks by oneself versus working with others
- "I can do it better and faster" syndrome
- Unwillingness to transfer responsibility/authority to untrained or inexperienced staff
- Insecurity
- Inability to delegate
- Unwillingness to let others determine project methods and details
- Perfectionism
- Risk aversion
- Organizational instability
- Lack of resources
- Poorly defined accountability

TABLE 11.7 Strategies for Reducing Conflict

- Rotate leadership at least every two years to address conflicts that arise from unequal sharing of power.
- Separate individuals from the problem; let individuals voice their differences and work together to resolve them.
- Use formal group process techniques to address conflict arising from lack of or over-participation in meetings.
- Distribute information relative to the coalition or its issue as it becomes available.
- Rotate meeting sites to reduce "turf" battles.
- Do not allow "either-or" thinking. Require that dissenting parties generate an alternative to "my way" or "your way."
- Rule out the use of "you" messages and personal accusations. Engage members in a joint effort to locate the source of the problem.
- Rotate seating to promote or reduce communication. Creatively seat parties next to (as opposed to across from) each other.
- Search for areas of agreement and trust.
- Take a break from the topic until emotions have cooled.

▶ Expected Outcomes

Many outcomes are associated with community coalition efforts. To be embraced and supported by its community, a coalition must show it has influenced the ultimate health behaviors and health status it seeks to address. Over time, positive coalition outcomes should occur such as reduced rates of youth smoking, increased immunization rates, reduced hospital and emergency room admissions of people with asthma, or earlier detection of cancer. Some coalition outcomes, however, are related to the *process* of coalition building and maintenance. Examples of these include:

■ *Partnerships and relationships are established among community agencies, individuals, and influential people.* These relationships are developed through networking and collaboration and may be useful in focusing on other community issues in the future.

■ *Relationships are developed with the media.* As coalition staff and members strive to accomplish their goals, they may have frequent contact with reporters, write letters to the editors of local papers, and speak on local radio or television. A relationship is built in which the coalition and members become recognized by the media as experts on the issue. As a result, the media will take the initiative to contact someone from the coalition the next time the issue surfaces.

■ *Public awareness is raised and community and social change is initiated.* Creating community awareness of an issue may lead to changes in individual beliefs and personal habits as well as public policy. Many times, changes in public policy precede changes in personal habits. For example, businesses that establish tobacco-free policies influence employees to quit smoking.

■ *Legislators and local policymakers become aware of the coalition and its potential influence.* Coalitions tend to be highly visible in communities and can easily draw the attention and interest of legislators and local policymakers. These individuals are interested in having their names

associated with initiatives that lead to positive changes in their communities.

■ *Coalition members and community members are empowered from their experiences.* The process of implementing coalition strategies creates a sense of accomplishment and a "can make a difference" attitude for coalition members, priority audiences, and the whole community.

■ *Each person or organization within a coalition becomes part of a greater whole.* Members speak to the problem with a combined power and a unified voice.[7] This combined power is much greater than what each organization could accomplish alone. Issues are solved because individuals and agencies in the community begin to talk to each other and take ownership of the community problem.

■ *A community standard of acceptability is developed.* A coalition that addresses an issue and creates awareness of the risks, benefits, and possible solutions can help change the community norm of what is and is not acceptable. Coalition efforts become a process of setting the community standard of beliefs and behavior.

A coalition serves as a catalyst to engender community involvement and build capacity. Innovative strategies that are carefully planned, executed, and evaluated by a diverse, collaborative group have a strong chance of succeeding.[19–21] Coalitions should pride themselves on the fact that they do not develop strategies with the intent of owning them. Instead, they are developed to help empower the community to solve its own health problems. Strategies should be based within community organizations and agencies, as the material and personnel resources the coalition brings serve as seeds to generate future ownership of these strategies and other spin-offs.

A coalition's job is to use resources fairly and wisely so it is regarded as a partner in the change process and not as the owner. Ultimately, traditional healthcare providers and grassroots groups must recognize that this collaborative approach is effective in changing behaviors and health status before they embrace it. The best compliment a coalition can receive is to see a strategy begun in the community still thrives or has been adapted to fit changing circumstances. For example, partners who help develop new standards of care for managing pediatric asthma must feel ownership of the process and product. If so, the standards will be easily embraced as routine for institutions such as schools and hospitals instead of being imposed by an outside authority (i.e., the coalition).

ⓘ DID YOU KNOW?

When coalitions *exceed* the expectations of both their members and the community, success in reaching outcomes is inevitable.

▶ Conclusion

Coalition building can be challenging and time consuming. The benefits to communities and health professionals, however, usually far outweigh these drawbacks. Community benefits derived from coalitions are numerous, including the ultimate reduction of the community health problem or issue. As reinforced in this chapter, the skills required to build or maintain a coalition can be learned. A variety of manuals, textbooks, and web-based references and tools are available (see Additional Resources). Many foundations and professional organizations offer coalition technical assistance and training opportunities for health education specialists. Serving on coalitions can expand professional networks, enhance personal knowledge and experiences in community organizing, and assist in achieving professional health promotion and disease prevention goals. It is no longer a question of whether a health education specialist will be asked to join or form a coalition, but rather when. Preparing for that opportunity will be well worth the effort.

Key Terms

Action plan The written plan that outlines how the coalition will carry out its mission, including goals, objectives, strategies, resources, member responsibilities, budget, and measurable outcomes.

Bylaws Rules or procedures developed to self-regulate an organization.

Capacity A community's ability to sustain a level of action needed to accomplish coalition goals.

Community coalition A formal, long-term alliance among a group of individuals representing diverse organizations, factions, or constituencies who agree to work together to achieve a common goal.

Community organizing The coordinated efforts of a group of citizens to promote an issue in their community.

Memorandum of understanding (MOU) A formal agreement between two or more parties.

Steering committee A committee that decides on the priorities of an organization and oversees its operations.

References

1. Feighery, E. & Rogers, T. (1990). *How-to guides on community health promotion: Guide 12. Building and maintaining effective coalitions*. Palo Alto, CA: Stanford Health Promotion Resource Center.

2. Butterfoss, F. D., Goodman, R. M., & Wandersman, A. (1993). Community coalitions for prevention and health promotion. *Health Education Research*, 8, 315–330.

3. Whitt, M. (1993). *Fighting tobacco: A coalition approach to improving your community's health*. Lansing, MI: Michigan Department of Public Health.

4. McLeroy, K., Kegler, M., Steckler, A., Burdine, J., & Wisotzky, M. (1994). Community coalitions for health promotion: Summary and further reflections. *Health Education Research, 9*, 1–11.

5. Butterfoss, F. D. (2007). *Coalitions and partnerships in community health*. San Francisco, CA: Jossey Bass Publishers, Inc.

6. Dowling, J. D., O'Donnell, H. J., & Wellington Consulting Group. (2000). *A development manual for asthma coalitions*. Northbrook, IL: The CHEST Foundation and the American College of Chest Physicians.

7. Butterfoss, F. D. (2013). *Ignite! Getting your community coalition fired up for change*. Bloomington, IN: Author House.

8. Berquist, W., Betwee, J., & Meuei, D. (1995). *Building strategic relationships*. San Francisco, CA: Jossey-Bass Publishers, Inc.

9. Kreuter, M. W., Lezin, N. A., & Young, L. A. (2000). Evaluating community-based collaborative mechanisms: Implications for practitioners. *Health Promotion Practice, 1*, 49–63.

10. NAACHO. *First things first: Prioritizing health problems*. Retrieved August 9, 2017, from http://archived.naccho.org/topics/infrastructure/accreditation/upload/Prioritization-Summaries-and-Examples.pdf

11. Butterfoss, F. D., Morrow, A. L., Rosenthal, J., Dini, E., Crews, R. C., Webster, J. D., & Louis, P. (1998). CINCH: An urban coalition for empowerment and action. *Health Education and Behavior, 25*, 215–225.

12. Foster-Fishman, P. S., Berkowitz, D., Lounsbury, S., Jacobson, S., & Allen, N. (2001). Building collaborative capacity in community coalitions: A review of an integrative framework. *American Journal of Community Psychology, 29*(2), 241–261.

13. Butterfoss, F. D., Goodman, R. M., & Wandersman, A. (1996). Community coalitions for prevention and health promotion: Factors predicting satisfaction, participation and planning. *Health Education Quarterly, 23*, 65–79.

14. Ontario Healthy Communities Coalition. (2002). *From the ground up: An organizing handbook for healthy communities*. Toronto: The Search Institute. Retrieved August 9, 2017 http://www.ohcc-ccso.ca/en/from-the-ground-up

15. Bataan, M. F., Butterfoss, F. D., Jaffe, C., & LaPier, T. (2011). *The Sustainability planning guide for healthy communities*. Atlanta, GA: CDC Division of Adult and Community Health, Healthy Communities Program. Retrieved August 9, 2017 http://www.cdc.gov/healthycommunitiesprogram/pdf/sustainability_guide.pdf

16. Kegler, M. C., Steckler, A., McLeroy, K., & Malek, S. H. (1998). Factors that contribute to effective health promotion coalitions: A study of 10 Project ASSIST coalitions in North Carolina. *Health Education and Behavior, 25*, 338–353.

17. Kaye, G. & Wolff, T. (1995). *From the ground up: A workbook on community development and coalition building*. Amherst, MA: AHEC Community Partners.

18. Wolff, T. (2001). A practitioner's guide to successful coalitions. *American Journal of Community Psychology, 29*, 173–191.

19. McKenzie, J. F., Neiger, B. L., & Thackeray, R. (2017). *Planning, implementing and evaluating health promotion programs* (7th ed.). New York, NY: Pearson.

20. Wolff, T. (2010). *The power of collaborative solutions*. San Francisco, CA: Jossey Bass Publishers Inc.

21. Butterfoss, F. D. & Kegler, M. C. (2013). A coalition model for community action. In M. Minkler (Ed.), *Community organizing and community building for health and welfare* (3rd ed.). New Brunswick, NJ: Rutgers University Press.

Additional Resources

Print

Amherst H. Wilder Foundation. (1977). *The collaboration handbook: Creating, sustaining and enjoying the journey.* St. Paul, MN: Author.

Bobo, K., Kendall, J., & Max, S. (2001). *Organizing for social change: Midwest academy manual for activists* (4th ed.). Santa Ana, CA: Seven Locks Press.

Butterfoss, F. D. (2007). *Coalitions and partnerships in community health.* San Francisco, CA: Jossey-Bass Publishers Inc.

Butterfoss, F. D. (2013). *Ignite: Getting your community coalition fired up for change.* Bloomington, IN: Author House.

National Business Coalition on Health and the Community Coalitions Health Institute. (2006). *Community health partnerships tools and information for development and support.* Retrieved from http://www.nbch.org/nbch/files/cclibraryfiles/filename/000000000353/community_health_partnerships_tools.pdf

National Commission for Health Education Credentialing, Inc. (NCHEC), & Society for Public Health Education (SOPHE). (2015). *A Competency-Based Framework for Health Education Specialists-2015.* Whitehall, PA: National Commission for Health Education Credentialing, Inc. (NCHEC) and Society for Public Health Education (SOPHE).

Fetterman, D. & Wandersman, A. (2005). *Empowerment evaluation: Principles in practice.* New York, NY: The Guilford Press.

Kretzmann, J. P. & McKnight, J. (1993). *Building communities from the inside out: A path toward finding and mobilizing a community's assets.* Chicago, IL: ACTA Publications.

Kreuter, M., Lezin, L., Kreuter, M., & Green, L. (1998). *Community health promotion ideas that work: A field-book for practitioners.* Sudbury, MA: Jones and Bartlett.

The National Network for Collaboration. (1996). *Collaboration framework: Addressing community capacity.* Fargo, ND: Author.

Turning Point Social Marketing National Excellence Collaborative. (2003). *Social marketing and public health: Lessons from the field.* Seattle, WA: Turning Point.

W. K. Kellogg Foundation. (1998). *W. K. Kellogg Foundation Evaluation Handbook.* Battle Creek, MI: Author.

Wolff, T. (2010). *The power of collaborative solutions: Six principles and effective tools for building healthy communities.* Hoboken, NJ: Jossey-Bass Publishers Inc.

Internet

America's Health Rankings. *United healthcare.* Retrieved from http://www.americashealthrankings.org/learn/reports/2015-annual-report

BoardSource. *Resources and solutions for nonprofit leaders.* Retrieved from http://boardsource.org/resources-solutions/

Centers for Disease Control and Prevention (CDC). *Best practices for tobacco control and prevention programs user guides. coalitions: State and community interventions.* Retrieved from ftp://ftp.cdc.gov/pub/fda/fda/user_guide.pdf

Centers for Disease Control and Prevention (CDC). Atlanta, GA. Coalitions to promote immunizations; 5-a-Day nutrition programs; diabetes control; asthma control and management; HIV/AIDS community planning; breast, cervical, and prostate cancer control; and unintentional childhood injury prevention, among others. Retrieved from http://www.cdc.gov

Coalitions Work. *Tools and resources.* Retrieved from http://coalitionswork.com/resources/tools/

Community Anti-Drug Coalitions of America. *Resources.* Retrieved from http://www.cadca.org/resources

Community Commons. *Data, tools and stories to improve communities and inspire change.* Retrieved from http://www.communitycommons.org/

County Health Rankings and Roadmaps. *What works for health.* Retrieved from http://www.countyhealthrankings.org/roadmaps/what-works-for-health

Health Services Resource Administration (HRSA). Bethesda, MD. Agency of U.S. Department of Health and Human Services for improving health and achieving health equity through access to quality services, skilled health workforce, and innovative programs. Retrieved from http://www.hrsa.gov

National Coalition for the Homeless. Washington, DC. Retrieved from http://nationalhomeless.org/

Substance Abuse and Mental Health Services Administration. Center for Substance Abuse Prevention. *Tobacco-free schools and communities.* Rockville, MD. Retrieved from http://www.samhsa.gov/

The Prevention Institute. *Developing coalitions: An eight-step guide.* Retrieved from http://www.preventioninstitute.org/publications/developing-effective-coalitions-an-eight-step-guide

University of Kansas Work Group on Health Promotion and Community Development. *The community toolbox.* Retrieved from http://ctb.ku.edu

CHAPTER 12

Advocating for Health Policy

Cicily Hampton, PhD, MPA
Sue Lachenmayr, MPH, CHES

▶ Author Comments

Today, when a single tweet can spread across the world in a matter of seconds and we are bombarded with nonstop information and misinformation, it is more important than ever for health education specialists to develop their own effective advocacy skills and provide these skills to individuals they serve. As President Barack Obama said in his farewell speech, "Change only happens when ordinary people get involved, and they get engaged, and they come together to demand it."[1]

As a former state government employee whose job was implementing public policy and a government relations and policy professional responsible for shaping policy, we know how important it is to hear from frontline people who deliver programs, from the individuals who receive services, and most importantly from people who cannot get the services they need. Whether you are happy with current programming and services or you think changes need to be made, your advocacy efforts make a difference. Speaking to your elected officials, testifying at a public hearing, and sharing your personal experiences can have tremendous impact. If you do not speak out about what makes good public health policy, legislators and other policymakers will assume either no one cares about the issue, so funding can be cut, or no changes are needed. If special interest groups want funding for another cause and they are the only ones who speak out, legislators may assume there is only one point of view. *Healthy People 2020*, the comprehensive planning document for ensuring the health of the public, provides multiple advocacy calls to action that challenge all health education specialists to work to "achieve health equity, eliminate disparities, and improve the health of all groups" and the website includes a *Healthy People in Action* section to add stories about successful advocacy.[2]

🔍 *CHES COMPETENCIES*

1.6.2   Identify policies related to health education/promotion.
1.6.4   Assess social, environmental, political, and other factors that may impact health education/promotion.
2.1.1   Identify priority populations, partners, and other stakeholders.
2.1.2   Use strategies to convene priority populations, partners, and other stakeholders.
2.1.3   Facilitate collaborative efforts among priority populations, partners, and other stakeholders.
7.2.1   Identify current and emerging issues requiring advocacy.
7.2.2   Engage stakeholders in advocacy initiatives.
7.2.3   Access resources (e.g., financial, personnel, information, data) related to identified advocacy needs.
7.2.4   Develop advocacy plans in compliance with local, state, and/or federal policies and procedures.
7.2.5   Use strategies that advance advocacy goals.
7.2.6   Implement advocacy plans.
7.2.7   Evaluate advocacy efforts.
7.2.8   Comply with organizational policies related to participating in advocacy.
7.3.1   Assess the impact of existing and proposed policies on health.
7.3.2   Assess the impact of existing and proposed policies on health education.
7.3.3   Assess the impact of existing systems on health.
7.3.4   Project the impact of proposed systems changes on health education.
7.3.5   Use evidence-based findings in policy analysis.
7.3.9   Use media advocacy techniques to influence decision-makers.
7.3.10   Engage in legislative advocacy.

Reprinted by permission of the National Commission for Health Education Credentialing, Inc. (NCHEC) and Society for Public Health Education (SOPHE).

▶ Introduction

At times, the health education profession has been a follower rather than a leader in public policy development, but today, advocacy is an essential component of the *Code of Ethics for the Health Education Profession*[3,4] and a required competency for health education specialists.[4,5] Health education specialists have a personal right and a professional responsibility to become effective policy advocates; not only is it fairly easy, but also it is rewarding. Learning about local, state, and national issues can be a starting point to developing laws and regulations to support and ensure effective health promotion efforts for individuals and communities.

Becoming involved in the political process has been identified as a key function of health education specialists since the late 1970s.[5] Practitioners can be involved in the legislative process in many ways not only to influence the kind and amount of resources allocated for health education programs, but also to affect the larger policy framework that defines public health. When it comes to shaping policy, nothing is more effective than a well-educated, unified voice. Effective advocacy and influencing policy require a long-term commitment. Building relationships with policymakers at every level is essential for success.

Health education specialists have skills that **policymakers** need that can assist them in crafting legislation and gathering support for an issue. They are experts in gathering data; assessing individual and community needs; consensus building; and in planning, implementing, and evaluating programs. In addition, health education specialists know how to define a problem using the facts and can frame it through personal stories. This

COMMUNITY CONNECTIONS 12.1

Erica is a Masters of Public Health student who just got elected as the Advocacy Chair for her chapter of Eta Sigma Gamma (ESG). She was unfamiliar with the word advocacy until one of her professors gave a lecture on advocacy and the political process. When she learned that an advocate is someone who speaks on behalf of others, Erica recognized she had previously acted as an advocate when she petitioned the university administration to make her campus smoke free. After the campus went smoke free, she realized that she enjoyed the process of advocating for change.

expertise can assist policymakers in moving an issue from an idea to a **law**.

To be effective advocates, health education specialists can start with what they do best: assess social, environmental, political, and other factors that impact health; identify current and emerging issues that indicate gaps in services or possible health risks, especially in areas related to health education/health promotion; and use this information to educate elected officials or other policymakers. By sharing relevant data with policymakers, objective information can be used to make decisions about new legislation or policies or about changes needed in existing regulations. This process, known as **legislative advocacy**, involves making contact with a policymaker or legislator to discuss a social or economic problem on behalf of a particular interest group or population, as long as no specific bill number is mentioned.[6] While nonprofit organizations need to follow specific guidelines as defined in the U.S. tax code, as a private citizen, anyone has the right to engage in these activities without restrictions. Both *lobbying* and *grassroots activities* are legal strategies frequently utilized by for-profit and nonprofit organizations to support or change policy.

A health education specialist just becoming involved in advocacy might consider identifying policy changes needed at an academic institution, professional organization, or workplace. Experiences learned in making changes within organizations/institutions can be used to advance changes at the local, state, or national level. There are many practical advocacy strategies readily available for health education specialists to use, many of which will be discussed in this chapter.[7]

For most people, it is empowering to share their opinion about a social or economic problem with their elected official or advocate for an issue that is important to them. Although people may have a negative reaction to the term lobbying or lobbyist, lobbying is a very effective way to ensure an issue becomes a law. **Direct lobbying** is defined as communicating about specific legislation with a legislator or communicating a specific position on that legislation. In other words, asking a legislator to support (or veto) a specific bill. Providing a policymaker with factual, nonpartisan information on an issue or sharing information with the public without asking them to urge their legislator to vote in a certain way is *not* considered lobbying. **Grassroots lobbying** is when a group or organization appeals to the general public and asks them to take action to influence specific legislation. For example, a letter to parents of schoolchildren asking them to call or write their congressperson to support a bill to increase funding for a new school program is considered grassroots lobbying. In this instance, instead of a direct appeal to a legislator, people in the community are asked to take action to contact their elected officials and ask them to support the bill.

A health education specialist should be prepared to answer "Why should the government be involved in the solution?" Many legislators prefer to let private industry address a problem. If, however, the best solution is for government (at any level) to take an active role to, for example, address market failure or reverse perverse incentives, advocates need to be able to make the case that private industry has not and cannot address the problem and why government action is needed.

▶ Steps for Advocating Legislation

Understanding the legislative process will increase the likelihood of success. Seven crucial steps to legislative involvement include: (1) identifying the issue and developing a fact sheet, (2) understanding the steps needed to enact legislation, (3) identifying potential partners and forming or joining coalitions to strengthen the likelihood of success, (4) establishing a relationship with policymaker(s), (5) building grassroots support, and (6) introducing and tracking legislation.

Identify the Issue and Develop a Support Fact Sheet

In legislative advocacy, the health problem and who is affected should be defined. How many people are affected? Are some people affected more than others (or at greater risk)? What would be the cost if the problem is not addressed? What policy or law could help resolve the problem? Who else might be concerned about the problem? Answering these questions can help clarify the issue and determine where to start. The economic, human, and opportunity costs must be considered. Several cost-accounting metrics are available to help calculate these costs when considering prevention and public health programs or chronic disease burden, including quality adjusted life years.

A fact sheet about the issue could be developed to share with potential advocates and legislators. The key points identified in the above section such as a statement of the problem, the number of people affected, the cost of the problem, and strategies to lessen the problem should be included. A personal story about a community member who has experienced the problem (or been helped by a program that needs more funding) is a worthy addition to the fact sheet. Fact sheet examples can be found in many nonprofit organizations and federal agencies (see Additional Resources).

Most health issues can be addressed at many different levels. **Voluntary policies** are implemented without government direction. **Local ordinances** or regulations are enacted by township or county governmental entities. **State laws** are enacted by the vote of state legislators and signed into law by the governor. Senators and representatives at the federal level pass bills that are then signed into **federal law** by the president. **Policies** often start as voluntary practices, become local regulations, and then eventually become state or federal law. For example, many community organizations have established no-smoking policies. These policies gained favor and communities began to make public buildings smoke-free, which in turn influenced enactment of some state and federal policies to ban smoking in public places and places where people work.

Policies can be implemented at worksites or in community settings by choice rather than by law. For example, a magazine publisher can enact a policy not to accept alcohol or tobacco advertising. Governmental bodies such as township committees, local boards of health, local school boards, boards of chosen freeholders, or boards of county commissioners or supervisors enact ordinances at the municipality, township, or county level. A county board of commissioners may mandate smoke-free buildings in private worksites for businesses registered within the county. Elected **legislators** enact state and federal laws. For example, individual states enact specific penalties for driving under the influence. In general, state and federal laws are more difficult to change, so identifying influential partners and increasing media attention can increase success.

Groups or organizations that have never engaged in advocacy should start by identifying a "winnable issue" (**TABLE 12.1**). A small success or several small successes can build confidence to tackle more difficult issues. This strategy also provides an opportunity for people to work together to develop larger advocacy strategies. Encouraging the adoption of a voluntary policy, such as encouraging restaurants to go smoke-free on their own rather than advocating for a city ordinance to ban smoking in restaurants, can start the process. Encouraging voluntary policy gains allies who will support the issue at the regulatory level, especially if they have benefited from a voluntary policy. For example, the restaurant owner whose business increases as a result of being smoke-free may encourage other restaurants to adopt similar policies.

---

⑦ DID YOU KNOW?

Recent Gallup poll indicates Americans say they are most concerned about jobs, dissatisfaction with the government, the economy, and health care. You have a real opportunity to educate legislators if you are advocating about anything other than the top four issues.

Data from Riffkin, R. (2014, March 13). Gallup: Americans cite jobs, economy, gov't as top U.S. problems. *Gallup News*. Retrieved from http://www.gallup.com/poll/167873/americans-cite-jobs-economy-gov -top-problems.aspx

Understand the Steps Needed to Enact Legislation

Health education specialists can educate policymakers about an issue or even better persuade a legislator to **sponsor** (or author) a bill to address the problem. It is important to remember that if working in a governmental agency, no lobbying can take place! In this case, the health education specialist would either advocate and educate the policymaker as part of work duties or lobby for a health issue or change on time outside work hours. If allowed to lobby, identifying **bipartisan** sponsors (sponsors from each political party) can increase the likelihood a bill will gain broad support. A legislator who sponsors a bill can be a champion for the health issue.

There are several steps before a bill becomes law at the local, state, or federal level. It is important to remember that only about 3% of the bills introduced each year make it through the process and are signed into law.[8] Persuading a legislator to sponsor a bill is only the start. Advocating for action at each step in the process increases the likelihood for success.

Local policy issues are fairly easy to introduce. First, a member of the local governing body

---

TABLE 12.1 Choosing an Advocacy Issue

- Why is this issue important? Who is affected?
- What will be gained or lost by supporting or opposing the issue?
- What is the experience and level of commitment of the advocacy group?
- Are there sufficient staff and volunteers to implement a legislative campaign?
- What funding is available to support the campaign? (Some funding agencies and grant funds have specific guidelines about legislative involvement. This should be determined beforehand in case alternative funding is needed.)
- What community resources (e.g., money, space, and materials) are available?
- Who are the advocacy group's allies and adversaries on this issue?
- Who else (groups or individuals) shares this problem?
- What would those groups who share the problem gain or lose by joining the campaign?
- What laws, if any, already exist to deal with the issue of concern?
- What are the rules and regulations that govern involvement in legislative advocacy?
- What stories, metaphors, and facts can be used to make your case?

Data from Alcohol Justice. (1994). Advocating for policy change. San Rafael, CA: Author.

in which the policy is to be introduced should be contacted to determine the best approach. This might be the city council or the local zoning board, or other appointed or elected group.

At the state level, a policy issue can be introduced either in the State Assembly (House of Representatives) or the Senate, or both simultaneously (**TABLE 12.2**). A member of the advocacy group or the group's **lobbyist** proposes the issue to a legislator, who then introduces the issue to the legislature. The President of the Senate or Speaker of the House (or Assembly) must agree to have the bill introduced (also known as *dropped* or *posted*).

Once introduced, the issue will be processed as a bill. The bill is then referred to all committees that have jurisdiction over the issues presented

---

TABLE 12.2 How a Bill Becomes a Law (State Level)

1. A bill is introduced in either the Senate or the House. Sometimes identical bills are introduced simultaneously. The bill receives a FIRST READING in the House and a FIRST AND SECOND READING in the Senate (at which time the title is read). Then, either the Majority Leader of the Senate or the Speaker of the House refers the bill to an appropriate standing committee (Education, Commerce, Health Policy, etc.). If the bill is a budget bill or has fiscal implications, it will be referred directly to the Appropriations Committee or to an appropriate standing committee, and then to the Appropriations Committee.

2. In committee, the bill is discussed and debated. Public hearings may be held. Not every bill in the committee will be considered. The committee may take several different actions:
   - Report the bill with favorable recommendation.
   - Add amendments and report the bill with favorable recommendation.
   - Report the bill with the recommendation that a substitute be adopted.
   - Report the bill with adverse recommendation.
   - Report the bill without recommendation.
   - Report the bill with amendments but without recommendation.
   - Report the bill with the recommendation that the bill be referred to another committee.
   - Take no action on the bill.
   - Refuse to report the bill out of committee.

3. If a bill is reported out favorably or a substitute is offered, the bill is returned to the Senate or House where it receives a GENERAL ORDERS status in the Senate and a SECOND READING status in the House. The Senate resolves itself into the Committee of the Whole and the House assumes the order of SECOND READING. At this time, committee recommendations are considered and amendments may be offered and adopted. The bill then advances to THIRD READING.

4. Upon THIRD READING in the Senate, an entire bill is read unless unanimous consent is given to consider the bill read. In the House, the bill is read in its entirety on THIRD READING unless four-fifths of the members consent to consider the bill read. At THIRD READING, the bill is again subject to debate and amendment. At the conclusion of THIRD READING, the bill is either passed or defeated by a roll call vote of the majority of members elected and serving OR one of the following options may be used to delay final action:
   - Refer bill back to committee for further consideration.
   - Postpone bill indefinitely.
   - Make the bill a special order of business on THIRD READING for a specific date.
   - Table the bill.
   Following either passage or defeat of a bill, a legislator may move to have the bill reconsidered. In the Senate, the motion must be made within the next two session days; in the House, within the next succeeding day.

(Continues)

TABLE 12.2 (*Continued*)

5. If the bill passes, it goes to the other house where the same procedure is followed. If the bill is passed in the same form by both houses, it is ordered "enrolled" in the house in which it originated. It then goes to the governor for his or her signature.

6. If the bill is passed in a different form by the second house, the bill is returned to its house of origin. If this house accepts the changes, the bill is enrolled and sent to the governor. If the changes are rejected, the bill is sent to a conference committee which tries to resolve differences. If the first conference report is rejected, a second conference committee may be appointed.

7. The governor has 14 days after receiving a bill to consider it. He or she may:
   - Sign the bill. The bill becomes law either 90 days after the legislature adjourns or at a later date specified in the bill. If the bill has been given immediate effect by a 2/3 vote of the members elected and serving, it becomes law upon the governor's signature.
   - Veto the bill (which would then require a 2/3 vote to override; see No. 8.).
   - Neither sign nor veto, in which case the bill becomes law 14 days after reaching the governor's desk, unless the legislature adjourns sine die within the 14 days. In that case, the bill does not become law.

8. If the governor vetoes a bill while the legislature is in session or recess, one of the following actions may occur:
   - Legislature may override the veto by a 2/3 vote of the members elected and serving in both houses.
   - Bill may not receive the necessary 2/3 vote, and thus the attempt to override the veto will fail.
   - Bill may be tabled pending an attempt to override veto. Bill may be re-referred to a committee.

Reproduced from Michigan State Legislative Council. (2015–2016). *A citizen's guide to state government*. Lansing, MI. Retrieved February 12, 2017 from www .legislature.mi.gov/documents/Publications/CitizensGuide.pdf

in the bill. For example, if the bill requests a new health screening and funding to cover it, both the Health Committee and the Appropriations Committee must hear the bill. The bill is then reviewed by committee members and marked up (additions, deletions, or amendments) to be heard by the full house. If passed by both the House and Senate, the bill goes before the governor. When the governor signs the bill, the bill becomes a law.

The process for passing a bill into law at the federal level is similar (**TABLE 12.3**). Each step that is taken to affect legislation should also be used to target the executive branch of government, regardless of whether the goal is to enact new legislation, establish regulations, or implement and enforce the new law. The U.S. website, www. congress.gov, has detailed information and videos describing the legislative process and the introduction and referral of bills.[9]

Identify Potential Partners

People usually feel more confident and willing to tackle legislative issues when they are part of a group that has similar beliefs. Forming a group to advocate for or against an issue can be more effective than an individual voice because the group can share responsibilities and complete more tasks. These groups are commonly known as **coalitions**. For example, when groups like the American Cancer Society, American Lung Association, and the Society for Public Health Education join forces in Washington, D.C., they represent hundreds of thousands of individual voices. Policymakers listen because they know some of their constituents are part of these groups.

TABLE 12.3 How a Bill Becomes A Law (Federal Level)

Legislation is Introduced. Any member can introduce a piece of legislation. **House**: Legislation is handed to the Clerk of the House or placed in the hopper. **Senate**: Members must gain recognition of the presiding officer to announce the introduction of a bill during the morning hour. If any Senator objects, the introduction of the bill is postponed until the next day.

Committee Action. The bill is referred to the appropriate committee by the Speaker of the House or the Presiding Officer in the Senate. Most often, the actual referral decision is made by the House or Senate parliamentarian. Bills may be referred to more than one committee and it may be split so that parts are sent to different committees. The Speaker of the House may set time limits on committees. Bills are placed on the calendar of the committee to which they have been assigned. Failure to act on a bill is equivalent to killing it. Bills in the House can only be released from committee *without* a proper committee vote by a discharge petition signed by a majority of the House membership (218 members).

Steps in Committee:
1. Comments about the bill's merit are requested by government agencies.
2. Bill can be assigned to subcommittee by chairman.
3. Hearings may be held.
4. Subcommittees report their findings to the full committee.
5. Finally, there is a vote by the full committee—the bill is "ordered to be reported."
6. A committee will hold a "markup" session during which it will make revisions and additions. If substantial amendments are made, the committee can order the introduction of a "clean bill" which will include the proposed amendments. This new bill will have a new number and will be sent to the floor while the old bill is discarded. The chamber must approve, change, or reject all committee amendments before conducting a final passage vote.
7. In the House, most bills go to the Rules committee before reaching the floor. The committee adopts rules that will govern the procedures under which the bill will be considered by the House. A "closed rule" sets strict time limits on debate and forbids the introduction of amendments. These rules can have a major impact on whether the bill passes. The rules committee can be bypassed in three ways:
   • Members can move rules to be suspended (requires 2/3 vote).
   • A discharge petition can be filed.
   • The House can use a Calendar Wednesday procedure.

Floor Action
1. Legislation is placed on the Calendar.
2. *House*: Bills are placed on one of four House Calendars. The Speaker of the House and the Majority Leader decide what will reach the floor and when. (Legislation can also be brought to the floor by a discharge petition.)
3. *Senate*: Legislation is placed on the Legislative Calendar. There is also an Executive calendar to deal with treaties and nominations. Scheduling of legislation is the job of the Majority Leader. Bills can be brought to the floor whenever a majority of the Senate chooses.
4. Debate occurs.
   • *House*. Debate is limited by the rules formulated in the Rules Committee. The Committee of the Whole debates and amends the bill but cannot technically pass it. Debate is guided by the Sponsoring Committee and time is divided equally between proponents and opponents. The Committee decides how much time to allot to each person. Amendments must be germane to the subject of a bill—no riders are allowed. The bill is reported back to the House (to itself) and is voted on. A quorum call is a vote to make sure that there are enough members present (218) to have a final vote. If there is not a quorum, the House will adjourn or will send the sergeant at arms out to round up missing members.

(Continues)

TABLE 12.3 *(Continued)*

- *Senate.* Debate is unlimited unless cloture is invoked. Members can speak as long as they want and amendments need not be germane—riders are often offered. Entire bills can, therefore, be offered as amendments to other bills. Unless cloture is invoked, Senators can use a filibuster to defeat a measure by "talking it to death."
5. *Vote.* The bill is voted on. If passed, it is then sent to the other chamber unless that chamber already has a similar measure under consideration. If either chamber does not pass the bill, then it dies. If the House and Senate pass the same bill, then it is sent to the president. If the House and Senate pass different bills, they are sent to Conference Committee. Most major legislation goes to a Conference Committee.

Conference Committee

1. Members from each house form a conference committee and meet to work out the differences. The committee is usually made up of senior members who are appointed by the presiding officers of the committee that originally dealt with the bill. The representatives from each house work to maintain their version of the bill.
2. If the Conference Committee reaches a compromise, it prepares a written conference report, which is submitted to each chamber.
3. The conference report must be approved by both the House and the Senate.

The President

The bill is sent to the president for review.

1. A bill becomes law if signed by the president or if not signed within 10 days and Congress is in session.
2. If Congress adjourns before the 10 days and the president has not signed the bill, then it does not become law ("Pocket Veto").
3. If the president vetoes the bill, it is sent back to Congress with a note listing his/her reasons. The chamber that originated the legislation can attempt to override the veto by a vote of two-thirds of those present. If the veto of the bill is overridden in both chambers, then it becomes law.

The Bill Becomes a Law

Once a bill is signed by the president or his veto is overridden by both houses, it becomes a law and is assigned an official number.

Identifying nontraditional allies and partners can significantly strengthen the likelihood of success. By looking for common ground among unlikely groups (e.g., mothers opposing gun violence in schools and gun retailers, public health professionals and tobacco farmers), strong coalitions with expanded resources can be developed. Understanding the values, needs, and concerns of perceived opponents to an issue and identifying areas of common ground can result in broader, more realistic options that will create additional advocates.

COMMUNITY CONNECTIONS 12.2

As the ESG Advocacy Chair, Erica became aware of a state movement to raise the age of tobacco product purchases to 21 years old. How could she make a difference? She took her concerns to her ESG chapter and they agreed to sign a resolution with other state public health organizations. She even discussed the issue with two other state ESG chapters and got them to sign the state level resolution.

Establish a Relationship with Policymakers

Policymakers are the elected officials who enact policy, laws, and ordinances. At the local, state, and federal levels, they are responsible for creating and enacting policies that guide and influence the activities and actions of individuals and organizations (**TABLE 12.4**).

Developing a relationship with legislators requires more than an occasional meeting or letter about an issue. Building a relationship means a long-term commitment that involves an ongoing exchange of information such as letters or phone calls congratulating legislators when they support important issues. Local officials are accessible and there are many opportunities to meet with them. For instance, many policymakers hold town hall meetings at local establishments in their districts. This allows constituents to meet with their policymakers without an appointment. Knowing the civic groups in which the official is a member (e.g., Lions Club, Rotary Club) can provide insight into personal interests and community commitment and may help determine allies or opponents for legislative concerns. Attending hearings before

---

TABLE 12.4 Levels of Policymakers

- *Local officials.* County, city, township, or village elected officials such as commissioners, council members, supervisors, mayors, and village presidents. A list of local policymakers can be obtained from any city, township, or county office. The office addresses and telephone numbers, office hours, and committee assignments (e.g., budget and finance, health policy, transportation) of each elected official are also available.
- *State officials.* Elected individuals, such as the governor, members of the state assembly and state senate, and other elected or appointed government officials (e.g., judges, lieutenant governors, attorneys general, commissioners, assistant commissioners, deputy commissioners). A legislative directory may be available from organizations such as the League of Women Voters. The directory includes state and federal legislators' mailing addresses, telephone and fax numbers, legislative aides, and committee assignments. The guide also lists addresses for state and federal executive branches. In addition to this type of directory, many legislators can be reached through the Internet via state or federal legislative web pages.
- *Federal officials.* The president, vice president, members of the U.S. House of Representatives and Senate, and appointed policymakers such as representatives of governmental agencies or cabinet members. Directories of federal elected officials are available from many nonprofit organizations and federal and legislative web pages.

COMMUNITY CONNECTIONS 12.3

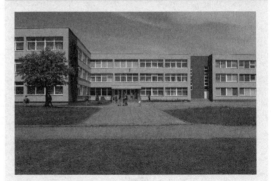

© giedre vaitekune/Shutterstock.

As part of a class assignment, Erica had to identify her state policymakers and find out the type of government in her town. Finding out about her state representatives was easy—she went to her state's legislative webpage, put in her zip code, and the names of her representative and state senator appeared. Each of them had a webpage, so she could find out their party affiliations, assigned committees, and sponsored bills.

Identifying her city's governing body was just as easy. She just went to her city's webpage to learn the names of the council members and the mayor. One of her classmates made a trip to her town's municipal building, where all of the information was available to the public. This information helped her in determining whom she would contact about the T21 issue.

local boards of health, township committees, and other local committees helps identify priority issues at the local level and provides the opportunity to meet policymakers prior to a formal appointment. Legislators can also be invited to visit one's place of work or attend a local event.

Elected officials are often treated with a level of respect that seems to place them at a different level from the ordinary citizen, but their claims to the positions they hold are the result of the votes cast by ordinary citizens. Politicians are people, too. In fact, their primary job is to respond to the concerns of their **constituents** (voters and residents of their district). Although legislators listen to their party, special interest groups, and lobbyists, their greatest allegiance is to the residents of their district—those who voted them into office (or might vote for or against them in the next election).

A health education specialist's experience as a person who works in the community to improve its health can be an asset to legislators. By providing well-documented facts, stories, and statistics to policymakers, good public health laws and regulations will be developed and supported.

The appropriate level for policy change (local, state, or federal) will help determine which elected official to contact. Staff and legislative aides of elected and appointed officials can be key allies, as all correspondence and appointments go through these individuals. Because legislators cannot be experts on all the myriad issues that come before Congress, they employ legislative aides who have expertise in certain policy areas. These staff provide background information that will shape the legislator's position on an issue. Health education specialists advocating for an issue should not be disappointed when meeting with a staff member rather than a legislator, because the aides listen carefully, gather pertinent information, and read the materials they are given. A series of actions can be taken to increase the likelihood of gaining a legislator's attention (**TABLE 12.5**).

In order to meet with a legislator, an organized health education specialist must determine when committee meetings and general legislative sessions are scheduled. Any official's office staff or legislative aide can assist with this information.

Newspapers usually print or post committee and board meeting information one week in advance. These meetings are open to the public, and can provide an opportunity to meet policymakers before introducing a legislative issue. State legislators divide their time between the state capitol and their individual districts. In Michigan, for example, legislators are typically in their respective districts on Monday and Friday, while the rest of the week is spent at the capitol working on legislative issues. It is usually easier to speak with legislators when they are in their local districts. If at the capitol, however, do not miss an opportunity to meet legislators and their staff. Even though a scheduled appointment is best, one may visit an official's office without an appointment. If the official is not available, a meeting with one of the legislator's staff members can be requested. At the very least, information can be left for the legislator.

⑦ DID YOU KNOW?

When you ask a legislator to sponsor new legislation or support a bill that is already introduced, the worst that can happen is that the legislator will say no. Remember that each policymaker has certain issues that he or she is passionate about and will never change position; but for the majority of legislation, your policymaker will more likely be influenced to support your request if you are a constituent in the district and have accurate information and other advocates who support your views.

Developing a plan for legislative visits will help to increase support for an issue. To address state-level issues, health education specialists should start with their own Assembly or House representative, as being a constituent from his or her local district provides the greatest likelihood for success. It will also be important to determine the committee that might hear the issue. For example, if the issue is related to health and the legislator is not on the Health Committee, ask him or her to write a letter of support to the chair of the Health Committee. Plan to meet with the chair or another member of the Health

TABLE 12.5 Steps for Advocating Legislation

- *Make a monetary donation.* A financial contribution, even a small one, puts your name on the legislator's list of contributors. Consider contributing to two opposing candidates—this is what major corporations do to ensure they are seen as a "friend" regardless of who is elected. *Caution:* This is a good strategy for an individual or a for-profit organization; however, there are strict rules regarding nonprofit organizations and direct campaign contributions and **electioneering** (supporting or opposing a candidate for public office).
- *Provide policymakers with objective, factual information about key issues.* Supply that information periodically (even when there is not an immediate issue for which a legislator's help is needed).
- *Visit legislators when they are at home in their district, attend their town meetings or other public appearances, and make an appointment to visit them when they are at their government office.* Let the legislator know you are a constituent of the legislator's district. If you are not a constituent, identify local residents to make the visit with you and encourage them to share how this issue affects them. Always provide written information about the issue and the legislative action that should be taken.
- *Invite legislators to a community site so they can see a program in action and meet people who are benefiting from the program.* These site visits can be particularly useful if you are asking for continued or increased funding for the program. *Note:* Nonprofit organizations that invite elected officials for a site visit near the time of an election should also invite opposition candidates for a site visit, so the organization is not seen as electioneering.
- *Recognize legislators when they introduce or vote for a bill on an issue that is important to you.* Write letters of appreciation or send a press release to the local newspaper.
- *Involve constituents and community members who have been affected by the issue.* An advocate's personal story can demonstrate the potential consequences of legislation or funding decisions in ways that a fact sheet cannot.
- *Criticism of or opposition to a bill is fine, but plan to provide a solution so that the legislator can work to rectify the situation.* Providing realistic solutions to the problem you are advocating on behalf of ensures that your policy solution is considered and you are considered a credible advocate. Be prepared to offer several policy solutions or funding levels. Remember that incremental changes still give you a foundation to build from.

Committee to discuss the issue. If the issue will need funding to implement (nearly every issue requires some funding), an additional meeting with members of the Appropriations Committee should be scheduled. Whenever possible, members of the organization or coalition who are constituents of the policymaker should be identified, so they can also attend. Each of these steps will need to be repeated to identify a legislative sponsor and gain support for that legislation in the legislature.

When the appropriate committee for the issue has been identified, a meeting with officials from the state health department (or other agency) should be considered in order to enlist their support. This is an important step because the governor (if a state issue) will want the department's

endorsement before the bill will be signed into law. It is important to develop a positive working relationship with individuals in the state or local health department (depending on the level of the issue), because they may be able to provide supporting information about the need for the proposed legislation.

Meetings with staff members of the minority and majority legislative offices will identify support and opposition and will provide the opportunity to educate additional policymakers about the issue. Additional meetings with members of the governor's cabinet to discuss the legislation should also be considered. Local officials should also be enlisted for support as they can reinforce the need for legislation and describe how local citizens will benefit from the new legislation.

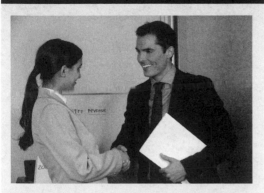

© Robert Kneschke/Shutterstock.

Erica and some of her classmates organized a free advocacy webinar for the three ESG chapters that was to be held on her campus. To her surprise, an employee of the state health department's tobacco unit agreed to present on the webinar. One local council member even agreed to attend. She also called her state representative's office to invite him to the event. Although his legislative aide said he could not attend the webinar, she was excited to find out that, as a physician, he was a big proponent of T21 legislation. The aide asked her to send him a letter with facts about T21 as he considered sponsoring a state-level bill.

Build Grassroots Support

Grassroots movements are alliances of local people, usually volunteers, working together toward a common goal. Mobilizing local support for an issue greatly increases the likelihood a policymaker will be interested in the group's position. Through grassroots initiatives, health education specialists have the opportunity to not just advocate for those who need better policies, but also empower members of the public to become their own advocates. When current services are not available, the people who are directly affected can be the most powerful advocates for change.

Motivating individuals for a grassroots movement is more likely if the issue affects many community members. Helping new advocates articulate the issues will increase their confidence

when they have the opportunity to voice their concerns before policymakers. Grassroots advocates can increase confidence by providing facts about the issue and giving examples of the experiences of others. Health education specialists should encourage advocates to share their stories by providing a guide for the type of information they should share, and asking them to practice their stories to increase their confidence.

Even a grassroots effort that is loosely organized requires a leader and a shared decision-making process. Key community leaders, organizations, and community members who have the ability to create change should be recruited. These individuals often have the skills and resources (e.g., experience and political connections) to help make the initiative a success.

A grassroots group can formulate either a short- or long-term **legislative initiative**. The goals of the group will help determine the strategies needed for success. Activities might include developing an information campaign, polling policymakers to identify potential legislative support, contacting government offices to determine the procedure to introduce policy issues, creating a media campaign, or developing a budget. Each group member's previous experience with legislative committees, reputation in the community, personal or professional experience with the issue, and association with the group should be considered. For example, in introducing a policy on maintenance and safety checks for park equipment, a parent of a child injured in a poorly maintained playground would be an effective spokesperson.

One example of grassroots advocacy is the backlash against the manufacturer of the EpiPen (Mylan). After having a conversation with a friend about the high cost of the life-saving epinephrine injection to those suffering a life-threatening allergy attack, a New York woman created an online petition that garnered signatures from more than 80,000 people and generated more than 121,000 letters to Congress.[10] After receiving these letters, the House Oversight and Government Reform Committee invited the CEO of Mylan to testify as to why the price of the EpiPens increased more than $500 in seven years and the Department of Justice launched an investigation into whether Mylan overbilled Medicare, which was subsequently settled. As a result of this, Mylan introduced a generic version of their EpiPen that was less than half the price of the original version and competitors said they would also bring an epinephrine injector to the market.

In any group's advocacy movement, progress should be reviewed to determine (1) if objectives are being met, (2) whether members feel satisfied with their involvement, (3) what barriers continue to exist, and (4) the future direction of the initiative. Asking members about their achievements and challenges, listing policymakers' stands on the issue, assessing changes in policy or community opinion, and identifying what still needs to be done and what is not working will provide important information about the potential success or failure of the grassroots campaign.

As suggested earlier, policy issues should reflect the problems identified by the local community or coalition. If the issue will impact the community, others should be asked to identify people affected by the issue who are not part of the legislative efforts and invite them to join (**TABLE 12.6**).

TABLE 12.6 How to Recruit Grassroots Advocates
■ *Meet with or write to potential advocates.* Ask for their help and outline the issue, describing how new legislation can benefit members of the community or group.
■ *Develop an online communication to recruit like-minded individuals.* Using relevant social media hashtags can greatly increase visibility of messages and recruit like-minded advocates.
■ *Ask volunteers to write, fax, or phone their legislators.* Provide fact sheets and sample letters to use as a guide. Include information about how to ask legislators for services. Share examples of personal stories and how the impact of personal stories can help change legislation.
■ *Support first-time advocates.* Identify others who have had similar experiences and ask them to describe their contact with legislators.
■ *Share success stories from other advocates as a model.* Legislators respond to personal stories of constituents. Including personal stories with information sent to new advocates will illustrate how someone's personal experiences can influence policymakers.

Introduce and Track Legislation

The steps required to introduce legislation have been previously described. Remember, just introducing legislation does not ensure it will become law. A diligent health education specialist will meet with various local and state officials to build support for the issue. When a representative agrees to sponsor a bill, both Republican and Democratic cosponsors from the appropriate committee should be found so the bill will have bipartisan support. Bills and policies are often stalled in committee or never brought up for a hearing, so tracking the bill is the best way to monitor the process. The GovTrack site can be used to get automatic alerts on the status of bills at the federal level. This site provides information on legislation, committees, votes, members of

Congress, and will send alerts on the status of the bills being tracked.[8]

Frequently, legislation does not move because of partisan views. If bipartisan sponsors have been identified for a bill, contacting both the minority and majority offices will help to enlist their aid in moving the bill forward. When a bill is stalled, the chair of the committee should be contacted for information as to why the bill has not progressed. It may even be appropriate to request the Speaker of the House or Senate President to refer the bill to another committee for consideration. Bills that have not been referred to another committee may have to be reintroduced to the committee during the next session. It may also be possible to add a bill onto another bill that has already passed the committee. The bill's sponsor should be contacted to determine if this is a viable strategy. If both houses of Congress do not pass the bill during a current session, the bill's sponsor should be asked to refile the bill for a hearing in the next session. An upcoming election may change the balance of power and the bill can be reintroduced during the next session. Bills introduced often get caught up in the reelection cycle. If a bill is introduced late in an election cycle, there may be no follow-up. The best strategy is to plan to introduce legislation early and recognize that it may need to be reintroduced.

---

⑦ DID YOU KNOW?

Elected officials serve you, whether you vote for them or not. You are a constituent and have the right to ask for their support or to take action on issues that matter to you.

Once a bill has been posted (or dropped), letter-writing campaigns (described in the next section) should be initiated to committee members, requesting both the bill be heard and support for the legislation. Maintaining regular contact with staff of the sponsoring legislator will help to monitor the need for additional letters or visits.

Health education specialists should understand the legislative process and carefully monitor bills as they progress through the system. Amendments, which are a normal part of building support, can often weaken or strengthen legislation.

▶ Tips and Techniques for Successful Legislative Advocacy

All too often, legislation is enacted, changed, or dissolved without the public's knowledge. Elected officials need to know how their constituents feel about the issues. If policymakers do not hear from their constituency, their votes may not reflect the opinions of the community, which could result in passing laws that will hurt rather than help the people of their district. Health education specialists can provide useful ways for the public to get involved and increase the likelihood of legislative advocacy success. Strategies include developing legislative alerts, instituting letter-writing, email, and telephone campaigns, meeting with legislators, testifying at hearings, and initiating media advocacy. These activities will educate the community and policymakers about the issue and move the public to action.

Develop Legislative Alerts

Legislative alerts are notices to a group's members about upcoming votes, needed action (e.g., letters or phone calls to officials), committee meetings, or hearings. An effective alert contains a summary of the issue, the position of the group, background information, and the action needed by the individual or group receiving the information. To make contacting a policymaker easier, the official's name, address (including email and other social media contacts), and phone number should be strategically placed on the alert. A simple message, accompanied by a specific action, will help ensure that the alert is understood. The specific time period needed for action should be included and members should record the action taken. Legislative alerts can be distributed to members via mail, fax, or email (see **FIGURE 12.1** for an example legislative alert). Faxes and emails are the fastest way to get a legislative alert to a policymaker. Due to mail security, letters sent to congressional offices can take up to five weeks to be delivered to the office.

Initiate Letter-Writing, Emails, and Telephone Call Campaigns

Letter-writing campaigns are used to educate policymakers and urge them to take action. A successful campaign encompasses the information

ACTION ALERT

Don't Repeal Prevention and Public Health

February 27, 2017

In early January, Congress passed a budget resolution kicking off the budget reconciliation process intended to repeal major portions of the Affordable Care Act. While the initial deadlines have slipped, SOPHE has learned that the House Energy & Commerce Committee (E&C) plans to mark up their budget reconciliation bill beginning next week. A legislative draft dated in early February that has been circulated in recent days eliminates the Prevention & Public Health Fund (PPHF) in its entirety beginning in 2019.

The Prevention & Public Health Fund, established by the Affordable Care Act, funds nearly $1 billion in prevention activities from the Centers of Diseases Control (CDC) to states, counties, cities, public health oriented nonprofit organizations, and tribal organizations across the United States.

Eliminating the Prevention & Public Health Fund constitutes an extreme threat to public health and puts many core public health programs and services at risk, as funds from the PPHF make up 12 percent of the CDC overall budget with some programs funded entirely by allocations from the PPHF.

SOPHE encourages all members to contact their members of the House, particularly if those members are on the House Energy & Commerce Committee and oppose repeal of the Prevention & Public Health Fund.

Prevention & Public Health Fund Resources

Background Information on the Prevention & Public Health Fund
Prevention & Public Health Fund State Allocations
Prevention & Public Health Fund State One-Pagers

View the E&C Committee Members

FIGURE 12.1 Sample Action Alert
Courtesy of the Society for Public Health Education.

found in a legislative alert, but with more detail. It is important to find out how a legislator prefers to be contacted (i.e., telephone, direct contact, emails, or letters). For example, some legislators view email as an acceptable method of communication, whereas others do not. All legislative offices, however, routinely tally issues mentioned by constituents, regardless of how the message is received.

A letter-writing campaign can begin before or after the issue has been introduced as a bill. A sample letter to legislators should include opportunities for individuals to personalize the letter with their own thoughts (**TABLE 12.7**).[7] Often, community response to letter-writing campaigns is small because people are unaware of what to do. Names should be spelled out and the letter proofread prior to mailing. Letters from constituents

---

TABLE 12.7 Writing a Letter to a Policymaker

- *Properly address the letter.* Use the legislator's full name and the following format:

For a U.S. Senator:	For a State Representative:
The Honorable (full name)	The Honorable (full name)
United States Senator	State Representative
Address	District
	Address
Dear Senator (last name):	Dear Representative (last name):

- *Include your name and address and telephone number in the letter.* A letter cannot be answered if no return address exists or the signature is not legible.
- *Use your own words.* In general, legislators do not like form letters. These are identified as organized pressure campaigns and are often answered with form replies. As stated previously, however, sending sample letters to members helps organize thoughts. If time is of the essence, a form letter is better than no letter.
- *Know your deadline!* Write the legislator and the chair of the committee in which the bill is assigned while the bill is still in committee to request the bill be heard.
- *Identify the bill by number or by title.* For instance, "House Bill 2440" is a bill number, while "Healthy Michigan Fund" is a bill title. The Secretary of the Senate, Clerk of the House, or the sponsoring legislator's office will have information about the bill of interest.
- *Be brief and constructive.* State the facts and the group's issues, solutions, and personal positions on the matter. Keep the letter to one page, if possible. If you disagree with a bill or policy, be constructive and offer solutions, or state a better way to approach the issue.
- *Request a response.* Responses are not always sent. Asking for one in your letter, however, will increase the likelihood of receiving a response. Follow up with the legislator's office if a reply is not received.
- *Fax or email the letter to the legislator's office rather than mailing it.* The speed associated with faxing ensures swift receipt.
- *Send a thank you.* If legislators have taken action requested, thank them. Legislating can be a thankless job, so recognizing a legislator's efforts is all the more important to maintaining good relations.

Data from Centers for Disease Control and Prevention, Chronic Disease Prevention Programs and Campaigns. Retrieved January 26, 2017 from www.cdc.gov /chronicdisease/resources/campaigns.htm

---

that are individually authored have more impact than form letters. A personal letter shows that time and thought went into the letter. When time is of the essence, however, a signed form letter or email is better than no correspondence at all. Telephone or email campaigns should follow the same suggestions as letter-writing campaigns. It may be better to fax or email rather than mail letters to U.S. Representatives and Senators. Check with the legislator's staff to determine the most effective method for delivering letters.

Meet with Legislators

Contact by members of the policymaker's constituency is crucial. Policymakers are elected by their local residents to represent them in a larger arena (e.g., city, county, state, federal). Writing, calling, and meeting with legislators reminds them that local constituents support the issue. Legislators also learn that someone is concerned and watching their actions (**TABLE 12.8**).

TABLE 12.8 Visiting a Policymaker

- *Look for advocates who have personal contacts with policymakers.* Being on a first-name basis improves access to officials, and personal and professional relationships with policymakers can be an advantage.
- *Know the facts.* Before contacting the policymaker, all sides of the issue should be researched for a clear understanding of the facts about the issue. If possible, find out the legislator's position on the issue ahead of time so advocates can persuasively argue. Although expertise is not required, the group should be well informed.
- *Know when and how to contact policymakers.* Advocates should be aware of when policymakers are at the capitol or in their respective districts prior to initiating a meeting. If the policymaker is unavailable, a meeting should be arranged with a legislative aide. Staff members are often more accessible, and they will share your concerns with the official.
- *Send a letter or fax or call to request an appointment.* Submit your request to the district office or to the legislator's office at the capitol, depending on where you want to meet with your legislator. Identify yourself as a constituent.
- *Follow-up by phone, email, or fax to confirm the appointment.* It may take several calls to arrange for a visit, but do not give up.
- *Be an expert.* Expertise on an issue should be shared with a policymaker. Policymakers cannot be experts on everything, so they will welcome additional information. Share your fact sheet on the issue.
- *Arrive on time.* If you are meeting with a staff member, be sure you have the correct contact name and arrive at the time you said you would be there.
- *Send other advocates to talk with policymakers.* A crowd is not necessary to get a message across. A few advocates who represent the group can be effective. A primary spokesperson should be identified to keep the meeting focused on the issue.
- *Keep it simple.* Select pertinent information about the issue and present it to the policymaker during a face-to-face meeting. Be sure to ask the policymaker for a specific action (e.g., support for a bill, contacting a fellow policymaker, or sponsoring legislation). A cover letter providing a brief overview of the group's position and a business card for follow-up should be left for the policymaker.
- *Remain calm.* If the legislator disagrees with the group's position on an issue, advocates should remain calm and polite. Listen to arguments and take notes to help in developing counterarguments.
- *Be patient.* Once information is presented, give the policymaker a few days to review the issue. The bill or policy must be tracked as it moves through the legislative process, because legislators may need to be approached several times to increase support for the issue.
- *Follow up with a letter.* Thank your legislator for meeting with you; ask for a response to your request.

Data from Centers for Disease Control and Prevention. Chronic disease prevention programs and campaigns. Retrieved January 26, 2017 from www.cdc.gov/chronicdisease/resources/campaigns.htm

COMMUNITY CONNECTIONS 12.5

After Erica sent her representative a letter about T21, she received a response from him stating that he supported the issue. Although Erica was becoming more proficient as an advocate, being a health education specialist she knew she was not an expert on the T21 issue. She decided to have ESG collaborate with her state health department's tobacco unit and a state-level coalition, as their unified voice would be stronger with policymakers. Together, they developed materials to assist her representative and others interested in T21 policy.

Testify at a Legislative Hearing

The purpose of a committee hearing is to obtain written and oral testimony on a bill (**TABLE 12.9**). Before the start of the hearing, audience members usually submit testifying cards, which include the individual's name, organization, and position on the bill. Even if not testifying, a card indicating support or opposition to the bill should be completed because all completed cards are filed and tabulated for the record.

Use Media and Social Media for Legislative Advocacy

The media can strengthen the public's desire to see changes made and can help promote an issue. Media can educate policymakers, other members of the media, and the general public. Effective media campaigns require planning similar to the steps required to have a bill introduced. If possible, relationships with media personnel should be established before providing information on an issue (**TABLE 12.10**).

In recent years, social media has revolutionized who is an advocate and the ways in which advocates interact with policymakers and influence change. Social media can be used to create viral advocacy campaigns, recruit and organize advocates around the globe, and contact local, state, and federal policymakers. Social media campaigns are a relatively low-cost way to energize and mobilize people from around the globe on an important issue. The use of relevant and meaningful hashtags is an incredibly important part of social media advocacy as users can search the hashtag to find and connect with the advocacy issue. There is often an opportunity for social media campaigns to cross over and be recognized in traditional media, particularly the cable news cycle, if a social media campaign gains enough followers and garners support among advocates.

TABLE 12.9 Developing Effective Testimony

- *Prepare a written statement in advance.* Keep it brief. Usually, each person testifying is allotted two to three minutes. Comments should be practiced ahead of time. Before testifying, a person's name, organization, and position on the bill should be stated.
- *Use sound bites.* Legislators will remember sound bites and the press will quote them. For example: "The number of tobacco-related deaths each year is equal to two jumbo jets crashing every day for a year."
- *Use personal experiences to enhance testimony.* For instance, personal insight on how drunk driving has affected families or how barriers to health care have diminished a child's health may be helpful. Avoid overly emotional testimony and inflammatory words that might alienate committee members.
- *Listen to prior speakers.* By taking notes, those testifying can avoid repeating previously stated facts. When it is time to speak, offer highlights of your prepared testimony and ask that the full written testimony be placed in the record.
- *Observe the members of the committee.* Watch officials' body language and their comments to one another and other speakers. Change testimony if needed, or reinforce a previous point made with additional facts.
- *Do not be disappointed if members of the committee are not attentive.* Frequently, members may talk during testimonies or they may be called out of the session. In this situation, continue presenting the testimony. Those who did not hear it will receive a written copy or can listen to a recorded version.
- *Expect questions or comments.* When answering a question, do not improvise. This is not the time for misinformation. Offer to provide written comments later to avoid misinformation. If a hostile response is received from committee members, stay calm and cool. Stop and think about the appropriate answer before responding.
- *Testifying in opposition to a bill.* If a bill will be opposed, research the facts, consult with other professionals, and provide alternatives to the bill. Stay focused on solving the problem.

Data from Americans for Nonsmokers' Rights. *Tips for testifying.* Retrieved February 12, 2017 from http://www.no-smoke.org/document.php?id=240

TABLE 12.10 Using Media Advocacy to Support a Legislative Advocacy Campaign

- *Develop an effective message that identifies the problem, the solution, and who can make the solution possible (i.e., whose support is needed to make the solution happen).* The message should be simple and clear; it should state why people should be concerned with the problem in persuasive and compelling terms.
- *Identify a local person who has been personally affected by the problem and ask that individual if he or she would be willing to tell the story to the press.* Help the person "rehearse" the story, and ask the individual permission to share his or her contact information with the press.
- *Create a media list, including local papers and television and radio stations.* Identify the audience a station or paper reaches. Create a list of media contacts and find out how reporters like to receive information (fax, email, social media, or phone).
- *Select a spokesperson who is comfortable with speaking to the media and answering questions and who is knowledgeable on the issue.* This is an excellent opportunity for someone who has been personally affected by the issue to tell their story in a compelling, heartfelt way.
- *Write editorials stating the issue and the solution. Meet with newspaper and magazine editors to ask for advice on editorials.* In order to increase the chance of your op-ed or editorial being picked up by media outlets, ask someone with name recognition to consider authoring the piece.
- *Write news and social media releases about the issue.* Make sure to spread your message across the social media platforms using the same hashtags. Be sure to create different media for the different social media and traditional media platforms. While posting the whole news release may work for Facebook, a message shorter than 140 characters must be crafted for Twitter and an infographic or picture capturing the issue must be created for Instagram. All these can be tied together with the issue hashtag. Many media personalities as well as policymakers are active on social media platforms and can be contacted this way.
- *Involve members of the media in training advocates about effective media communication.* This strategy informs advocates how to utilize the media, and it provides an opportunity to educate the media about issues.

Data from American Public Health Association. *APHA media advocacy.* Retrieved February 12, 2017 from www.action.apha.org/site/PageNavigator/Advocacy

▶ Overcoming Challenges in Advocating for Legislation

Barriers to being an effective advocate exist; some are easier to overcome than others. Following are strategies for overcoming some of the more common barriers to legislative involvement and action.

Prepare for Opposition

It is important to be prepared for opposition to any issue, because opponents are just as determined as advocates to ensure their voices are heard. Preparation starts by researching the facts and becoming familiar with the perspectives and plans of those who may not support the issue. Becoming a member of opposing organizations might also be considered. For example, in the tobacco arena, many tobacco-reduction advocates have signed up for smokers' rights mailing lists to gather information. This tactic was used to alert advocates about upcoming legislative initiatives the opposition was proposing, so that effective strategies for countering their actions could be planned.

Mobilize Community Support

Lack of community interest is a barrier for most groups. Even the largest, best-facilitated groups struggle to keep the public aware of their issue. The group, organization, or coalition should continually strive to provide clear, concise information and identify tasks for members and the community constituency to perform. Too often, people are unaware of their elected and appointed officials and are unsure of how to communicate with policymakers. Health education specialists should continue to assess community needs and be certain those needs align with the issues. Updates on progress should be provided and accomplishments of group member must be recognized. Social media provides an excellent way to keep a community engaged, as it can be used for everything from contacting and interacting with policymakers, to creating advocacy and/or fundraising events. It also can inform community members that may not be as familiar with an issue using a twitterchat (i.e., a group of Twitter users meet at a prearranged chat to discuss a specific topic that uses a designated hashtag), "Ask Me Anything" (a.k.a. AMA, which is an Internet interview that occurs between one user who hosts it and all the other users who want to ask questions), or a Storify (i.e., a social network service that lets the user create stories or timelines using social media such as Twitter, Facebook, and Instagram) that illustrates a problem from start to finish in a compelling way.

Prevent Volunteer Burnout

Advocates need to be provided with short, time-specific activities for involvement to combat volunteer burnout. People are more likely to get involved if they are educated about the process and have specific tasks to complete. Because burnout is bound to occur, new ways to encourage members must be strategized. Additionally, new members must be recruited to replace those who are no longer active. Small successes should be celebrated and the hard work of advocates must be recognized at every opportunity.

Deal with Internal Politics

Organizations may limit the types of activities and amount of resources that can be used for advocacy. If limitations exist, ways to participate in the legislative process other than advocacy or lobbying should be determined. For instance, an organization could write a letter of support to a policymaker. The organization might also identify individuals who support the issue and encourage them to bring the issue to the policymaker's attention. Adequate funding to promote legislative issues is often a major limitation for many organizations and coalitions.

It is often difficult to predict the outcome of legislative involvement and action because many internal and external factors can influence the outcome. If the goal has been successfully achieved, there will be more work to do following the celebration. Any new policy should be continuously reviewed and enhanced, because legislation can be overturned or be made less effective by other policies.

If the policy was not adopted, the original plan should be reviewed to determine areas for improvement. It is important to build on the positives of the effort, especially if community members were mobilized around the issue. Additional advocates should be identified and alliances with other groups who may have similar positions must be built. There *is* strength in numbers. Most important, do not give up! It can take two or three years to move a bill through committees, house votes, and eventual signing into law. Regardless of the outcome, the process itself provides invaluable experience that will be an asset when taking on the next issue.

⑦ DID YOU KNOW?

Even if a pro-health law is passed, the administrative rules and regulations can often greatly alter the law (and its intent). Health education specialists must be diligent in following the process through the regulatory stage once a bill is passed and signed.

▶ Expected Outcomes

By following the suggestions in this chapter, health education specialists can increase their legislative advocacy skills. More important, they will find they have taken steps to affect public health policy. The legislative process moves slowly; two or three

COMMUNITY CONNECTIONS 12.6

Erica, her ESG chapter, and their state-level public health professionals found out that Erica's representative would be sponsoring legislation to limit the sale of tobacco and tobacco-related products to those over 21 years. This was a complex for their state, but because her representative was part of the majority party, everyone felt confident that with additional advocacy, T21 legislation would eventually become law.

years may pass before legislation is written, introduced, and passed into law. Interim goals should be celebrated and advocates must remain active and engaged in social media. These can serve as inspiration for the additional commitment needed to reach the next level of success. New legislation should be monitored and reviewed to determine its effects. Any legislation can be overturned or watered down by other policies, making it much more difficult to enact changes in the future.

When the proposed policy is not adopted into law, efforts should be reevaluated and challenges reviewed to find areas to improve. All experience should be viewed as opportunity to incorporate "lessons learned" and to identify legislators who will be more supportive in the future, and any successes are building blocks for upcoming issues and community mobilization efforts.

▶ Conclusion

Advocating for personal and community health is an essential responsibility of health education specialists.[3,11] The efforts of advocates, health education specialists, and other health-related professionals have resulted in important legislative changes such as changes in healthcare coverage for most Americans and increasing the purchase age of tobacco to 21 years in many cities, counties, and even some states.

Health education specialists need to take a leadership role in policy development and enactment, as they are uniquely qualified to provide input into public health policy. With an understanding of public policy, health education specialists can use their unique skills to help assess the needs of the community to determine key issues and motivate community members to action. They are a bridge between policymakers and constituents because they are in daily contact with community members directly affected by regulations or by the lack of legislation that provides protection or access.

The principles presented in this chapter can guide a community through the legislative process. Advocacy groups, facilitated by a knowledgeable health education specialist, should choose legislative issues important to the community and issues that can be improved by legislative advocacy efforts.

Key Terms

Bipartisan Supported by members of both major parties. Such support increases the likelihood that a bill will be posted into committee and passed into law.

Coalition An alliance of various groups that temporarily come together around a common goal.

Constituent Any person who is entitled to vote for a representative of a specific district (a House member's district is a defined portion of a state, while a Senator's district is the entire state).

Direct lobbying Support for or opposition to certain legislation; the attempt to influence specific legislation.

Electioneering Any attempt by a nonprofit or public organization to influence an election by mentioning a candidate running for office (including such words as "vote for," "vote against," "elect," "defeat," "support," or "oppose").

Federal law Laws enacted at the national level such as the U.S. Constitution, laws enacted by Congress, or Supreme Court decisions.

Grassroots lobbying An initiative that reaches out to community members, members of an organization, or the general public and contains a call to action such as asking people to call or write their legislators to urge them to support or reject specific legislation.

Grassroots movement Collective action by ordinary people at the local level to effect change using a bottom-up approach.

Law A principle governing action or procedure that has been approved by a legislative body has been published to notify the general public and is enforced by representatives of the local, state, or federal governments.

Legislative advocacy To speak for those who have no voice or representation. Effective advocacy works to create a shift in public opinion, money, and other resources and to support an issue, policy, or constituency.

Legislative alert A notice to group members or constituents about upcoming votes, needed action, committee meetings, hearings, or the like.

Legislative initiative An action or set of actions undertaken to change policy or put pressure on an institution to enforce existing policies.

Legislator A citizen who is elected to represent the local, state, or federal level and enact laws. Also referred to as a policymaker or official; includes commissioners, township supervisors, and so on.

Lobbyist A person who works to promote the passage of specific legislation by influencing public officials.

Local ordinance A policy or law in a locality that applies to that community but not the state or nation.

Policy A law, regulation, procedure, or administrative action made by governments and other institutions.

Policymaker Anyone who sets policy such as Rotary committees, college administrators, and PTA members. Every institution makes policy, so every institution has policymakers.

Sponsor A legislator who writes or submits legislation is known as the prime sponsor or author of the legislation. Additional legislators or cosponsors may sign on to the bill to indicate their support.

State law A law passed by a State legislature and signed by the governor.

Voluntary policy Policy initiated through agreement, but not bound by law.

References

1. *President Obama's farewell address*. Retrieved January 13, 2017, from http://www.nytimes.com/2017/01/10/us/politics/obama-farewell-address-speech.html?_r=0

2. U.S. Department of Health and Human Services, Office of Disease Prevention and Health Promotion. *Healthy People 2020*. Retrieved January 13, 2017, from http://www.healthypeople.gov

3. *Code of ethics for the health education profession*. Retrieved January 20, 2017, from http://www.nchec.org/assets/2251/coe_full_2011.pdf

4. Tappe, M. K. & Galer-Unti, R. (2001). Health education specialist's role in promoting health literacy and advocacy for the 21st century. *Journal of School Health*, *71*, 477–482.

5. National Commission for Health Education Credentialing. (2015). *Responsibilities and competencies for health education specialists*. Retrieved January 20, 2017, from http://www.nchec.org/responsibilities-and-competencies

6. Vernick, J. S. (1999). Lobbying and advocacy for the public's health: What are the limits for nonprofit organizations? *American Journal of Public Health*, *89*, 1425–1429.

7. Galer-Unti, R. A, Tappe, M. K, & Lachenmayr, S. (2004). Advocacy 101: Getting started in health education advocacy. *Health Promotion Practice*, *5*, 280–288.

8. *GovTrack*, Retrieved February 13, 2017, from http://www.govtrack.us/

9. *Overview of the legislative process.* Retrieved February 13, 2017, from http://www.congress.gov/legislative-process/introduction-and-referral-of-bills

10. Parker-Pope, T. (2016, August 26). Parental revolt on a drug price. *New York Times*, p. A1.

11. Wooley, S. J., Balin, S., & Reynolds, S. (1999). Partners for advocacy: Non-profit organizations and lobbyists. *Health Education Monograph Series, 17,* 45–48.

Additional Resources

Print

Guo, C. & Saxton, G. D. (2012, January 8). Tweeting social change: How social media are changing nonprofit advocacy. *Nonprofit and Voluntary Sector Quarterly, 43*(1), 57–79.

Kidwai, S. & Imperatore, C. (2011). How to use social media as an advocacy tool. *Techniques: Connecting Education and Careers (J1), 86*(6), 36–39.

National Commission for Health Education Credentialing, Inc. (NCHEC), & Society for Public Health Education (SOPHE). (2015). *A Competency-Based Framework for Health Education Specialists-2015.* Whitehall, PA: National Commission for Health Education Credentialing, Inc. (NCHEC) and Society for Public Health Education (SOPHE).

Neiger, B. L., Thackeray, R., Burton, S. H., Giraud-Carrier, C. G., & Fagen, M. C. (2012). Evaluating social media's capacity to develop engaged audiences in health promotion settings: Use of Twitter metrics as a case study. *Health promotion practice, 14*(2), 157–162.

Obar, J. A., Zube, P., & Lampe, C. (2012). Advocacy 2.0: An analysis of how advocacy groups in the United States perceive and use social media as tools for facilitating civic engagement and collective action. *Journal of information policy, 2,* 1–25.

Thackeray, R., Neiger, B. L., Smith, A. K., & Van Wagenen, S. B. (2012). Adoption and use of social media among public health departments. *BMC public health, 12*(1), 242.

Internet

#SocialCongress 2015: Perceptions and use of social media on capitol hill (Rep.). (2015, October 15). Retrieved from http://www.congressfoundation.org/storage/documents/CMF_Pubs/cmf-social-congress-2011.pdf

American Public Health Association. Retrieved from http://www.apha.org/policies-and-advocacy/advocacy-for-public-health

American Public Health Association. *APHA media advocacy.* Retrieved from http://action.apha.org/site/PageNavigator/Advocacy

American Public Health Association. *Tips for effective advocacy.* Retrieved from http://www.apha.org/legislative/Writingtips.htm

CDC community guide. Retrieved from http://www.thecommunityguide.org/home_f.html

Centers for Disease Control and Prevention. *Chronic disease prevention programs and campaigns.* Retrieved from http://www.cdc.gov/chronicdisease/resources/campaigns.htm

Coalition of National Health Education Organizations. *Health education advocate.* Retrieved from http://healtheducationadvocate.org

National Conference of State Legislatures. Retrieved from http://www.ncsl.org

Research! America. Retrieved from http://www.researchamerica.org/advocacy-and-action

THOMAS: Legislative information on the Internet. Retrieved from http://thomas.loc.gov

U.S. Census Bureau. Retrieved from http://www.census.gov/

U.S. House of Representatives. Retrieved from http://www.house.gov/

U.S. Senate. Retrieved from http://www.senate.gov/

The White House. Retrieved from http://www.whitehouse.gov/

CHAPTER 13

Using Media Advocacy to Influence Policy

Lori Dorfman, DrPH, MPH

Michael Bakal, MPH, MEd

▶ Author Comments

Media advocacy is exciting because it is one of the few public health education tools we have that allow us to work "upstream" to address the conditions and inequities that harm the public's health. Media advocacy, used as a tool to accelerate and amplify community organizing and policy advocacy, can direct public and policymaker attention to the policies that can reshape our social and physical environments so public health problems can be effectively addressed.

We can learn a great deal from the successful development of media advocacy in the field of tobacco control. Since the first Surgeon General of the United States' report linking tobacco with cancer and heart disease, we have seen an incredible shift in attitudes about smoking in public. Much of this is due to information on the toxicity of secondhand smoke, the health effects associated with smoking, and the emergence of the nonsmokers' rights movement. News coverage of public debates about tobacco has contributed to the number of smoke-free worksites, restaurants, and public places by influencing institutional policy changes, local ordinances, and state and federal laws. As a result, we have seen a decrease in adult tobacco use in communities and states that have policies restricting public smoking. Media advocacy has since helped public health advocates enact policies on issues as varied as alcohol, firearms, nutrition, childhood lead poisoning, children's oral health, injury control, community violence, early childhood education, and other public health issues.

This chapter will help you think strategically about working with the news media. This means switching from thinking about using mass media solely as a tool for getting information to health consumers to thinking about the news media as a mechanism for informing and engaging residents to pressure decision makers to transform environments. By learning the skills presented in this chapter and acting on them, you will help yourself and others focus on mass media in its most powerful form.

🔍 CHES COMPETENCIES

1.4.1	Identify and analyze factors that influence health behaviors.
1.4.2	Identify and analyze factors that impact health.
2.2.1	Identify desired outcomes using the needs assessment results.
2.3.3	Apply principles of evidence-based practice in selecting and/or designing strategies/interventions.*
2.3.4	Apply principles of cultural competence in selecting and/or designing strategies/interventions.
2.3.7	Tailor strategies/interventions for priority populations.
2.4.1	Use theories and/or models to guide the delivery plan.
2.4.6	Select methods and/or channels for reaching priority populations.
3.3.7	Use a variety of strategies to deliver plan.
6.1.1	Assess needs for health-related information.
6.1.4	Adapt information for consumer.
6.1.5	Convey health-related information to consumer.
7.1.1	Create messages using communication theories and/or models.
7.1.3	Tailor messages for intended audience.
7.1.6	Assess and select methods and technologies used to deliver messages.
7.1.7	Deliver messages using media and communication strategies.
7.1.8	Evaluate the impact of the delivered messages.
7.2.5	Use strategies that advance advocacy goals.
7.2.6	Implement advocacy plans.
7.3.9	Use media advocacy techniques to influence decision makers.

*Advanced level competency

Reprinted by permission of the National Commission for Health Education Credentialing, Inc. (NCHEC) and Society for Public Health Education (SOPHE).

▶ Introduction

The history of public health is clear: Social conditions and the physical environment are important determinants of health. The primary tool available to public health for influencing social conditions and environments is **policy**. Policies define the structures and set the rules by which we live. If public health practitioners are to improve social conditions and physical environments in lasting and meaningful ways, they must be involved in policy development and policy advocacy. Furthermore, being successful in policy advocacy means paying attention to the news.

The reach of the news media is intoxicating. In society, the news media largely determine what issues society collectively thinks about, how they are thought about, and what kinds of alternatives are considered viable, which in turn influences key policy decisions pertaining to health. The public and policymakers do not consider issues unless they are visible, and they are not visible unless the news has brought them to light. Naturally, health education specialists want to take advantage of the vast audience the news media reach.

Nonprofit organizations and community activists often are unhappy with the way their issues are presented in the news, and typically respond by criticizing the media, ignoring it, or even becoming hostile. These responses are nonproductive because they cede power over the public portrayal of their issues to journalists and widen the gulf between journalists and advocates. Media advocacy addresses this problem. It is an approach to health communication that differs from traditional mass communication approaches. **Media advocacy** helps people understand the importance and reach of news coverage, the need to participate in shaping such coverage, and the methods to effectively do so.

News portrayals of health issues are significant for how they influence policymakers and the public regarding who has responsibility for health. If public health-oriented solutions are to be given full consideration, then advocates talking to journalists and journalists themselves must understand how to frame issues from the perspective of shared accountability so news coverage is not exclusively focused on individual responsibility. This shared accountability recognizes health and social problems will only be adequately addressed when all sectors of society—not just the individual—share responsibility for solutions. Media advocacy emphasizes **social accountability**, which typically receives less attention from the news than individually oriented solutions.

Public health practitioners tend to overlook the power of the news media to influence change. Journalists themselves, even when committed to covering social problems, often produce stories that emphasize individual behavior and treatment rather than social factors and prevention. Despite the media's enormous reach and potential as a tool for change, public health professionals rarely use mass media to its full advantage. Rather, they tend to use it in its least effective capacity: to convey personal health information to consumers.[1] By contrast, media advocacy harnesses the power of the news to mobilize advocates and apply pressure for policy change.

▶ Steps for Developing Effective Media Advocacy Campaigns

Before public health advocates can harness the power of the news, they have to be clear and precise about why they want to use media advocacy. Four layers of strategy organize the approach to communications campaigns. The first is the *overall strategy*—the ultimate goal of the campaign. Next is the *media strategy*—chosen based on appropriateness for the overall strategy. This chapter focuses on one media strategy: *media advocacy*. Once they have selected a media strategy, advocates need to determine the specifics of what they want to say, who will say it, and to

whom. That is the *message strategy*. Finally, once the other layers of strategy are in place, advocates can figure out how to attract news attention—the *access strategy*. Unfortunately, many groups begin by trying to attract journalists' attention without figuring out first why they want that attention, and what they will say after they have it.

Develop an Overall Strategy

The most important part of a media strategy does not concern media at all. Rather, it is the clarification, articulation, justification, and operationalization of the desired change. The media advocacy *prime directive* is: "You cannot have a media strategy without an overall strategy." It makes sense for advocates to develop a media strategy only after they know what needs to be accomplished overall and how it will be done. In practical terms, this usually means determining the policy that needs to be enacted, changed, or enforced. The following four questions can help guide the development of an overall strategy:

1. What is the problem or issue?
2. What is a solution or policy—the desired outcome?
3. Who has the power to make the necessary change?
4. Who must be mobilized to apply the necessary pressure?

What Is the Problem or Issue?

Defining the problem is often not as simple as it seems. It is a process rife with social and political tension because different stakeholders will offer competing definitions of the problem. This process is important because the ultimate definition of the problem will fundamentally determine the solution. For example, increases in the incidence of type 2 diabetes among children might be explained by various factors related to nutrition and physical activity such as too much time watching TV or playing video games; the $2 billion spent annually on sophisticated food marketing targeting children; eating encouraged in places it never was before such as cars and bookstores; soda and fast food available in schools; a decline in physical education; urban "food deserts" and "food swamps" where it is easy to find cheeseburgers but hard to find fruits and vegetables; and social conditions that have sped up contemporary life, putting a premium on time and creating a huge demand for fast foods that are high in salts, fat, and sugars. News attention to one or the other of these factors helps determine the saliency of various policies and, ultimately, which ones will prevail.

Articulating the problem is important because it will need to be concisely conveyed to a reporter. Public health is often very problem oriented. This means those from health departments or social service agencies can endlessly discuss the problem. Indeed, health officials often feel they have a moral and professional obligation to tell journalists everything they know anytime they are asked about the problem because they know their issue is of such vital importance. The realities of news today, however, demand that health education specialists identify only the most critical aspect of the problem that is to be addressed now and be able to describe it well in just a sentence or two.

⑦ DID YOU KNOW?

Television news stories that focus on individuals or events without context may do more harm than good. Experiments have demonstrated that people use explanations of personal responsibility as their default. That is, in the absence of an explanation that explicitly involves forces outside the individual, audiences will blame the victim. News stories that focus on the plight of individuals without bringing in the larger social or environmental context distance viewers from the problem. From a public health perspective, a news story framed this way may be worse than no news story at all.

Advocates must isolate the piece of the large public health problem that will be specifically addressed. For example, alcohol is related to more than 80,000 deaths a year in this country and is the number one drug of choice for young people.

COMMUNITY CONNECTIONS 13.1

Public Health Advocates (PHA; formerly the California Center for Public Health Advocacy) is a nonprofit organization that works to prevent diabetes and obesity in young people, among other public health goals. While the organization recognized that diet-related disease is related to both individual choices and environments, it made the strategic choice to define the problem in terms of environments. This broad problem definition allowed the group to hone in on strategies that could have a population-level impact.

One way advocates can narrow the problem is by focusing on how alcohol creates problems on college campuses, particularly when it is consumed in large quantities over a short period of time. The problem of binge drinking on college campuses might be narrowed further and defined in terms of price specials at bars nearby that encourage those who are drinking to get drunk. Cheap alcohol is not the only factor leading to alcohol problems on campuses, but it is probably an important one. It is also a problem that can be remedied by a clear policy solution that would affect the overall alcohol environment. Rather than educating reporters about the extensive range of alcohol problems, public health advocates would be more effective by narrowing the focus of their discussion with reporters to the details relevant to a specific policy goal; in this example, the elimination of price specials that encourage binge drinking.

What Is a Solution or Policy— The Desired Outcome?

Sometimes, advocates are so concerned about focusing attention on the problem they give inadequate attention to the solution. Or, they may not have identified a clear solution. Public health advocates need to identify a solution or policy—not necessarily one that will solve the entire problem, but something that can make a difference. Typical inadequate responses tend

COMMUNITY CONNECTIONS 13.2

The goal of PHA was to develop policies that would reduce the number of individuals entering population at risk for diet-related diseases, which it knew would require implementing policies to create healthier environments such as marketing restrictions on junk food in schools and taxes on sugary beverages. In a 2009 report, *Bubbling Over: Soda Consumption and Its Link to Obesity in California*, PHA and the University of California, Los Angeles, Center for Health Policy Research presented strong evidence linking soda to the obesity epidemic. A day after the release of the report, the *San Francisco Chronicle* announced in a front-page story that the then San Francisco mayor Gavin Newsom was considering "a fee on soft drinks." While the fee did not gain immediate political traction, it fueled a national discussion about sugary beverages that has since ignited. PHA's specific definition of the problem—that soda consumption contributes to obesity— supported its mayor's policy recommendation to introduce fees on sugary drinks.

to be statements such as "This is a very complex problem with multifaceted solutions," "There is no magic bullet," "Children are our future and we must do something," or "The community needs to come together." Unfortunately, none of these responses provides any concrete direction. Public health advocates need to be clear about what they want to happen: Is a new law necessary? Is more enforcement required? Does the budget need to be changed? Does someone need to take responsibility to do something to protect the community's health? If so, who? What should they do?

In the example of problems related to alcohol on campuses, one solution was to eliminate happy hour price specials that encourage quick consumption of large quantities of alcohol. Public health problems are complex, so advocates may be working on only one salient part of the problem or one policy solution at a time or more, depending on what resources are available, the maturity of the campaign, and other factors.[2]

Who Has the Power to Make the Necessary Change?

The next step is figuring out what person, group, organization, or body has the power to make the desired change. This question identifies the **target**, but reflects a fundamental change in what that term means. In this context, there is a difference between traditional use of mass media in public health as a vehicle for public information campaigns to change personal behavior and integrating media as an advocacy tool to change policy. In the former, the person with power to make the change is the one with the problem, for example, the person who drinks too much, smokes, does not exercise, or has a poor diet. When using media advocacy to change, implement, or enforce policy, the target is different because the power may reside with a legislator, other elected official, regulatory agency, small business owner, or corporate officer. In addition, the individual or group in power—or target audience—is likely to change over time. For example, changing a regulation may require focusing on different targets depending on the stage of development of the issue. The **primary target** is the person or body (e.g., school board or city council) who has the power to make the necessary change. The **secondary targets** are those groups and individuals who can be mobilized to put pressure on the primary target.

The primary target for a media advocacy campaign to reduce alcohol problems on and around campus would not be the students who are drinking. Instead, it would be the alcohol vendors and those who regulate them. Eliminating happy hours, to use the policy example previously mentioned, is not in the power of the students. Once happy hours are gone, there will be a beneficial effect regardless of the knowledge and attitude of student drinkers—one avenue for the dangerous behavior would be closed. News coverage generated by media advocacy activities can describe the problem and articulate the demands for solutions so the city government and campus community can more easily move ahead. Advocates must articulate to reporters the reason for the policy and what it will accomplish. In the process, the public learns about the problems alcohol causes on campus via the news, which is perceived as a highly legitimate and credible source.

Who Must Be Mobilized to Apply the Necessary Pressure?

Public health-oriented policies are often hotly contested. Fluoridating drinking water, distributing condoms, mandating bicycle or motorcycle helmets, or limiting the availability of junk food, alcohol, handguns, or tobacco brings out intense opposition to public health goals. Many legislators and other policymakers unlikely will support a controversial change unless constituency groups put pressure on them to do so. The pressure might consist of telephone calls, letters or emails, demonstrations, media coverage, and office visits. The role of news coverage here is twofold. First, media coverage of the issue will let policymakers know their vote or position is being watched and will be part of the public debate. Second, media coverage can help mobilize constituency groups to contact the policymaker or get involved in other ways, thus applying pressure.

Mobilizing supportive groups is important because public health policy efforts can often be prolonged struggles. The media can only provide periodic coverage, placing the spotlight on the issue at key times. Constituency groups need to apply pressure over time. For example, students and local merchants around campuses can put pressure on bar owners to change their policies about pricing alcohol. They also can put pressure on campus administration, city government, and alcoholic beverage-regulating agencies to take actions that will reduce the problems related to alcohol use. Additionally, they can strengthen and amplify those efforts by garnering news coverage at key moments such as prior to a policy decision or as students return to campus in the fall.

Paying attention to these four questions is a good start to creating an overall strategy. Once advocates have defined the problem, selected and developed a realistic and achievable policy objective, conducted an analysis to identify the locus

for change, and identified and mobilized groups to apply pressure, then they can determine the media, message, and access strategies.

Develop a Media Strategy

Traditional forms of mass media interventions emphasize the "information gap" or "motivation gap," which suggests health problems are caused by individuals with the problem or at risk for the problem who lack either information or sufficient desire to behave in a more healthful manner. Health education specialists then attempt to provide information to fill that gap. When people have the information and "know the facts," it is assumed they will adopt a positive attitude toward the health behavior and then accordingly act and the problem will be solved. The role of the media, in this case, is to deliver the solution (knowledge) to the millions of individuals who need it. Media advocacy, on the other hand, focuses on the "power gap," viewing health problems as arising from a lack of power to create change in social and physical environments.

Media advocacy can be defined as the strategic use of mass media to advance public policy by applying pressure to policymakers.[3] The use of media advocacy has evolved as the definition of health problems has shifted from the individual level to the policy level. What distinguishes media advocacy from traditional health promotion and educational efforts is the goal of the effort (**FIGURE 13.1**).[4]

Media advocacy differs in many ways from traditional public health campaigns. It is most marked by an emphasis on:

- Linking public health and social problems to inequities in social arrangements rather than to flaws in the individual.
- Changing public policy rather than personal health behavior.
- Primarily focusing on reaching opinion leaders and policymakers rather than on those who experience the problem (the traditional audience of public health communication campaigns).

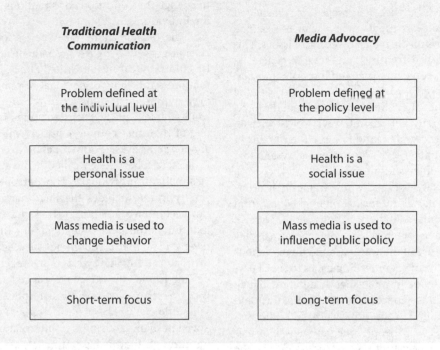

Traditional Health Communication	Media Advocacy
Problem defined at the individual level	Problem defined at the policy level
Health is a personal issue	Health is a social issue
Mass media is used to change behavior	Mass media is used to influence public policy
Short-term focus	Long-term focus

FIGURE 13.1 Traditional Health Communication versus Media Advocacy.

- Working with groups to increase participation and amplify their voices rather than providing health behavior change messages.
- Having a primary goal of reducing the **power gap** rather than just filling the information gap.[1]

In practice, media advocacy uses some of the same media relations techniques that practitioners of social marketing or public information campaigns might use: sending out news releases, pitching stories to journalists, monitoring the media and keeping a list of media contacts, and paying attention to what is newsworthy. But these practices alone are not media advocacy, though they are frequently used by media advocates and may be the most visible part of a media advocate's process. Because media advocacy's target is the power gap, it attempts to motivate social and political involvement rather than changes in personal health behavior.[3] It is the best media strategy choice when the overall strategy involves changing policy.

Develop a Message Strategy

A message strategy identifies the message, the messenger, and the target audience. The message is what is said to the target. The overall strategy determines the target audience: a single person or a small group, perhaps the CEO of a company, or a legislative committee. Selected messengers through the news media deliver the message to the target. Other mechanisms for delivering the message are used at the same time because media advocacy is used in combination with community organizing and policy advocacy. Media advocacy adds power and amplification to those strategies by harnessing the news media's reach and credibility. It is a mechanism for thrusting the discussion with the target into the public conversation.

Framing

Because media advocacy messages are transmitted through the news media, it is useful to examine how the news media typically represent issues. This process is called **framing**. Framing, in general, is about how people interpret and integrate information they receive from the outside world with the understanding they already possess about the topic. People are only able to interpret words, images, actions, or text of any kind because their brains fit those texts into an existing conceptual system that gives them order and meaning. Just a few cues—a word, an image—trigger whole frames that determine meaning.[5] The information might come from pictures, words, sounds, or actions people witness. People's brains organize the information so they can make sense of the world around them. Various disciplines, from cognitive linguistics to social psychology, describe framing slightly different, but all the explanations concern how people extract and absorb meaning from experience and information. Frames help people integrate new information into their existing understanding of how the world works, which helps them determine what is important and how to act.

The Default Frame. Social psychologists have shown that a pervasive frame people use to understand the world emphasizes personal motivations, not the situations influencing personal decisions. Over the years, hundreds of experiments have demonstrated that people tend to "see the actors and miss the stage." When explaining others' behavior, people in the United States tend to emphasize personal attributes such as skill, desire, or work ethic; their explanations tend to ignore the influence of the situation surrounding the person. Much like a spotlight illuminates an actor onstage but leaves the rest of the set in shadows, this tendency to focus on people's motivations renders the surrounding elements almost invisible, reinforcing the idea of personal responsibility and minimizing the role of larger structural forces. This default frame—that people's behavior is determined by personal motivation, not by the situations in which they find themselves—makes advocating for health policy challenging, because many policies are designed to change the conditions or situations surrounding individuals.

The default frame taken to its logical conclusion gives us "rugged individualism," a popular cultural ideal in the United States. The frame reinforces the value of personal responsibility for overcoming harsh odds, as in the Horatio Alger "pull yourself up by your bootstraps" myth. It is one of the most common stories Americans tell about themselves. Former Labor Secretary and Professor Robert Reich called it the story of the "triumphant individual." The personal responsibility frame includes the idea that individuals can accomplish anything if they put their mind to it. But at the same time, the frame includes the reverse idea: that if you do not succeed, it is your own fault. Both these ideas come together in the default frame. If you evoke rugged individualism, you also evoke personal responsibility and self-sufficiency. The default frame gets reproduced in many exchanges of information, including through the media. Journalists are subject to the default frame as much as any other group in society. In fact, because they are high media consumers, journalists may have even greater exposure to the default frame.

The Special Case of News Frames. News Frames are one particular type of framing that have evolved from the routine practices of journalism. Any message media advocates have will be filtered through the news frame. News is organized or framed to make sense of infinitely sided and shaded issues. Framing is the process of identifying how the issue will be depicted; it is "the package in which the main point of the story is developed, supported, and understood."[6] Inevitably, some elements of a story are left out while others are included. Similarly, some arguments, metaphors, or story lines may be prominently featured, while others are relegated to the margins of the story. News frames are important because the facts, values, or images included in news coverage are accorded legitimacy, while those not emphasized or excluded are marginalized or left out of public discussion. The coverage will significantly contribute to how the issue is "felt" and talked about by the public.

Traditions and routines exist in journalism that result in consistent frames, almost like story lines or scripts reporters gravitate toward such as heroes and villains, overcoming adversity, and the unexpected or ironic twist of the protector causing harm. Stories have characters, characters have roles, and characters carry out their actions on location in recognizable circumstances within a range of predictable outcomes. Television, in particular, with its two-minute storytelling, uses compact symbols to tell a familiar story. By studying the patterns of news storytelling, advocates can determine the implications for public health.

Portraits versus Landscapes: Typical News Frames and the Challenge for Framing Public Health Issues

Most news, especially television news, tries to "put a face on the issue." The impact of an issue on an individual's life is often of more interest to news reporters than the policy implications of an issue, in part because they believe readers and viewers are more likely to emotionally identify with a person's plight. News stories tend to focus on specific, concrete events, using good pictures to tell a short, simple story. Unfortunately, research on television's effects has shown that when viewers see individually focused, event-oriented stories (which researcher Shanto Iyengar calls "episodic framing") and then are asked what should be done about the problem depicted, the viewers will respond in ways that tend to blame the victim.[5,6] Stories about isolated episodes do not help audiences understand how to deliberate and solve social problems beyond demanding that individuals take more responsibility for themselves. "Following exposure to episodic framing," notes Iyengar, "Americans describe chronic problems such as poverty and crime not in terms of deep-seated social or economic conditions, but as mere idiosyncratic outcomes."[5,6] Alternatively, when stories are more issue oriented, audiences respond

differently—they include government and social institutions as part of the solution. That is usually the type of response sought by public health advocates.

A simple way to distinguish between the two story types is to think of the difference between a portrait and a landscape. In a news story framed as a **portrait** (or as an episode, in Iyengar's terms), one may learn a great deal about an individual or an event, with great drama and detail. But it is hard to see what surrounds that individual or what brought him or her to that moment in time. A **landscape** pulls back the lens to take a broader view. It may include people and events, but must connect them to the larger social and economic forces. The challenge for media advocates is to make stories about the public health landscape as compelling and interesting as the portrait.

To focus attention on the landscape, media advocates try to frame the *content* or underlying message of a news story. **Framing for content** focuses on how the story gets told, not on whether it gets told in the first place. Attracting news coverage entails another type of framing, "framing for access," described later in this chapter. When framing for content, advocates shift the focus of stories from individual problems to social issues. For example, attention to problems related to childhood nutrition has prompted calls for parents to make good nutrition choices for their children. But parents do not choose what is stocked in grocery stores. Parents do not control pricing strategies that make 20 ounces of soda cheaper than 20 ounces of milk. Parents do not decide whether a grocery store will be located in their neighborhood. Parents do not blazon cartoon characters on sugary cereals and salty snacks. Personal responsibility matters, but so does the environment in which those decisions are made, and it is the involved industries and the policy-makers who support them who largely determine the nature of that environment. Framing for content, in this example, makes the industry's role in causing the problem better understood, and then advocates can articulate why it is reasonable to assign responsibility for changing practices to the industry.

Components of a Message

The **message** is what is to be said to the target audience—those who have the power to make the change being sought. But the message is going to be delivered in the context of a news story, so it must conform to the needs of journalists for clear, concise statements. Therefore, it is important to keep it simple.

To improve reporting from a public health perspective, advocates will need to be well versed in social factors and other contextual variables related to the issue so they can inform journalists of those links. They should be able to fill in the blanks in the following statement. Similarly, advocates should understand how typical news stories might connect to particular health issues and be able to complete the reverse of the same statement.

> Every time there is a story on _____, it should include information about _____.

For example, asthma rates began rising in the late 1980s, and studies began to define risk factors such as outdoor pollutants and secondhand smoke.[7] Advocates working to prevent asthma need to determine whether news stories reflect this understanding. If they do not, advocates will know how to focus their discussions with journalists. Given what is now known from epidemiologists, it is reasonable to expect that whenever there is a story on children's health, it mentions rising asthma rates. Similarly, whenever there is a story on asthma, it should mention children's rates going up, prevention measures for parents, potential environmental policy protections, and the health department as a community resource. It would also be appropriate to include an angle on asthma in stories on environmental tobacco smoke or air quality, such as:

> Every time there is a story on asthma, it should include information about secondhand smoke.

> Every time there is a story on secondhand smoke, it should include information about asthma.

Advocates can use the same formula to think through other public health issues, their risk factors, and important aspects of prevention that should regularly be included in news stories. So, for example, if advocates' policy goal is focused on reducing air pollution from idling diesel trucks, as was the case for asthma prevention programs in Long Beach, California, the message in news stories can be thought of as follows:

> Every time there is a story on _asthma_, it should include information about diesel trucks and air pollution.

> Every time there is a story on _diesel trucks or air pollution_, it should include information about _asthma_.

Advocates can collect the materials that clearly and simply solidify their point of view so they are available to send to reporters on short notice when an article on the topic appears. Advocates need to have data and examples at the ready to explain why the reporters should include this information in their story.

The message an advocate delivers is often in the context of an answer to a journalist's question. Journalists will usually ask at least two questions: "What is the problem?" and "What is the solution?"[8] In the authors' experience working with organizations throughout the country, it is common for public health professionals and their community allies to spend about 80% of their time talking about the problem and 20% talking about the solution. Strategically, it is important to reverse the ratio. Advocates should briefly identify the problem, but emphasize more what needs to be done to solve it.

Levels of a Message

Cognitive linguist George Lakoff described three levels of messages.[5] The first level is the articulation of core values such as fairness, justice, or human dignity. The second level refers to the issue being discussed such as access to healthy foods, housing, or the environment. The third level refers to the details of the issue such as a policy proposal to provide healthy foods in school lunches. According to Lakoff, it is at the values level that people most deeply connect with a message. Therefore, to motivate audiences to act, messages must activate these core values.

Understanding Lakoff's levels provides insight into how to construct effective messages. By concisely stating a problem, advocates can connect with their audiences without miring them in details. By providing a feasible solution, they can present their issue in a way that shows it is solvable. Most importantly, by including core values, advocates can help audiences understand why the solutions are consistent with deeply held moral beliefs and the society they want to create together.

A practical rule of thumb derived from Lakoff's levels is that a good message uses concise, direct language to convey at least three elements.[9] One component is the clear statement of concern, for example, the fact that there are too many alcohol-related problems on campus. The second component represents the value dimension such as the threat to healthy student life and a nurturing learning environment. The third component elucidates the policy objective, for example, the elimination of happy hours in bars near campuses. The components need not always fall in that order, but usually are all present.

For example, when a study was released on drinking on college campuses, reporters sought comments from those who were concerned or affected by the problem. At the University of Iowa, a coalition had formed to try to reduce alcohol problems on and around campus. The coalition had several specific policy goals as its prime directive and had been trained in media advocacy. When the time came to respond to the study, the president of the university told reporters, "Of course, students who drink too much must be responsible for the problems that they cause. But students are not responsible for manufacturing and marketing alcoholic beverages. Students are not responsible for the excessive number of bars within walking distance of our campuses. Students are not responsible for the price specials that encourage drinking to get drunk."[10] In that statement, the university president was able to acknowledge the personal responsibility of students, but also paint a picture of the landscape surrounding those students that helps illustrate why the policies she seeks are both necessary

and reasonable. She cannot say everything in one small media bite, but her example goes a long way to define the problem, illustrate the landscape surrounding the problem, and effectively point to the solution.

Media advocates can develop all the story elements reporters need to tell the public health side of the story. Media bites, like that shared by the University of Iowa president, are essential. In addition, media advocates can prepare compelling visuals to help illustrate their point of view, calculate "social math" so large numbers can be made meaningful, identify "authentic voices"—those advocates who can effectively "put a face on the issue," as reporters might put it—and identify and use evocative symbols in their descriptions of the problem and solution (see Tips and Techniques for Successful Media Advocacy). Having ready story elements that portray the public health frame will make it easier for journalists to cover the story.

Develop an Access Strategy

Once an overall strategy has been determined, a media strategy selected, and the message crafted, it is ready to attract journalists' attention. At this point, it is important to think of what parts of the issue will make a good story. By emphasizing those elements of that issue, advocates will be **framing** the issue, which is called **framing for access**.

Journalists likely will not think of the public health aspects of their stories, but they are always eager for new and interesting angles. Public health practitioners can offer ideas to journalists by suggesting stories on the topics and by thinking about how the public health angle fits into the news of the day.

Monitoring the News and Building Relationships with Journalists

In order to work well with journalists, advocates need to understand how they define and report news. Advocates can do this by watching television news, reading newspapers and blogs, and listening to the radio. Advocates should regularly scan all sections of the local print or online newspaper for articles that directly or indirectly relate to their advocacy issue. For instance, the sports page may cover a rodeo that is tobacco sponsored. This may provide an opportunity for a group working on a policy to ban tobacco-sponsored sporting events. Members of the group could respond to the article with a letter to the editor or an invitation to the reporter who covered the event to learn more about sponsorship. Copies of the article can be sent to other community activists and appropriate legislators.

⑦ DID YOU KNOW?

Reporters often use silence to get their sources to speak. If there is an awkward silence during an interview with a reporter that you feel compelled to fill, ignore it and wait for the next question. If you feel you must speak, repeat what you have just said. Or find another way to say the same thing. Do not be pressured into saying something you do not want to say.

Monitoring means listening and paying attention to the local and relevant national media outlets. For each of the outlets, advocates will have to determine how often they cover the issues of concern. To **monitor** means they will notice what the coverage says about the issue. Does it tell the whole story? Advocates need not do a detailed study of the media, but they need enough information to inform their media advocacy efforts. To do this, advocates should read and critically watch the news from a public health perspective. When reading the newspaper, questions to think about include: Does the article include everything it should given the topic it covers? Are there important aspects missing? Is there a public health aspect to this story that should have been included? Monitoring can help advocates evaluate the comprehensiveness of a news story and determine the specifics to bring to the attention of the journalist, who may do similar stories in the future.

By paying attention to news stories about an issue, advocates can identify which journalists are interested in a specific topic and what aspect of the topic interests them most. Advocates will also start to see how different symbols and journalistic conventions are used to tell the story. This is the

COMMUNITY CONNECTIONS 13.3

PHA knew the release of its report *Bubbling Over* report would not earn media coverage on its own. Therefore, PHA also prepared brief documents and tool kits that reporters and advocates could use in either writing stories or talking to the media. These included news releases, Spanish-language materials, a media kit, contacts for spokespersons familiar with the study, fact sheets, and a list of policy recommendations that highlighted the environment and role of key decision makers, not just individuals. PHA's media bites included social math to illustrate the quantity of sugar adolescents were consuming, "39 pounds of sugar each year in soda and other sugar-sweetened beverages." The resulting media coverage was dramatic. Prominent news coverage appeared in the *New York Times, Sacramento Bee, San Francisco Chronicle, Los Angeles Times*, and *Fresno Bee*, among other periodicals. PHA also prepared a video television outlets used to talk about the study and policy recommendations. Finally, PHA used its email network to disseminate the report to public health professionals and other allies. Because PHA fact sheets included clear specifics about the story for their region, including breakdowns of consumption by legislative district, local news reporters could localize the story so it was relevant to the audience of their papers as well as the local policy targets. This extensive media coverage helped raise the profile of PHA's issue, and increased pressure on decision makers to enact policies to create healthier environments.

foundation from which they can approach journalists about the aspects of the story that are not receiving attention.[9]

Advocates will have greater success attracting journalists to the story if they have built a relationship with them. The first step is to compile a list of local media contacts. Each entry on the list should include: (1) the name of the reporter; (2) telephone and fax numbers; (3) email and mailing addresses; (4) the name of the newspaper, blog, magazine, television station, or radio station; (5) the best time to be reached; (6) sections or *beats* in which the reporter writes or reports (e.g., sports, columnist, lifestyle, health); and (7) any notes pertaining to interactions to date. Advocates should meet with the reporters who may have an interest in their issue or those whose beats intersect with the issue. The advocate should introduce self, explain the interest for having a meeting, and get to know them. Advocates need to regularly update the media list because there is a high rate of turnover in the news business. It is, therefore, important to keep track of contacts as they move onto other news outlets. A relationship at a local television station today may be a relationship at a national news program tomorrow.

Newsworthiness

Framing the issue for access involves making the issue newsworthy. The following questions can help determine newsworthiness[3]:

- Is the issue controversial (e.g., freedom of choice versus restricting the sale of sweetened beverages in schools)?
- Is there a milestone event (e.g., a major study on childhood obesity)?
- Is there an anniversary (e.g., the date the first school district in the country banned the sale of sodas in schools)?
- Can irony or outrage be used (e.g., schools "pushing" soda on students in the face of a rising obesity rate)?
- Can a local issue be connected with a larger, national event (e.g., local school district efforts to improve nutrition in schools tied to state or federal policy campaigns)?

Identifying newsworthy components can help turn an issue into a story. Stories have action, plot, and characters. What are they in relation to the topic of interest? Why is it a story *now*? Why does it matter to the people who read that newspaper or watch that television station?

General Strategies

There are five general strategies for getting in the news: creating news, piggybacking on breaking news, paying for advertisements, editorial strategies, and social media and digital strategies. Each is detailed in this section.

Creating news. Tobacco control advocate Russell Sciandra said, "To gain the media's attention, you can't just say something; you have to do something."[9] That "something" need not be elaborate, but it must be newsworthy. Creating news can be as simple as releasing new data or announcing a specific demand. The important part is that it be publicly done and that someone alerts the news media, emphasizing why the story is newsworthy. For example, if advocates know an important document will be released, they could plan a briefing for journalists so they will be prepared or issue a statement with the group's reaction to it.

Piggybacking on breaking news. When advocates identify a connection between an issue and news of the day, they should make the story known to journalists. Labor organizers could use wall-to-wall coverage of the swine flu epidemic to advocate for a bill that would expand paid sick time for workers. Domestic violence advocates could use the release of a study about high school students' desire for more adult guidance on romantic relationships to advocate for policies that would include healthy relationships in middle and high school health curricula. Piggybacking on breaking news can be achieved in a letter to the editor, with a news conference, or by other actions.

Paid advertising. Buying space is sometimes the only way to be sure a message gets out unadulterated. The truth° Campaign, a nationwide, multi-million dollar tobacco prevention and cessation initiative that was supported by funds garnered from a lawsuit against tobacco companies,[11] does this through paid television advertisements. In 2017, truth aired a 40-second advertisement during the Grammy's, a music award show popular among young people, featuring the well-known African American comedian, actress, and musician Amanda Seales. Set to a visual backdrop of liquor stores plastered with tobacco advertisements, Seales looks directly into the camera and tells her viewers, "Big Tobacco is really trying to make friends with black folks... So much that in the past Big Tobacco called us a 'market priority,'" as her hands draw out exaggerated quotation marks in the air. Bold typeface then spells out

Seales' next sentence: "It's not a coincidence. It's profiling."[12]

The truth Campaign's use of paid advertising is an example of a powerful media advocacy strategy known as **counter-marketing**, an approach that aims to coopt the branding techniques used by tobacco, soda, and other industries to market harmful products to young people.[13,14] Emulating the successful youth marketing strategies of brands or companies such as Mountain Dew and Nike, Truth ads aim to turn symbols of teen rebelliousness and independence against the tobacco industry by revealing the predatory techniques the industry uses to attract young people, particularly young people of color, to use its addictive products. The Campaign's ultimate aim is to create a "counter-brand" that pries market shares away from the tobacco industry.

In reality, few public health organizations possess the resources necessary to purchase prime time television advertising slots. Given budget constraints, placing the right ad in the right outlet at the right time with a bit of creativity can go a long way. In 2004, the Campaign for Safe Cosmetics decided to take out a paid ad to publicly pressure cosmetic industry executives to eliminate toxins in their products.[15] On a day when executives were attending an industry conference in New York City, the advocates took out a full-page ad in the New York edition of the newspaper *USA Today*. Because the organizers knew that *USA Today* would be delivered to the doorstep of each room at the hotel where the conference was taking place, organizers felt certain their message would reach their target audience. Additionally, since *USA Today* is a national newspaper, industry executives would likely assume the ad was running across the country. Thanks to the organizers' clarity about their primary target, they were able to maximize the impact of their paid ad with limited resources. Their message dominated the conference that day.

Editorial strategies. Letters to the editor, editorials, and "op-eds" (opinion editorials or opinion pieces found opposite the editorial page) provide other opportunities for bringing attention to a policy solution. Letters are usually 200 words or less and can be written, faxed, or emailed to the editor of the newspaper. They are typically in response to a specific article or editorial the paper has published, offering a concise statement of support or objection.

Editorials (sometimes called *masthead editorials*) are unsigned and written by the editorial board of the newspaper. Advocates can make an appointment to talk with the editorial board to ask them to take a position and make a statement about an issue or a pending policy. The meeting is usually attended by the newspaper staff responsible for writing the editorial and those who will make the decision about whether the newspaper will take a position on the issue. The advocates may have two or three people there who can speak to various aspects of the issue or represent different perspectives.

If the newspaper decides not to do an editorial, the advocates can ask if the paper would publish an op-ed. An op-ed is an opinion piece that appears opposite the editorials. Op-eds are typically 600–800 words, written from a personal point of view. They describe the problem, solution, and its relevance to the readers. Monitoring should include reviewing op-eds, both to keep tabs on how an issue is being argued and to identify the style the news outlet prefers.

Newspapers often publish on the editorial pages or list on their websites the contact information and instructions for submitting letters and op-eds. Some radio stations and television news programs allow audience members to record commentaries that function like op-eds, though they are usually short (i.e., no more than a few minutes).

Social media and digital strategies. Organizations today use social media in one form or another. The novelty and potential reach of social media make them attractive, and indeed, they can serve an important function in the media advocacy toolkit. At the same time, using social media requires careful attention to strategy. Digital strategy goes deeper than merely posting information to social media in hopes of activating networks of supporters.

Social media should be embedded in a digital strategy, which just like media advocacy in general begins by establishing clear objectives. For example, an advocacy group may wish to gather online signatures to petition the local school board or to build a list of social media contacts who can respond on short notice to attend a demonstration. Digital strategies to support these goals entail gathering data on how best to communicate with secondary target audiences and move them to action.

Groups build large email lists so they can employ data-driven digital organizing by using information they collect about supporters to determine which messages and requests get the best response. For example, they might use "A/B testing," in which two otherwise identical emails with different subject lines are each sent to a random segment of the organization's email list to see which framing inspires the most actions such as opening the email, forwarding it, signing a petition, making a donation, or some other action. Similar research can be used to determine which visuals are most compelling to audiences or which calls to action are most likely to elicit responses and move primary target audiences to action. Over time, organizations can learn to personalize messages to their constituents based on past online behavior. Such information can help organizations tailor their communications and move their members and supporters to take action. While some organizations exclusively rely on online organizing, digital strategy is often used as a complement to other community organizing and communications activities.

---

⑦ DID YOU KNOW?

Media advocates have adapted their traditional tools as social media platforms like Facebook, Twitter, and YouTube have become popular. In addition to traditional news releases and media advisories, advocates also produce model Facebook posts and model Tweets that their coalition members can adapt and share with the their own social networks. Social media—Twitter in particular—has also become an important platform for reaching journalists. Advocates follow journalists on Twitter to learn about their interests and pitch stories to them through Twitter.

▶ Tips and Techniques for Successful Media Advocacy

Several techniques can enhance media advocacy's effectiveness: Focusing on health equity, calculating social math, localizing stories, cultivating authentic voices, and "reusing the news." Applying these can enhance media advocacy efforts.

Focus on Health Equity

Injustice and inequity are at the root of many of today's health problems. U.S. history is replete with policies—from the Chinese Exclusion Act to Jim Crow to "redlining" to the dumping of toxic waste in communities of color, to many others—that have damaged the health of specific groups based on gender, sexual preference, race, ethnicity, ability status, language, religion, or social class. Although the passage of civil rights legislation in the 1960s ended many legalized forms of discrimination, a large body of evidence shows institutional and structural racism and discrimination continue to harm the health of a great many individuals and communities today.[16] Given that discrimination and injustice are key determinants of population health, how can media advocacy help us work upstream to address them?

According to many leading public health experts, the answer lies in the practice of health equity, defined by the WHO as "the absence of avoidable or remediable differences among groups of people, whether those groups are defined socially, economically, demographically, or geographically."[17] While health equity policies and practices can—and often do—benefit society as a whole, their primary aim is to eliminate disparities affecting marginalized groups. Examples of health equity interventions and policies include expanding educational and career opportunities for marginalized people of color; providing opportunities for immigrants to integrate into society without sacrificing their language or cultural identity; reforming the criminal justice system; protecting communities of color against displacement; ensuring access to healthy foods; and creating inviting spaces for physical activity.[18] What unites these seemingly disparate initiatives as health equity interventions is an explicit intent to benefit groups that experience the brunt of the health harms resulting from social injustices.

Because health equity approaches specifically seek to benefit marginalized groups, communicating their importance to the general public and to policymakers entails unique challenges. As scholar john powell describes, one of the foremost challenges in communicating about health equity is the perception that policies aimed at promoting the well-being of specific groups will necessarily detract from the welfare of others.[19] While there is no single, definitive means of overcoming such communications challenges, there are several broad strategies that can be useful when framing health equity messages: (1) connecting disparities to specific injustices; (2) naming and identifying privilege; and (3) describing how equitable policies benefit all of society. It is important to bear in mind, however, as with all strategic communications, health equity messages are most effective when they are aligned with an overall strategy and are tailored to specific target audiences and messengers.

Connect Disparities to Specific Injustices

It is common in public health to draw attention to health disparities; indeed, the identification of disparities is a key function of public health research. Merely identifying a disparity, however, is insufficient to make the case for an equity-based solution. One reason for this is audiences that heavily subscribe to the default frame of rugged individualism may rationalize disparities by attributing them to poor choices made by individuals. To avoid this pitfall, advocates must go beyond identifying disparities to articulate how disparities came to be in the first place.

For example, in Cuyahoga County, Ohio, public health leaders identified health equity as a priority. They knew that to work toward achieving equitable outcomes, they would need to ensure that their public communications efforts were framed through a health equity lens. In the department's Community Health Improvement Plan, a core document that guides their programmatic and communications efforts, public health leaders described stark racial and ethnic disparities across a variety of health outcomes. They then pointed to *redlining*, a policy of restricting home loans to residents of color, as a key factor that led to segregation and poverty, which in turn were key causes of health disparities observed. By explicating the causal chain linking unjust policies to disparities, the agency primed audiences to understand the need for equity-based policy solutions. Ensuring that the health equity was at the forefront of their framing helped the health department staff more effectively communicate about and address racialized health disparities.

Discuss Privilege

Understanding how injustice produces disparities is necessary to avoid victim blaming, but it may not be sufficient. When attention is focused on how inequity affects marginalized groups, audiences can overlook its inverse effect: *privilege*. john powell describes privilege as "a system by which groups of people actively acquire or passively attach to reward without earning it, simply by membership in privileged groups such as whites, heterosexuals, males, able-bodied persons, or a combination of these or other categories."[19] Competence in communicating about privilege is vital to advancing a health equity agenda because it draws attention to *systems* and *structures* that confer unfair advantage, thereby weakening the frame that suggests individuals are to blame for their own marginalization. Media advocates can contribute to this dialogue when they bring history, structures, and privilege into their framing and messages.

Discussing privilege helps build audiences' understanding that advantaged groups are just as implicated in systems of racism and discrimination as marginalized groups. From this perspective, addressing health inequity is not merely a matter of aiding those who have been marginalized, but also of undoing social and ideological structures (e.g., white supremacy) that produce inequity in the first place. To this end, members of dominant groups are authentic voices (described in the next section) who can explain how privilege has granted them unearned advantage. Multiple spokespeople talking about racism and discrimination from diverse vantage points can help elevate these important determinants of health in the public conversation—a necessary step toward addressing them.

Describe How Equitable Policies Benefit All of Society

Unfortunately, despite ample evidence that targeted policies often lead to benefits that span society, the perception is often to the contrary. Because the default frame of individualism implies problem solving through self-reliance, it is important for advocates to use language that reinforces values of interdependence and shared responsibility. After all, the goals of working upstream in public health are geared to improve the conditions in which people live together.

John Powell uses the term "targeted universalism" to describe the idea that by meeting the needs of the most vulnerable members of our society, we in fact can help all of society.[19] The "universal" in " targeted universalism" refers to the end goal of universal health and well-being. The "targeted" refers to the fact that the means of achieving universal goals will vary from one group to the next based on their starting points or current conditions. For example, targeted universalism might take the form of policies to invest in the local infrastructure, commerce, and housing of the African American communities who were harmed by redlining. In the context of their policy, media advocates will need to convey the importance of the targeted universalist policy to groups who may not immediately see themselves as beneficiaries of the initiative.

One key to communicating the importance of targeted universalism lies in Lakoff's levels, described earlier. Advocates can invoke fundamental values like fairness to explain why it is important that historical injustices be rectified. The majority of Americans believe all people should be fairly treated, so advocates might express

fairness by explaining that those who contribute to the economy or neighborhood deserve to enjoy its benefits. Advocates can also explain that when the impacts of discrimination are addressed, all members of society benefit because a fair society is a universal goal.

Calculate Social Math

Social math is the art of making large numbers meaningful, usually by breaking them down and making a relevant, vivid comparison. Calculating social math can illustrate a message. Raw numbers assume the audience already knows something about the issue and why the numbers are important or revealing. Comparisons, on the other hand, can highlight a specific point of view at the same time they deliver basic information.

Calculating social math involves restating large numbers in terms of time or place, personalizing numbers, or making comparisons that help bring a picture to mind. Examples of social math using comparisons include:

- A children and youth advocacy group wanted to increase county spending on prevention of violence. To make their point, they said, "In San Francisco, there is one police officer for every 18 young people and only one school counselor for every 500 kids."[20]

- To illustrate persistent racial disparities in wealth, columnist Ta-Nehisi Coates wrote, "We now know that for every dollar of wealth white families have, black families have a nickel."[21]

- Public health education professor Meredith Minkler noted, "In a single year one company spent more than $30 million advertising a single sugar-coated cereal. During the same year, the amount spent by the U.S. government on nutrition education for school children was just $50,000 per state."[22]

- The UCSF national Center of Excellence on Women's Health published on its website: "Each year, more than 12.7 million people are physically abused, raped or stalked by their partner, which is approximately the population of New York City and Los Angeles combined."[23]

■ A victim's right's advocate used irony to point out society's skewed priorities and illustrate the need for more resources when he said, "We have more shelters for animals than we have for human victims of abuse."[24]

Localize Stories

Every day, there is a multitude of news from which to choose. News outlets are tuned in to satellite broadcasts from around the world that operate 24 hours daily. Assignment editors, city desk editors, reporters, and producers read several newspapers every morning, listen to news radio and police scanners, subscribe to and follow social media channels, and monitor wire services. One way advocates can break through clutter is to alert news contacts about the local relevance of a story. Questions to consider can include "Why does this story matter to people who live here?" and "Why would it matter to the listeners at this radio station; the viewers of this local television news; the subscribers to blogs, Twitter feeds, or other social media outlets; or this newspaper?" When advocates know the answers to those questions, they will know what to tell the reporter. Every reporter has to convince his or her boss why to select one story over another. If the story has local relevance, it is much more likely to be pursued.

Elevate Authentic Voices

Reporters populate their stories with characters. A common character in health stories is the "victim"—someone who has suffered from or who has direct experience with the problem, whatever it might be. If the story is about binge drinking on college campuses, reporters will want to talk to students. If the story is about gun safety in the home, reporters will want to talk to a parent whose child was hurt or killed by a gun in the home. If the story is about immunizations for children, they will want to show a toddler getting injected.

This is done for two reasons. First, the reporter needs to present evidence in the story that what happened was real and that it happened to a real person. Showing someone with direct experience in the story makes that clear. Second, reporters feel their audience will connect more with the emotion than the facts of a story. People who actually endured a trauma or other experience can be more compelling because they are speaking from experience. These individuals qualify as a "real person," in journalists' parlance.

Besides the usual questions—"What is the problem?" and "What is the solution?"—reporters will ask victims another question: "How do you feel about the tragedy?" The problem, of course, is if the story does not move much beyond the "victim"—if it is a portrait rather than a landscape—when audiences see the story, they are likely to distance themselves from the individual with the belief it will not happen to themselves or, in some cases, even blame the victim. Journalists cannot tell stories without characters, and victims can be powerful spokespeople for public health. A better approach, however, is to change the dynamic and think of victims as survivors or **authentic voices**. Authentic voices are survivors who have become advocates. They bring personal experience to the story, just like a victim, but tend to understand their role as advocates. For instance, if an authentic voice is asked "How do you feel about this tragedy?" he or she might respond with, "I feel angry because this tragedy could have been prevented," and then explain how.

Victims become authentic voices with training and experience as they move through their grief and put it to work for prevention. There are many authentic voices to thank in public health for opening up their lives to the public and becoming leaders for change in breast cancer, HIV/AIDS, tobacco control, and other diseases. For example, in 2000, Mary Leigh Blek became the first chair of the board for the Million Moms March; she lost her son Matthew to a "Saturday night special" handgun and has been advocating for reasonable gun laws ever since. In 1980, Mothers Against Drunk Driving was created by a small group of women in California after a drunk driver killed Candy Lightner's 13-year-old daughter. The national child abduction alert system, also known as the AMBER Alert, was named after 9-year-old Amber Hagerman, who was abducted and murdered in Arlington, Texas. Survivors have joined with public health advocates to advocate for safer baby cribs, drowning prevention, pedestrian safety, motorcycle helmets, mandatory CPR training, and auto safety, including interior trunk release latches.[25] All these authentic voices have selflessly shared their stories and been willing characters in news stories to help further policies that can save lives.

"Reuse the News"

Media advocacy uses mass communication to reach a very small target—sometimes just one person. The power comes from the fact that a vast audience has been privy to this conversation between the advocates and the target. It is a public conversation, not a private conversation. To ensure the target understands this, advocates can "reuse the news." If their op-ed is published, advocates can clip it, copy it, and send it to the target. They can have the target's constituents copy and send news stories and letters to the editor that have been published. They can also reuse the news to educate reporters who are just coming to the issue or use it to educate new advocates. They can share clippings and discuss them in order to become better at framing issues and anticipating the opposition's questions and challenges. News, simply by virtue of its having been published, confers legitimacy and credibility on issues. Media advocates reuse the news to remind the target the public is paying attention and knows what it wants done.

▶ Overcoming Challenges in Media Advocacy

The biggest barrier to successful media advocacy is in the development of a clear overall strategy, even before getting access to reporters is considered. Other barriers include institutional constraints, being distracted by the opposition, and not staying "on message." This section discusses strategies for overcoming these barriers.

Avoid a Murky Strategy

The most important part of media advocacy is developing strategy. If the strategy is not clear and the target has not been well defined, the media advocacy effort will be diffused and ineffective. Public health advocates sometimes resist the simplification necessary to carve out a viable strategy. Public health problems are complex, and that complexity needs to be addressed. Yet, at the same time, not everything can be done at once. Public health problems need to be prioritized into manageable "chunks" that can be addressed in specific time periods. The alternative—strategies that remain too large or overly vague—will be ineffective. Goals such as "raising awareness" are not specific enough for media advocacy campaigns. Instead, clear objectives must be stated that identify who must do what to create or change the rules that will ensure healthier social and physical environments.

Advocates must translate general principles into substantive demands. For example, in San Francisco, a campaign to seek justice for a man who unnecessarily died in police custody was transformed into a campaign to change police practices. Demanding justice was too vague and left the action up to others. So, the advocates asked themselves: What would justice look like? They decided the offending police officer should be fired and safeguards put in place to avoid future hires of officers with similar records of brutality. Advocates had then defined justice in tangible terms that could be put into practice, and used media advocacy to put pressure on the mayor and the police commission to enact the policy changes they desired.

Media advocacy strategies and targets can change over time. In fact, they *should* change. Targets and strategies will shift in response to circumstances and after the advocates achieve their objectives. Advocates can use the strategy development questions, discussed earlier, to refocus efforts and evaluate strategies. With every new activity, it should be asked: How will this help us achieve our objectives? And will this make a clear, positive change in the environment surrounding the people whose health we are concerned about? The answers to those questions can guide strategy and decisions throughout the media advocacy effort.

Alter Perceived Institutional Constraints

Media advocacy is about raising community voices to demand change. In most cases, policy change is the desired outcome. Sometimes, this will require lobbying that public and some nonprofit agencies are prohibited from conducting. In most cases, however, there is a lot those in both public and nonprofit agencies can do that is not considered lobbying. Unfortunately, advocates often stop short of what is allowed and needlessly limit their effectiveness. Organizations such as the *Alliance for Justice* provide training and consultation to nonprofit agencies to help them maximize their ability to legally participate in the policy process. Constraints are often not as prohibitive as some in the agency perceive.

Still, media advocacy can be confrontational. Thus, health education specialists in health departments or other institutions may not be comfortable being "out front" on media advocacy campaigns. Some have a preference for consensus when instead conflict is what is needed. In these cases, individuals can find roles for themselves in the media advocacy effort that place them more in the background than the foreground. For example, health departments can provide data, resources, meeting space, technical assistance, and other supports without compromise.

Avoid Opposition Distraction

While media advocates need to construct thoughtful, succinct answers to the questions their opponents will raise, their goal is not to convince the opposition. Media advocates can be distracted by the arguments their opposition puts forward, and may be tempted to answer those arguments point-by-point. Sometimes, that is necessary, but often it is a ploy by opponents to frame the issue on their own terms. Instead, media advocates' goals are to motivate and mobilize their supporters so those voices will be heard and attended to by policymakers. Everyone does not have to be convinced the proposal is worth supporting—only those who have decision-making power must be convinced. Media advocacy employs the mass media to make private conversations public, so decision makers can be held accountable for their decisions and the impact of those decisions on the public's health. Advocates should use the media to give credibility and visibility to their own arguments, so those who agree with them will know they are not alone.

Stay on Message

Media advocates need to be vigilant when defining the problem and the solution, and focus their attention on the clear and consistent articulation of what they want. *Staying on message* means whatever advocates may be asked, advocates do not stray from the key message they are trying to deliver. Staying on message is a skill that can be honed with practice. It is helpful to practice aloud, with colleagues. That way, advocates can anticipate what questions they might receive from reporters, decision makers, or the opposition, and craft answers that logically lead from the question to the outcome they seek. Practicing aloud is important because speaking is different from writing or thinking. The right words will more easily flow if they have been said before. At the same time, advocates should not memorize a script—that can sound stiff and forced.

▶ Expected Outcomes

When media advocacy is done well, healthy public policy is enacted and implemented. Enacting policies that benefit the public's health is a long-term process, however, with many contributing factors. Media advocacy cannot achieve that end alone, but can certainly amplify advocates' voices and accelerate the process. Properly applied, media advocacy can punctuate the advocacy process, add urgency to a campaign, and create visibility.

Media advocacy does this by increasing the salience of issues for the public and policymakers through agenda setting and framing. Practicing media advocacy can also improve relationships with journalists and increase the capacity of local groups to influence the rules that govern their environments.

Increased Skills and Power

Because policy advocacy is usually a long-term endeavor, it is useful to identify some interim effects and outcomes of media advocacy, most commonly the increases in skills and power of the groups using it. By developing and adapting strategy, advocates gain skills in critical thinking. By talking with journalists and others about the solutions they seek, advocates develop the confidence necessary to effectively speak in public. They become skillful at framing for content and understanding newsworthiness so they can frame for access. By participating in the policy process, either by meeting with decision makers or mobilizing supporters, advocates exercise their democratic power. These skills build on one another and transfer as advocates work together in a community setting to demand change.

Better Relationships with Journalists

An important outcome advocates can expect from media advocacy campaigns is better relationships with journalists. This tangible benefit develops over the course of a media advocacy campaign and from one campaign to another, because advocates bring good information and interesting stories to reporters. The mutually beneficial relationship helps reporters get what they need to do their job and eases advocates' access to and responsiveness from journalists. Simply, an expected outcome of media advocacy is that certain reporters and advocates end up in each other's contact list or email address book. For example, after their concerted media advocacy effort to generate news that reframed

alcohol as a policy issue, staff at the Marin Institute for the Prevention of Alcohol and Other Drug Problems, located in California, were frequent sources for journalists. Eventually, reporters would call the Marin Institute for comments on stories that had been generated elsewhere. The Marin Institute had become a required source on alcohol policy issues.

Increased Visibility and Influence

Advocates' increased skills and power, along with their better relationships with reporters, lead to increased visibility for the issue and more influence from advocates on how that issue is interpreted. If they are successful, advocates will have generated news that put their issue and solution on the policymaker's agenda. Advocates can expect to see their examples used in debate by themselves and eventually by others, shifting the debate toward the advocates' desired outcomes. Advocates' influence will increase with the increased visibility because news coverage confers legitimacy and credibility.

▶ Conclusion

Health education specialists can harness the power of the news media to advance healthy public policy. Their effectiveness can be increased by developing an overall strategy, learning about how the news media operate, developing a specific media strategy, developing a message that frames the issue from a public health perspective, and understanding how to attract journalists' attention. The news media are too important a resource to ignore. If health education specialists are serious about serving the public and improving its health, they need to be serious about the news and about learning how to better integrate it into prevention efforts.

Media advocacy, however, is not appropriate in every instance. The strategy requires a clear and precise plan for policy change and a constituency that can carry it out. It is a public strategy—on the record. Media advocates bring public attention to specific individuals.

At times, they may need to be confrontational and adversarial, depending on the situation. The policies being advocated for are usually controversial. If they were not, then there would not be a need for a pressure tool and publicity via media advocacy. Advocates should be clear with themselves and their colleagues about what is at stake when choosing to use media advocacy. Media advocacy is the right choice when public demands must be made and pressure brought to bear on decision makers to protect and promote the public's health.

Key Terms

Authentic voices They are individuals who by virtue of their own lived experience, knowledge, or credibility, are compelling spokespersons for an issue.

Counter-marketing A strategy that uses strategic communications to combat the influence of companies that sell harmful products, often by spoofing their marketing and branding, and highlight policy solutions to health problems.

Editorial A newspaper piece, written by the editorial board and usually unsigned that expresses the opinion of the news outlet.

Framing How an issue or idea is conceptualized, explained, and interpreted.

Framing for access Focusing on what is newsworthy about an issue.

Framing for content Focusing what is said about an issue regarding the desired outcome, the solution, or policy goal being sought. Framing for content focuses on institutional accountability rather than personal responsibility.

Landscape A news story that takes a broad perspective such that individuals and events are situated within a social, political, economic, or some other context (as contrasted to "portrait"). *Portrait* and *landscape* are modeled after Iyengar's research classifications for news *episodic* and *thematic*.[6]

Media advocacy The strategic use of mass media to enhance the effectiveness of community organizing and policy advocacy.

Messages Communications to the target audience that emphasizes a specific campaign theme.

Monitor To carefully listen and pay attention to relevant media outlets to understand how and how often they portray an issue of concern.

News frames The way an issue is defined and portrayed in the news.

Policy A policy is a deliberate system of principles to guide decisions and achieve outcomes. They define the structures and set the rules by which we live either formally (e.g., legislation) or informally.

Portrait A news story that focuses narrowly on individuals and events without providing a broader context (as contrasted to "landscape"). *Portrait* and *landscape* are modeled after Iyengar's research classifications for news *episodic* and *thematic*.[6]

Power gap The discrepancy in status and influence between groups in a society.

Primary target Primary targets are individuals and groups that have the power to institute desired policy and systems changes.

Secondary target Secondary targets are those individuals and groups who can influence the primary targets.

Social accountability The extent and capacity of people to hold state and service providers accountable and make them responsive to needs of constituents, residents, and beneficiaries.

Social math The art of making large numbers meaningful, usually by breaking them down and making a relevant, vivid comparison.

Target The person or body who has the power to make the desired change, usually the intended recipient of a message.

References

1. Wallack, L. & Dorfman, L. (2001). Putting policy into health communication: The role of media advocacy. In R. E. Rice & C. K. Atkin (Eds.), *Public communication campaigns* (3rd ed.). Thousand Oaks, CA: Sage Publications.

2. Dorfman, L., Ervice, J., & Woodruff, K. (Sept. 2006) Voices for change: A taxonomy of public communications campaigns and their evaluation challenges. *Nonprofit Online News*. Reprint of a paper prepared for the Communications Consortium Media Center, Media Evaluation Project, Washington DC, November, 2002. Retrieved July 15, 2017, from http://bmsg.org/sites/default/files/bmsg_report_voices_for_a_change.pdf

3. Wallack, L., Dorfman, L., Jernigan, D., & Themba, M. (1993). *Media advocacy and public health: Power for prevention*. Newbury Park, CA: Sage Publications.

4. Wallack, L. & Dorfman, L. (1996). Media advocacy: A strategy for advancing policy and promoting health. *Health Education Quarterly, 23*, 293–317.

5. Dorfman, L., Wallack, L., & Woodruff, K. (2005). More than a message: Framing public health advocacy to change corporate practices. *Health Education and Behavior, 32*, 320–336.

6. Iyengar, S. (1991). *Is anyone responsible?* Chicago, IL: University of Chicago Press.

7. California Center for Health Improvement. (2000, December). Joining forces to fight childhood asthma: A Prop 10 opportunity. *Field Lessons, 1*(5).

8. Dorfman, L. (1994). *News operations: How television reports on health*. Doctoral dissertation, University of California at Berkeley.

9. Wallack, L., Woodruff, K., Dorfman, L., & Diaz, I. (1999). *News for a change: An advocate's guide to working with the media*. Thousand Oaks, CA: Sage Publications.

10. Wilgoren, J. (2000, March 15). Effort to curb binge drinking in college falls short. *New York Times, A16.*

11. Hicks, J. J. (2001). The strategy behind Florida's "truth" campaign. *Tobacco Control, 10*, 3–5

12. Truth Initiative (2017). *#Stop Profiling | Market Priority | truth*. Retrieved July 14, 2017, from http://www.youtube.com/watch?v=2cfo4Nhlmp8

13. Palmedo, P. C., Dorfman, L., Garza, S., Murphy, E., & Freudenberg, N. (2017). Countermarketing alcohol and unhealthy food: an effective strategy for preventing noncommunicable diseases? Lessons from tobacco. *Annual Review of Public Health, 38*(1), 119–144.

14. Dorfman L. & Wallack L. (1993, Nov–Dec). Advertising health: The case for counter-ads. *Public Health Reports, 108*(6), 716–26,

15. *USA Today ad names cosmetics companies that won't commit to removing toxic chemicals from American products*, Retrieved July 16, 2017, from http://www.ewg.org/news/news-releases/2004/09/24/usa-today-ad-names-cosmetics-companies-wont-commit-removing-toxic#.WWn76tPysY1USA TODAY Ad Names Cosmetics Companies That Won't Commit To Removing Toxic Chemicals From American Products

16. Krieger, N. (2014). Discrimination and health. In L. Berkman, I. Kawachi, & M. Glymour (Eds.), *Social epidemiology* (2nd ed.). New York, NY: Oxford University Press.

17. World Health Organization. Retrieved June 20, 2017, from http://www.who.int/healthsystems/topics/equity/en/

18. Glover Blackwell, A., Kwoh, S., & Pastor, M. (2010). *Uncommon ground: Race and America's future*. New York, NY: W.W Norton & Company.

19. Powell, J. (2012). *Racing to justice*. Bloomington, IN: Indiana University Press.

20. Coleman Advocates for Children and Youth. (n.d.). *Youth time* [Brochure]. San Francisco, CA: Author.

21. Coates, T. (2016, January 24). Bernie Sanders and the liberal imagination. *The Atlantic*.

Retrieved July 14, 2017, from http://www
.theatlantic.com/politics/archive/2016/01
/bernie-sanders-liberal-imagination/425022

22. Minkler, M. (1999). Personal responsibility
for health? A review of the arguments and
the evidence at century's end. *Health Education and Behavior, 26,* 121–140.

23. UCSF National Center of Excellence in Wom-
en's Health. Retrieved July 14, 2017, from
http://coe.ucsf.edu/coe/spotlight/standing
_up.html

24. Stein, J., Deputy Director of the National
Organization for Victim Assistance, quoted
in J. Shiver, Jr. (1997, August 25). Home violence underreported, U.S. study says. *Los
Angeles Times,* p. A1.

25. McLoughlin, E. & Fennell, J. (n.d.). Channeling
grief into policy change: Survivor advocacy for
injury prevention. *Injury Prevention Newsletter,*
Vol. 13. San Francisco, CA: The Trauma Foundation. Retrieved July 14, 2017, from http://
www.traumaf.org/images/IPNweb.pdf

Community Connections

Babey, S. H., Malia, J., Hongjian, Y., & Goldstein, H.
(2009). *Bubbling over: Soda consumption and
its link to obesity in California.* Los Angeles,
CA: UCLA Center for Health Policy Research.

California Center for Public Health Advocacy.
(2009, September 17). *New research shows
direct link between soda and obesity.*

Dorfman, L. & Gonzalez, P. (2012). In M. Minkler
(Ed.), *Community organizing and community
building for health and welfare.* New Brunswick, Canada: Rutgers University Press.

Dorfman, L., Wallack, L., & Woodruff, K. (2005).
More than a message: Framing public health
advocacy to change corporate practices.
Health Education and Behavior, 32, 320–336.

Knight, H. (2009). "S.F. Looks at fee on soft drinks".
San Francisco Chronicle, September 18, A1.

Additional Resources

Print

Chapman, S. & Lupton, D. (1994). *The fight for
public health: Principles and practice of media
advocacy.* London, UK: BMJ Publishing
Group.

DeJong, W. (1996). MADD Massachusetts versus
Senator Burke: A media advocacy case study.
Health Education Quarterly, 23, 318–329.

Graeff, E., Stempeck, M., & Zuckerman, E. (2014).
The battle for Trayvon Martin: Mapping a
media controversy online and off-line. *First
Monday, 19,* 2–3.

National Commission for Health Education Cre-
dentialing, Inc. (NCHEC), & Society for
Public Health Education (SOPHE). (2015).
*A Competency-Based Framework for Health
Education Specialists-2015.* Whitehall, PA:
National Commission for Health Education

Credentialing, Inc. (NCHEC) and Society for
Public Health Education (SOPHE).

Ryan, C. (1991). *Prime time activism.* Boston, MA:
South End Press.

Shaw, R. (1999). *Reclaiming America: Nike, clean
air, and the new national activism.* Berkeley,
CA: University of California Press.

Shenker-Osorio, A. (2012). *Don't buy it: The trouble with talking about the economy.* Philadelphia, PA: PublicAffairs.

The Praxis Project. (2010). *Fair game: A strategy
guide for racial justice communications in
the Obama Era.* Washington DC: The Praxis
Project.

Thibodeau, P. & Boroditsky, L. (2011). Metaphors
we think with: The Role of metaphor in reasoning. *PLoS ONE 6*(2), e16782.

Internet

Allies for Reaching Community Health Equity. Retrieved from http://healthequity.global policysolutions.org

Alliance for Justice. Retrieved from http://www.afj.org

Berkeley Media Studies Group. Retrieved from http://www.bmsg.org

Dean, R. (2006, October). *Issue 16: Moving from head to heart: Using media advocacy to talk about affordable housing.* Retrieved from http://www.bmsg.org/pub-issues.php.

Dorfman, L., Sorenson, S., Wallack, L. (Eds.). (2009, February). *Working upstream: Skills for social change, a resource guide for developing a course on advocacy for public health.* Berkeley, CA: Berkeley Media Studies Group. Retrieved from http://bmsg.org /sites/default/files/bmsg_handbook_working _upstream.pdf

FrameWorks Institute. Retrieved from http://www.frameworksinstitute.org

Public Narrative. Retrieved from http://www.publicnarrative.org

Opportunity Agenda. Retrieved from http://opportunityagenda.org/

The Praxis Project. Retrieved from http://www.thepraxisproject.org

Seevak, A. (1997, December). *Issue 3: Oakland shows the way.* Berkeley Media Studies Group. Retrieved from http://www.bmsg.org/pub-issues.php

Spitfire Strategies. Retrieved from http://www.spitfirestrategies.com

Index